T0218328

SOCIAL SCIENCE PERSPECTIVES ON GLOBAL PUBLIC HEALTH

Approaching global health through a social justice lens, this text explores both established and emerging issues for contemporary health and wellbeing.

Divided into two parts, the book introduces key concepts in relation to global public health, such as ethics, economics, health disparities, and globalisation. The second part comprises chapters exploring specific challenges, such as designing and implementing public health interventions, the role of social enterprise, climate change, sustainability and health, oral health, violence, palliative care, mental health, loneliness, nutrition, and embracing diverse genders. These chapters build on, and apply, the theoretical frameworks laid out in part one, linking the substantive content to broader contexts.

Taking an inclusive, global approach, this is a key text for both undergraduate and postgraduate students of global health, public health, and medical sociology.

Vincent La Placa is Associate Professor of Public Health and Policy at the University of Greenwich and Senior Fellow of the Higher Education Academy (HEA). Previously, he was a Senior Research Consultant at the Department of Health (now DHSC), where he managed the qualitative strand of the Healthy Foundations Life-stage Segmentation Model, one of the largest pieces of qualitative research conducted across UK government. He co-edited the book *Wellbeing: Policy and Practice* with Anneyce Knight and Allan McNaught, published in 2014. Dr La Placa was recently appointed an Honorary Fellow of Eurasia Research's Teaching, Education and Research Association (TERA).

Julia Morgan is an Associate Professor for Public Health and Wellbeing. Her primary teaching and research interests focus on social justice and inequality; nomadic peoples; gender; global childhoods; international development; global public health; community development; and wellbeing amongst people who are imprisoned. She has carried out research with children whose parents have been imprisoned; Gypsy, Roma, and Traveller communities in the UK; Mongolian nomadic herders; and children who live on the street in Mongolia, Romania, and Zambia. She is currently researching ADHD late diagnosis in adult women in the UK.

SOCIAL SCIENCE PERSPECTIVES ON GLOBAL PUBLIC HEALTH

Edited by
Vincent La Placa and Julia Morgan

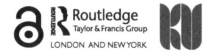

LONDON AND NEW YORK

An electronic version of this book is freely available, thanks to the support of libraries working with Knowledge Unlatched (KU). KU is a collaborative initiative designed to make high quality books Open Access for the public good. The Open Access ISBN for this book is 9781003128373. More information about the initiative and links to the Open Access version can be found at www.knowledgeunlatched.org.

First published 2023
by Routledge
4 Park Square, Milton Park, Abingdon, Oxon OX14 4RN

and by Routledge
605 Third Avenue, New York, NY 10158

Routledge is an imprint of the Taylor & Francis Group, an informa business

British Library Cataloguing-in-Publication Data
A catalogue record for this book is available from the British Library

ISBN: 978-0-367-65211-1 (hbk)
ISBN: 978-0-367-65209-8 (pbk)
ISBN: 978-1-003-12837-3 (ebk)

DOI: 10.4324/9781003128373

Typeset in Bembo
by codeMantra

Anneyce Knight (1959–2021) – Beloved Mum and Grandmother, inspiring writer and traveller, and much missed friend and colleague
Paul Farmer (1959–2022) – an inspiration to us all

CONTENTS

List of Contributors   *xi*
Acknowledgements   *xvii*

1 Introduction   1
   Vincent La Placa and Julia Morgan

2 Public Health, Theory, and Application to Policy and Practice   5
   Vincent La Placa

3 Globalisation and Global Public Health   17
   Vincent La Placa and Anneyce Knight

4 Economics and Global Health   28
   Julia Ngozi Chukwuma and Kevin Deane

5 Global Inequalities: The Impact on Health   38
   Kafui Adjaye-Gbewonyo and Ichiro Kawachi

6 Ethics and Global Public Health   50
   Nevin Mehmet

7 Engaging Critical Pedagogy within Global Health
   Teaching and Learning   59
   Jennifer Randall

8 Issues in Design, Implementation, and Evaluation of
Maternal Health Interventions in Low- and Middle-
Income Countries   68
Aduragbemi Banke-Thomas and Ejemai Eboreime

9 Social Entrepreneurship and Social Innovation in Global
Public Health Practice   78
Charles Oham, Maurice Ekwugha and Gladius Kulothungan

10 Planetary Health and the Anthropocene   88
Stefi Barna, Sonali Sathaye and Vanita Gandhi

11 The Climate Emergency and Zero-Carbon Healthcare   98
Vanita Gandhi and Stefi Barna

12 Violence and Global Public Health   109
Julia Morgan and Clare Choak

13 Every Child and Adolescent, Everywhere: Contemporary
Issues in Child and Adolescent Health   119
Abidemi Okechukwu, Babasola O. Okusanya, and John Ehiri

14 Armed Conflict and the Mental Health of Children   129
Julia Morgan and Constance Shumba

15 Agentic Dying: The Global Imperative to Acknowledge
Socio-Anthropological Aspects in Palliative Care Services
for All   139
*Carlos J. Moreno-Leguizamon, Marcela Tovar-Restrepo,
and Ana María Medina Chavez*

16 Nomadic Peoples and Access to Healthcare   149
Julia Morgan and Tumendelger Sengedorj

17 Living in a Foreign Land: Refugee and Migrant Health
and Related Health Inequalities   158
Floor Christie-de Jong

18 Unravelling Dietary Acculturation in the 21st Century   169
*Amanda Rodrigues Amorim Adegboye, Amanda P. Moore,
Claudia Stewart, and Gulshanara Begum*

19 Transgender, Genderqueer, and Non-Binary Identities:
   Social and Structural Inequalities in Public Health   179
   Danielle J. Roe, Jason Schaub, Jessica Lynn, and Panagiotis Pentaris

20 The Social Construction of Loneliness and Global
   Public Health   189
   Vincent La Placa and Julia Morgan

21 Global Oral Health and Inequalities   198
   Charlotte Jeavons and Bal Chana

22 Health Protection and Global Approach to Neglected
   Communicable Diseases   208
   *Maria Jacirema Ferreira Gonçalves, Anny Beatriz Costa Antony
   de Andrade, and Amanda Rodrigues Amorim Adegboye*

23 Conclusion: Social Sciences Perspectives on Global
   Public Health   220
   Vincent La Placa and Julia Morgan

Index   *225*

CONTRIBUTORS

Amanda Rodrigues Amorim Adegboye is currently Associate Head of School for Research at the School of Nursing, Midwifery and Health, Coventry University, UK. She is a PhD holder in Epidemiology with over 15 years' experience in the field of public health and nutrition. She has a strong background in intervention design, service evaluation, and evidence synthesis.

Kafui Adjaye-Gbewonyo is a Senior Lecturer in Public Health at the University of Greenwich. She is a Social Epidemiologist by training and has an interest in social and contextual determinants of health. She is particularly interested in chronic and non-communicable diseases in the African region.

Aduragbemi Banke-Thomas is a Physician, Public Health Practitioner, Health Policy and Finance Expert, Academic, and Researcher, with years of professional experience in clinical practice, development programme management, academia, operational research, monitoring, and evaluation in the maternal and new-born health in sub-Saharan Africa.

Stefi Barna is Director of Education Programmes at the Centre for Sustainable Healthcare and Associate Professor of Sustainability and Public Health at Azim Premji University, Bangalore.

Gulshanara Begum has over 15 years' teaching experience in Higher Education. She is currently a Senior Lecturer and Ethics Co-coordinator in the School of Life Sciences at the University of Westminster. Her research ranges from investigating health impact of nutritional ergogenic aids and nutraceuticals to public health nutrition.

Bal Chana is a Dental Therapy Tutor at Barts and the London Hospitals in London. She also works in General Dental Practice. She is currently a Council Member of the Dental Defence Union and an Education Associate with the General Dental Council. She is a former President of the BADT.

Ana María Medina Chavez is a Colombian Anthropologist, Specialist in family and community health, and a Doctor in Public Health, and she is currently pursuing a master's degree in thanatology. She is an Associate Professor at the Institute of Aging at the Faculty of Medicine of the Pontificia Universidad Javeriana in Bogotá-Colombia.

Clare Choak has been teaching and researching the lives of marginalised young people for two decades and has a particular interest in age, class, gender, race, and the ways in which they intersect. She has an interest in 'badness' and 'on road' cultures in relation to crime and violence.

Floor Christie-de Jong works as a Senior Lecturer in Public Health at the University of Sunderland, UK. Her research is focused on cancer screening, particularly for ethnic minority groups and migrant populations. She utilises community-centred and participatory approaches in order to improve uptake of screening and tackle cancer inequalities.

Julia Ngozi Chukwuma is a Lecturer in Economics at the Open University. Her research seeks to generate new insights into how social policy takes form in an African context, with a particular focus on the political economy of health policymaking and global efforts to achieve Universal Health Coverage.

Anny Beatriz Costa Antony de Andrade is a Nurse Graduate and obstetric nurse. Her specialism is in epidemiology applied to SUS services (FIOCRUZ Brasília). She has a master's in Living Conditions and Health Situations in the Amazon from the Leônidas & Maria Deane Institute (ILMD/FIOCRUZ Amazônia).

Kevin Deane is Senior Lecturer in economics at the Open University, UK. He is an Interdisciplinary Researcher, drawing on political economy, development economics, and global public health. His research focuses on the HIV epidemic in East and Southern Africa, malaria prevention, and the socioeconomic impacts of COVID-19.

Ejemai Eboreime is a Physician with postgraduate training and expertise in public health, implementation science, and health systems research. He has been Implementation Science Lead on several projects in sub-Saharan Africa and is one of the leading scientists who has published extensively on the subject in the sub-region.

John Ehiri is Professor of Public Health in the Department of Health Promotion Sciences, and the Associate Dean for Academic Affairs in the Mel and Enid Zuckerman College of Public Health, University of Arizona. He served as Chair of the Department of Health Promotion Sciences from 2009 to 2020.

Maurice Ekwugha is a Social Entrepreneur and Researcher with a background in National Health Service (NHS) property management. He is a Visiting Lecturer at the University of Greenwich. Maurice research interest is in healthcare management, social enterprise, and social innovation.

Vanita Gandhi is a Clinical Oncology Specialist Registrar in the National Health Service (NHS) and a National Medical Director's Clinical Fellow at Health Education England and NHS England in 2019–2020.

Maria Jacirema Ferreira Gonçalves is Associate Professor of the School of Nursing of Amazonas Federal University in Brazil. She is graduate in Nursing and Obstetrics at Manaus Nursing School, and Philosophy at Catholic University of Brasilia. She is a PhD holder in epidemiology with experience in researching and teaching in the field of Public Health.

Charlotte Jeavons is an Associate Professor of Public Health at Greenwich University. She is a qualified Dental Nurse and held dental public health and dental services management posts within the NHS. She has a master's in public health and a PhD in dental public health ethics.

Ichiro Kawachi is the John L. Loeb and Frances Lehman Loeb Professor of Social Epidemiology at the Harvard T.H. Chan School of Public Health. His research interests include social determinants of health, social capital and social cohesion, neighbourhood influences on health, income inequality, and population health.

Anneyce Knight retired in 2021 from her role as Associate Dean for Global Engagement and Senior Lecturer in Adult Nursing at Bournemouth University. Her esteemed national and international works and publications led significantly in developing concepts of health and wellbeing, giving them global impetus and relevance in teaching and research.

Gladius Kulothungan currently lectures in VIA University College in Denmark as a Visiting Professor and is the Programme Director at the University of Wales Trinity Saint David leading their MBA Programme. Dr Gladius has published extensively in international journals on social innovation and social entrepreneurship.

Vincent La Placa is Associate Professor of Public Health and Policy at the University of Greenwich. Previously, he was a Senior Research Consultant at the

Department of Health (now DHSC), where he managed the qualitative strand of the Healthy Foundations Life-stage Segmentation Model.

Jessica Lynn is a World-renowned Transgender Advocate, Educator, and Activist. Her experiences as a transgender woman and parent led her to dedicate her life to spreading awareness and acceptance for gender non-conforming communities around the world. Jessica is internationally considered one of the foremost transgender speakers.

Nevin Mehmet is a Senior Lecturer in Health Development. She has a background in complementary therapies, health and wellbeing, healthcare ethics, and public health ethics. She is currently part of a research group exploring simulations for ethical teaching and learning within health and paramedic science.

Amanda P. Moore is a Public Health Nutritionist and Researcher at King's College London. Her research focuses on health inequalities in UK minority ethnic communities, health behaviour change, and intervention design. Her work uses participatory methods.

Carlos Moreno-Leguizamon is an Associate Professor at the University of Greenwich. His research focuses on health inequalities and the provision of inclusive health services. His publications address the use of the Learning Alliance methodology and health services to BAME groups in the Southeast of England in the palliative care area.

Julia Morgan is an Associate Professor for Public Health and Wellbeing. She has carried out research with children whose parents have been imprisoned; Gypsy, Roma, and Traveller communities in the United Kingdom; Mongolian nomadic herders; and children who live on the street in Mongolia, Romania, and Zambia.

Charles Oham is a Senior Lecturer in Social Enterprise at the University of Greenwich, London, United Kingdom. His specialisation is in the fields of social entrepreneurship, social innovation, community development, and entrepreneurship. Charles's career in the public and third sector has included remits in community development, social entrepreneurship, and innovation.

Abidemi Okechukwu, MBBS, MPH, is a Physician and Public Health Epidemiologist with experience in designing and evaluating large-scale maternal and child health. She is currently a Doctor in Public Health and an MBA candidate at the Mel and Enid Zuckerman College of Public Health and Eller College of Management, University of Arizona.

Babasola O. Okusanya is an Associate Professor of Obstetrics and Gynaecology, University of Lagos, Nigeria, and a Global Health expert. He manages high-risk pregnancies like preeclampsia and eclampsia, and medical conditions in pregnancy, including HIV infection. Dr. Okusanya generates and synthesizes evidence for many health conditions in low and middle-income countries.

Panagiotis Pentaris is an Associate Professor of Social Work and Thanatology at the University of Greenwich, London, UK, where he is also a member of the Institute for Lifecourse Development. He has researched and published on death, dying, bereavement, culture and religion, social work, social policy, and LGBTQIA+ issues.

Jennifer Randall is a Senior Lecturer in Global Health at Queen Mary University of London (QMUL). She is an Award-winning Educator with a 20-year career spanning China, the US, and the UK. Her anthropological research explores harm reduction, drug policy reform, and community engagement through participatory action research.

Danielle J. Roe (she/her/hers) is a gay/queer, cisgender, PhD Researcher at the University of Birmingham studying gender diversity and online cis/homonormativity. She is a trans-inclusive feminist and current member of the International Queer Youth Resilience Student Training Network working with collaborators across Canada, the US, the UK, Mexico, and Australia.

Sonali Sathaye, QMUL, is an Anthropologist who teaches planetary health for QMUL and designs climate change education programmes in India.

Jason Schaub (he/him/his) is a Lecturer in Social Work at the University of Birmingham. He is a qualified Social Worker. His work focusses on gender and sexuality, particularly improving the lives of LGBTQ+ young people. Before entering academia, he was a Social Worker in the US, Ireland, and the UK.

Tumendelger Sengedorj is an Associate Professor in the Department of Social Sciences at Mongolian National University of Education. She teaches the courses of sociology, social stratification, and gender and society. Her research interests focus on inequality issues, especially gender and inclusive social services, children's rights, and nomadic access to services.

Constance Shumba is a Global Public Health Practitioner and Academic with experience in leading the design and delivery of complex gender responsive and high-quality health and nutrition programs in low- and middle-income countries with evolving demographic, economic, and disease contexts in Africa and Asia.

Claudia Stewart is a Public Health Consultant postgraduated in higher education teaching from Faculdades Metropolitana's Unidas. Since 2014, she has been working with academic research and research analyses, and as a Lecturer in Public Health, besides working for the NHS since 2004 within the Business Intelligence Unit.

Marcela Tovar-Restrepo is Lecturer at Hunter College and Columbia University in New York. She obtained her PhD in anthropology from the New School for Social Research and her master's from University College of London. She conducts research on diversity, gender, and development in Latin America, NY, and Europe.

ACKNOWLEDGEMENTS

Thank you to all the authors who have contributed to this edited book. Thanks also to Grace McInnes and Evie Lonsdale, from Routledge, for all your support; to Olivia Morgan for checking all the references; and to the copy editors for ensuring consistency throughout.

1

INTRODUCTION

Vincent La Placa and Julia Morgan

Social Science and Global Public Health

Traditionally, global public health has often been associated with the biomedical approach to medicine, with a focus upon, for instance, disease, the physical, and external observations of, for instance, illness, sanitation, and health services. Public health was rarely touched by social sciences and its rich plethora of perspective, theories, and capacity for insight. Where traditional public health did intertwine with the social sciences, it was often with the discipline of economics and the development of, for instance, health economics and the focus on supply, demand, and cost-effectiveness of public health interventions and the quantitative benefits, or otherwise, that their implementation generated. Even within health economics, traditional positivist approaches were adhered to, often overlooking, for instance, other socio-economic determinants, individual lifestyles and agency, and the broad social structures, generated through the direct or indirect organisation and patterning of societies.

However, a shift has occurred towards centring the social and behavioural sciences at the heart of global public health among, for example, international organisations, governments, policy makers, and practitioners worldwide (Shelton et al., 2018). This can be seen within, for instance, health inequalities, and protection of people from violence and forms of social injustice. Social science is an academic discipline concerned with the complex relationships between individuals and the wider society, often predicated on empirical approaches; it is also concerned with how individuals construct wider behaviours, relationships, and structural contexts, which then provide further impetus to enable or constrain action and agency over time. Given this, it is not surprising that public health itself should not be included within the social sciences or that it is critical in investigating

DOI: 10.4324/9781003128373-1

and transforming individual and population health, and the vast array of healthcare systems and challenges, in the light of, for instance, the global pandemic.

This shift has engendered a realisation that public health, as a discipline, is far less narrow than one might have assumed, and that global public health challenges range from traditional ones such as preventing obesity and smoking through prevention and cure to more recent ones highlighted through a social sciences perspective such as wellbeing, loneliness, transgender health, or the health of the planet. Other emerging and important global public health challenges, as a result, are, for instance, health inequalities, violence, the health of marginalised groups, social enterprise, the globalisation of health and illness, and the health and wellbeing of migrants and refugees. These issues challenge us to reflect upon the fact that global public health is often more sociological, anthropological, and behavioural than medical in nature.

This perspective perceives global public health as requiring more than a medical focus, but one that assumes an integrated approach, concentrating upon individuals, communities, and social structures (La Placa et al., 2013). This draws in, for instance, disciplines such as sociology, psychology, social policy, environmental science, economics including political economists, pedagogy, and anthropology (Public Health England, 2018). As a result, new perspectives and methods have been applied to illuminate these issues and challenges through a broad social sciences lens.

The Aims and Content of the Book

This book has been put together to illuminate and enhance the processes mentioned above and generate an enhanced social sciences perspective on global public health. It aims to ensure the importance of social sciences with public health (and vice versa) and its continued contribution by locating and establishing global public health within the context of society, structural realities, and human lived experience. It also advances understanding of how these influence and mould individual and population health.

For example, by assuming a social sciences perspective on global public health, the book sheds light on the role of social theory and theoretical frameworks and how they provide a more detailed and sociological illustration of health and illness. For example, issues around loneliness, stigma, violence, palliative care, and children's health are considered through social sciences theory and literature. Another theme emerging throughout the book is health inequalities, and how social sciences can illustrate important aspects around health inequalities and inequities. It has also enabled authors to keep in mind public health through a globalist perspective, emphasising the importance of how public health is affected by events and interconnections globally, especially the effects of COVID 19, often referred to throughout the book. The aim of the book is to provide a diverse and eclectic range of perspectives and approaches of interest to enable students, researchers, and practitioners to engage with debates, select areas of research interest, and think of a range of applicable perspectives.

The book chapters are arranged in two parts. Part I (Chapters 2–7) deals with key theoretical principles and challenges that underpin the social sciences perspective. Part II (Chapters 8–23) puts theory into practice by addressing a range of contemporary global health issues, relevant to an increasing diverse world, peoples, and communities.

In Chapter 1, Vincent La Placa examines the role of social sciences theoretical frameworks for potential use in global public health. In Chapter 3, Vincent La Placa and Anneyce Knight explore the concept of globalisation and 'wellbeing', arguing for a less foundationalist and structuralist approach to globalisation (as well as the concept of 'globalisation through equilibrium'), and develop the already significant work of La Placa et al. (2013) around wellbeing. Chapter 4 sees Julia Ngozi Chuckuoma and Kevin Deane examine alternatives to classical liberal approaches to health economics and Chapter 5, written by Kafui Adjaye-Gbewonyo and Ichiro Kawachi, considers current approaches to health inequalities and their global effects. Nevin Mehmet explores the theoretical and empirical implications of applying ethics frameworks to global public health in Chapter 6. Jennifer Randall's Chapter 7 ends Part I of the book, with an exploration of radical pedagogy in teaching and learning in global public health.

Part II opens with Aduragbemi Banke-Thomas and Ejemai Eborieme's chapter on designing, implementing, and evaluating global public health interventions, with an emphasis on maternal health. In Chapter 9, Charles Oham et al. focus on the roles of social enterprise in global public health. In Chapter 10, Stefi Barna et al. examine how social systems impact upon planetary health. Vanita Gandhi and Stefi Barna follow on with this by looking at intersections between the social determinants of health, health inequities, and the effects of a warming climate on health including an examination of how health systems can become more sustainable in Chapter 11. In Chapter 12, Julia Morgan and Clare Choak probe the impacts of structural violence on global health utilising examples of men's violence towards women and girls as well as youth violence, whilst Abidemi Okechukwu et al. focus on contemporary issues in child and adolescent health in Chapter 13. In Chapter 14, Julia Morgan and Constance Shumba explore armed conflict and children's mental health highlighting the socially constructed nature of trauma and healing. Part II continues with Chapter 15 whereby Carlos Moreni Leguizamon et al. detail dying and palliative care through a socio-anthropological approach.

In Chapter 16, Julia Morgan and Tumendelger Sengedorj investigate access to healthcare by nomadic people, and Chapter 17 sees Floor Christie-de Jong explore refugee and migrant health inequalities. Chapter 18 has Amanda Rodrigues Amorim Adegboye et al. writing on dietary acculturation and health impact; and in Chapter 19, Danielle J. Roe et al. highlight social inequalities in global public health for transgender, genderqueer, and non-binary people and how they translate into health inequalities.

In Chapter 20, Julia Morgan and Vincent La Placa consider the social construction of loneliness as a global public health issue, followed by Charlotte

Jeavons and Bal Chana, in Chapter 21, exploring global oral health and inequalities. In Chapter 22, the focus is on health protection and a global approach to neglected communicable diseases (NCDs) by Maria Jacirema Ferreira Gonçalves and Amanda Rodrigues Amorim Adegboye.

Finally in the conclusion, which forms Chapter 23, Vincent La Placa and Julia Morgan attempt to draw together the findings based on the knowledge and evidence base in the preceding chapters, and emergent themes. They conclude that applying the social sciences to global public health not only diversifies it but also strengthens it through processes which illustrate the social, cultural, and economic realities of health, healthcare, and health inequalities and assists in development of global public health skills and competencies. Without this approach it is difficult to know the contexts, ways, and means of encouraging people to change, for instance, health-related behaviour, but also the cultural and structural contexts which need to be altered to enable this action (La Placa, McVey et al., 2013).

References

La Placa, V., McNaught, A. and Knight, A. (2013). "Discourse on Wellbeing in Research and Practice". *International Journal of Wellbeing*, 3 (1): 116–125. https://doi.org/10.5502/ijw.v3i1.7

La Placa, V., McVey, D. MacGregor, E., Smith, A. and Scott, M. (2013). "The Contribution of Qualitative Research to the Healthy Foundations Life-stage Segmentation". *Critical Public Health*, 24 (3): 266–282. https://doi.org/10.1080/09581596.2013.797068

Public Health England. (2018). *Improving People's Health: Applying Behavioural and Social Sciences to Improve Population Health and Wellbeing in England*. London: Public Health England.

Shelton, R. C., Hatzenbuehler, M. L., Bayer, R. and Metsch, L. R. (2018). "Future Perfect? The Future of the Social Sciences in Public Health". *Frontiers in Public Health*, 5, (357). https://doi.org/10.3389/fpubh.2017.00357

2

PUBLIC HEALTH, THEORY, AND APPLICATION TO POLICY AND PRACTICE

Vincent La Placa

Introduction

Global public health practice is understood to be the circulation of global health issues into the social and cultural sphere, which were traditionally perceived through a biomedicine perspective. This chapter will introduce readers to the significance of social theory in global public health and outline various theoretical frameworks which can be used. It will consider 'Critical Public Health', 'Feminism', 'Social Constructionism', and 'Structuration' theory, affording examples to emphasise thinking around theory and application. It concludes that the evidence base of global public health should be positioned more coherently within theoretical perspectives which reflect its increasing relevance in the social sciences.

Social Theories and Public Health

Global public health practice is understood to be the diffusion of global health issues into the social and cultural sphere, which were traditionally perceived within a biomedicine framework. This may assume a focus on the wider socio-economic determinants of health behaviour, cultural constructions of the body and health, lived experiences of illness; through to design of interventions to encourage individual behaviours within wider circumstances (which constrain or facilitate behavioural drivers). The drive towards social sciences has also encouraged research on 'wellbeing' as a new phenomenon, distinct from, but linked to health, and enabling a holistic approach to healthcare, physical and subjective states (La Placa et al., 2013a). As a result, global public health research and policy is increasingly lending itself to linkages with social theories to enhance explanations, locate empirical experiences to predict and explain phenomena in wider

DOI: 10.4324/9781003128373-2

contexts, and produce testable hypotheses in quantitative research. Increasingly, global public health links to issues around modernity, inequalities, and globalisation. Such large-scale phenomena can engender instability and disagreement, which can fragment policy responses to health conditions. However, theories pointing towards collective order, are required, when developing policy in an often-fragmentary environment, when assessing , for instance, social exclusion, and the disruption of local and national identities, often caused by increased globalisation.

Generally, social theories can be conceptualised as systematic, reflective, and holistic elucidations on how social systems and societies function, operate, and change. As such, they are founded upon abstract concepts, definitions, and relations (Allan, 2013). Theoretical definitions designate two significant components. 'Stipulative conditions' are explanations of what makes an idea or concept unique in its relation to other parts of the theory (Allan, 2013). 'Dynamic qualities' stipulate the active and effectual movements within the theory which explain change and reality. Traditionally, theory has functioned for the provision of the following. Firstly, it is 'deductive-nomological' (Hempel, 1965), a compilation of explanations, operations and conditions, which potentially generate hypotheses and ideas to be tested, and used within empirical research, whilst proving the validity of the theory. An example of this would be testing the relationship between class and health and explaining potential causes of the link. Secondly, theories are often used as 'representational' categories to broadly encompass and provide a general world-view perspective around research findings and which locate the research or policy within wider contexts. An example of this is the application of Feminism to broadly explain, for instance, the further marginalisation of women in the coronavirus pandemic (Branicki, 2020).

Of course, one can debate, for example, the quantity and quality of evidence to disprove or confirm a theory and how far it can be extrapolated across different populations. One might also question how representative a theory is of the social world and its influence on agreed outcomes i.e., does it bias research to specific findings? Nevertheless, social theory provides a link to navigating and explaining complex social phenomena in public health, to order its complexity, and seeking further explanations for a correlation or cause, in terms of why and how this occurs. It aids one to understand how the research or policy can be applied with reference to constraints and facilitators of social systems, structure, and actions. For example, theory often enables the organisation of the social world into 'collective order' i.e., the social structures and historical conditions that enable predictability and routine or the 'macro' approach. Explanations and causes of, for instance, globalisation, modernity, and inequalities are often placed within the collective orientated schema, for instance, Wallerstein's (1979) global systems theory or La Placa and Knight's (2017) conceptualisation of wellbeing as structured by late-capitalism. Theory can also enable insight into 'individual action' and the ways that individuals negotiate and re-organise lived experience and routinised structures in day-to-day practice or the 'micro' approach. Social theory, then, can guide one to the level of importance of order and action and the extent to which they may combine.

Applerouth and Desfor Edles (2016) assert that social theory also organises behavioural drives with reference to the 'rational' and 'non-rational'. Where structural determinants permeate, actions, behaviour, and ideas may primarily be rationally drawn from pre-existing external conditions. For instance, broad cultural and legal discrimination against women may prevent them from access to healthcare and limit means of circumventing these. From a non-rational perspective, they may be drawn from subjective states, unquestioned, even implied only, symbolic codes, values, uncertainty of meaning, or emotional desires, less amenable to rational organisation. Some theories accentuate one more than the other i.e., Marx (1848/1978) emphasised collective structure and rational action as social explanation and prelude to transforming society. Other contemporary theories may seek to revise or expand the schema and relations between structure and action, for instance, Giddens (1984).

Postmodernist and Foucauldian traditions question whether theory can organise and explain anything valid, given contemporary fluidity of meaning and identity politics (including healthy and non-healthy ones) and contingency of relations (for instance, medical professionals and lay people), usually based upon oppressed and oppressor. This explanation itself may become a fixed reference and schema, synonymous with collective and rational actions, like Marx, and questions the uses of applying Marxist categories to contemporary identity politics (in the health and non-health arena). The proceeding section will outline some of the current theories being applied in global public health. These are not exhaustive, and serve as examples to reflect upon, and put into the context of public health.

Critical Public Health

Whilst there is no identifiable single definition of Critical Public Health theory, it is part of a broad range of work referred to as 'critical theory'. Critical theory emerged through the work of the Frankfurt School in the 1940s, represented by, for instance, Marcuse (1941) and Horkheimer (1947) as a response to classical theoretical over concern with collective cohesion. Rather, the emphasis is on social systems as characterised by significant degrees of social and economic inequalities, and how dominant groups perpetuate oppression of minorities, the poor, and marginalised. Critical Public Health examines, for example, inequalities in health and illness within and between countries, and the social and healthcare systems that perpetuate health inequalities in terms of morbidity and mortality.

The theory itself comprises various sub-theories and perspectives, organised around explanations of power and inequalities. As a result, the theory is broadly subsumed under the collective/rational orientation, focusing on structural determinants such as poverty, discrimination in the form of, for example, racism and hetero-sexism, and barriers to healthcare. The 'social suffering' perspective

(Renault, 2017) explores how socio-economic and political conditions such as war and violence create suffering and contributes to compounding, for instance, pandemics and anti-biotic resistance. There is also an emphasis on how bureaucratic social institutions, such as hospitals and healthcare can exacerbate human suffering and inequalities. Foucault's (1978–1979/2010) theory of biopower is often subsumed under this perspective, due to its rational and institutional explanation of oppression. The growth of the political state leads to centralisation of power and institutions, which exert power and control over individuals' health, through rationalist instruments such as population data, healthcare systems, and social statistics. This enables the state to control the surveillance of oppressed groups in terms of access to healthcare and welfare. The approach is often applied to the One Child policy in China but could easily capture empirical studies into the near-complete abolition of abortion and contraception in Ceausescu's Romania.

Health research and policy generated within this perspective tend to accentuate empowerment of people and reflect upon how disease and illness are often the result of economics and social systems beyond human control. It is often criticised for lack of attention to the role of human agency and consciousness in negotiating and changing social systems and the opportunities afforded to enable change. Nevertheless, it assumes a critical perspective, with the ability to highlight health inequalities, power differentials, and barriers to healthcare, often neglected by classical critical theory.

Feminism

Like Critical Public Health, Feminist theories comprise a broad range of perspectives to research and policies of sex and gender inequality regarding negative health, illness, and wellbeing experiences and outcomes for women, for instance, 'Radical' and 'Liberal' Feminism (Oakley, 1974/2018; hooks, 2014; Leavy and Harris, 2019). Despite differences in perspectives, the unifying theme throughout is underlined by universal agreement that historical and contemporary societies are structurally arranged by men, to the benefit of male power and interest, and to the detriment and subordination of women, both socially and physically. Referred to as 'Patriarchy' (Walby, 1990), women are disproportionally socially and economically disadvantaged in the labour market, economy, domestic life, and healthcare system compared to men. Subordination is enforced through, for instance, deliberate confinement to low-paid work, childcare, and legal and cultural discrimination, through physical and sexual violence globally. According to the World Health Organization (2021), men's violence towards women and girls, especially intimate partner violence and sexual violence, constitutes a significant public health problem, and a violation of women's human rights. Globally, 30% of women have experienced either physical and/or sexual intimate partner violence or non-partner sexual violence in their lifetime (World Health Organization, 2021). As a result, women are much more likely to experience negative physical and mental health outcomes and are more at risk of, for instance, contracting HIV/AIDS, unintended pregnancies, and miscarriages. Men's violence often precipitates depression, post-traumatic stress, and other anxiety disorders, sleep difficulties, eating disorders, and suicide attempts. For Feminists, this reflects patriarchal organisation, reinforcing women's low status, and subjection to male interest (hooks, 2014).

Most recently, the UK Office of National Statistics (2021) found that during the coronavirus pandemic, women were more likely to spend less time working from home, and more time on unpaid childcare and housework, and to be furloughed, compounding existing inequalities. As a result, women experienced more negative health and wellbeing outcomes than men. Literally, all young women in the UK have been subject to sexual harassment, according to a survey from UN Women UK (2021). Among women aged 18–24, 97% reported sexual harassment, whilst 80% of women across all ages, reported sexual harassment in public spaces. For Radical Feminist, Rich (1980/2003), heterosexual relations are compulsorily imposed upon women as a method of sexual control and limit women's other potential for non-heterosexual intimate and sexual relations.

Similarly, Ehrenreich and English (2005) have explored the patriarchal foundations of biomedicine as a means of historically categorising women against a range of biological and psychological disorders, requiring strict adherence to marriage, housework, and childcare to overcome 'abnormal' deviations. Patriarchy has medicalised childbirth in men's interest, for example as witnessed in confinement to hospitals, induction of labour, and increased use of Caesarean births, to deny women experiences of natural birth, and ensure male/medical control of women's bodies. Narayan (2000) discusses how the economic hardship of globalisation affects health by transforming gender roles. For example, the inability of men to attain traditional male jobs not only induces stress and illness in men but also forces women to take up lower skilled and paid work to compensate, negatively impacting their health. Montgomery et al. (2006) focused on how global health changes affect gender roles. For example, her studies in South Africa discovered that men find it harder to accept and enter traditionally lower paid 'female-orientated lower status' work, although women are expected to do this as part of a traditional role. Even where men do participate in childcare and domestic work, the emphasis continues to be, that this is not a recognisably valid male role, reinforcing patriarchal sex roles. As a result, a globally structured gender regime may not change negative outcomes for women's health.

Whilst Feminism is often criticised for perpetuating essentialist categories of sex and gender, many feminists and gender researchers have turned to analyses of the detrimental impact of patterned patriarchal structures upon men, in terms of, for instance, 'toxic masculinity' and its effects on increasing increased male suicide and vulnerability (Crenshaw, 1991; Atkinson, 2008; Kimmel, 2009; Lester et al., 2014) and how consumer capitalism exerts pressure on men and women negatively in terms of health and wellbeing (Acker, 2004). It has also been further developed by dual systems Marxist/Feminist explanations that examine how the inter-relation of capitalism and patriarchy causes a negative dual effect on women in patriarchal societies (Bryson, 2006). Feminism remains an important theoretical lens to interpret and understand health inequalities in a changing global gender order, where despite radical transformations, women continue to bear the brunt of negative health outcomes and socio-economic subordination.

Social Constructionism

Social Constructionism has its origins in the 1960s, with Berger and Luckman's (1966) approach to the Social Constructionism of reality, and the nature of reality as grounded internally within language and relationships, which are symbolically produced and generate further creation of reality (McIntosh, 1968; Stein, 1992; Conrad and Barker, 2010; Burr, 2015). Overall, Social Constructionism breaks with the more rational and collective approach to reject the idea that social reality can be studied as external and objectively observable, independent of human relations and interactions. Reality and knowledge are, however, constructed through discourses, providing public health practitioners with a paradigm accentuating lived experience, and how individuals create health, illness, and wellbeing, on the micro-level through signs, symbols, and stocks of knowledge.

Discourses are practices, which form the objects of which they speak and describe, referring to sets of meanings, metaphors, symbolic images, and narratives, grounded within a subject, for instance, medical, scientific, and psychiatric discourses. These are referred to by people, within interaction with one another, both regulating and providing further regimes of references and actions, albeit, within the discursive framework. They are consistently used and produced through language and relationships and formed because of their use. Illness is not a phenomenon to be rationally discovered, but is created, and emerges through available language and discourse, for instance, homosexuality as a 'psychiatric illness' in the Nineteenth Century and a lifestyle/identity in the Twenty First. Even medical statistics and 'facts' are constructed and updated according to fluid changes in meaning and categorisation processes available at the time.

Public health discourse and disease are not a stable reality, but contingent upon the medical discourses and communities, who construct and reproduce them through their use. Atkinson (1988) ascertained, for example, that students were coached into interpreting signs of disease and that biomedical knowledge was socially accomplished, between patients, students, and teachers. Through social accomplishment, the process could change with the emergence of new forms of knowledge. Barry et al. (2009) explored how obesity metaphors, such as 'obesity as sinful' (gluttony), emerge and impact individuals' support for public policies aimed at reducing obesity. Similarly, conditions such as HIV/AIDs, and responses to them, are not primarily grounded in medical facts, but the discourses and language, available to respond, for instance, stigma, shame, and moral judgement

(Weitz, 1990; Epstein, 1996). Stigma is not medically intrinsic to illness but discursively constructed through meaning and metaphors of disease.

Social Constructionism has been criticised for failure to focus sufficient attention on wider structural and external constraints, and for assuming an overtly relativist stance, which also fails to account for power differentials. Struggles against global inequalities are undermined if they are only perceived as discursive, and if empiricist explanations of health and treatments are negated, as merely existing in language. However, it has proved useful in its application to illuminate issues around the power and legitimacy of biomedical discourse and their production within socio-political struggles and contexts of globalisation. Social Constructionism has also enabled global health issues and interventions to assume social significance, when focusing on how they are discursively articulated and presented, and may focus on tensions between different groups and ideas in global health policy and the contexts in which they are produced.

Structuration Theory

Less often used in public health research is Structuration theory, developed by Gidden's (1984; 1990a; 1990b; 1991), partly to surmount the micro/macro dualism, but to reflect the complexity of late-modern societies. Individuals and society form an inter-linking duality, referred to as the 'duality of structure'. Social structures are both the medium and outcome of the practices they organise. For instance, to communicate, one draws upon language (structure) to articulate meaning. As a result, employing the rules that govern language effectively reproduces it as an outcome/structure of communication, to be employed again over time. Resources represent the individual actions, consciousness, and agency one draws upon to bring about desired outcomes. Rules constitute the available patterns of behaviour and practices, which individuals draw upon to realise desired outcomes. Through individual action, social structures are reproduced, which assume the foundations for further actions (Giddens, 1984). Social structures are properties that exist only over the time and space that they are used and reproduced by agents. They do not automatically exist independent of agents as conceptualised by, for instance, Critical Public Health. If social systems exist beyond agents, it is because of consistently reproduced patterns of action and practice, which often, agents are aware of. Public healthcare practice and global health systems, then, only exist as systems of recurrent relations and practices, across the time and space, that they are produced and prolonged. Giddens' (1984; 1991) articulation of time and space has enabled further analyses of social relations in a modern globalised world, whereby global technology and communication creates 'time-space distantiation', as traditional modernity recedes. For instance, individuals do not need to be physically present to communicate with others globally, for example, telemedicine, and can construct and negotiate relations beyond immediate vicinities. Furthermore, the emptying of time and space in late modernity, and the reorganisation of relations, exposes one to increased risks and dangers. These impact upon physical and mental health, as humans seek 'ontological security', due to impersonal and dis-embedded relations, and multiple forms of knowledge and ideas to choose from.

Structuration theory is critiqued on the grounds that the action/structure dualism is a requisite aspect of theory and that collective structures, such as capitalism and global healthcare systems, cannot be reduced to rules and resources, if theory is to conduct a wider structural analysis (Stones, 2005). Neither does it suggest any methodology to test assumptions (Thompson, 1989; Archer, 2000). However, Stones (2005) has developed an empirical strategy involving a hermeneutics orientated approach to understanding (1) external social structures (conditions for action); (2) internal social structures (agents' capabilities and what they 'know' about the world); (3) active agency and actions; and (4) outcomes of actions as they become solidified for further use by others. Greenhalgh and Stones (2010), in a study of implementing large IT programmes throughout healthcare systems, found that agents constructed their own socio-cultural views of healthcare technology, but were also constrained and enabled by existing frameworks, navigated, and revised through the implementation of the programme.

La Placa et al. (2013b) framed the Healthy Foundations Life-stage Segmentation model within Structuration theory. This explored how stocks of knowledge, drawn from people's understandings, motivations, and contexts, affected health behaviour and provided a further framework around whether behaviour can be changed, and the resources required to motivate change, if necessary. The work enabled development, and piloting of person-centred healthcare interventions, and aligned with people's knowledge and motivations. Clearly, there is potential for more application of the theory in empirical public health studies, to articulate the interaction of structure and agency, and refocus upon, which level it is most significant. The chapter will now proceed to examine the role theory in global public health.

Conclusion

Social theories in global public health are at the heart of intellectual arguments about the workings of societies, social determinants, and policy responses. They are a statement of ontology i.e., how the world works in its current state of existence, and why that is, as well as assumptions as to what is 'real' (Inglis and Thorpe, 2019). For example, rationalist and structuralist theories see social organisation and structure as 'real' which heavily determine or structure behaviour. The knowledge comprising a theory also lends itself to the study of 'epistemology'. This entails thinking about how the theory intends to study reality, based upon ontological assumptions. For example, Social Constructionism tends to lend itself to more interpretivist, phenomenological, and qualitative traditions, given its concentration on how people construct what is 'real' through meaning, discourse, and interpretative relations. This may assume the form of in-depth interviews and ethnographies, through to visual and textual analyses, whereby historical meanings and relations can be gauged from texts and historical depictions of events. One can easily look at Hogarth's portrait of Eighteenth-Century Bedlam Hospital and interpret meanings and representation of asylums and mental illness during this time and contrast them with contemporary representations. This is because both emerge through social and discursive formations that find themselves in representations of events. They are there because they emerged through discourse and practice, not some external social fact. The depiction is the discourse represented.

As a rule, ontology is closely linked to epistemology and methodology, and often, one might precipitate the other. Researchers and practitioners, for example, may be asked to link policies, public health interventions, case studies, and research, to theoretical frameworks or vice versa, to demonstrate knowledge of inter-relations. The one which one starts with is usually not significant. One might identify a theory of interest and seek out research, which it encompasses, or achieve it, the other way around. The key element is to ensure ontological and epistemological/methodological associations link relevant ideas, concepts, and relations together in a firm bind, to ensure intellectual clarity and debate. Identifying theory can be perceived as challenging, given that global public health research and policy often needs to account for the social determinants of health and, for instance, local agents' mobilisation of change in health-related behaviour or society, for instance, La Placa et al. (2013b). Similarly, evaluations of policy and interventions, then, also need to understand and account for the theory, embracing the specific intervention under evaluation, and the epistemology and research methods, used in the process. Theory, then, is a significant thread, running throughout global public health research, and intervention design, both a starting and end point, signposting to further stipulative conditions and dynamic qualities.

Global public health has historically emerged partly due to the inadequacies of biomedical approaches to conceptualise the social, economic, and political dimensions of, for example, health experiences, morbidity, mortality, and social dimension of treatment. As a result, the use of social theory to reflexively explain, and question assumptions and communities (Baert and da Silva, 2010), is under-developed. Unlike biomedicine, global public health is required to focus on the political and social struggles, which define health and illness, and the health disparities which mark countries and communities, within and between them. It is about transforming lives, communities, and access to healthcare. As such, the evidence base of public health should be positioned more coherently within theoretical perspectives that reflect relevant questions, but which question previous assumptions, too. They should also address issues of structures and individuals and be able to suggest policy and practice, within and against current trajectories of globalisation, and its impact on health and healthcare.

Research Points and Reflective Exercise

With reference to any of the theories used in this chapter, begin to reflect upon the following:

- How does the theory challenge biomedicine?
- How can your own research or practice potentially link to theory?
- What, if any, relevance do theories have to current global public health research, practice, and policy development?

Further Resources and Reading

Applerouth, S. and Desfor Edles, L. (2016). *Sociological Theory in the Contemporary Era: Texts and Readings*, 3rd edn. London: Sage.
Jones, P. and Bradbury, L. (2018). *Introducing Social Theory,* 3rd edn. Cambridge: Polity Press.

References

Acker, J. (2004). "Gender, Capitalism and Globalization". *Critical Sociology*, 30 (1): 17–41. https://doi.org/10.1163/156916304322981668
Allan, K. (2013). *Contemporary Social and Sociological Theory: Visualizing Social Worlds.* London: Sage.
Applerouth, S. and Desfor Edles, L. (2016). *Sociological Theory in the Contemporary Era: Texts and Readings*, 3rd edn. London: Sage.
Archer, M. (2000). *Being Human: The Problem of Human Agency.* Cambridge: Cambridge University Press.
Atkinson, P. (1988). "Discourse, Descriptions and Diagnoses: Reproducing Normal Medicine". In M. Lock and D. Gordon (eds.), *Biomedicine Examined*. London: Kluwer Academic Publishers.
Atkinson, M. (2008). "Exploring Male Femininity in the 'Crisis': Men and Cosmetic Surgery". *Body and Society*, 14 (1): 67–87. https://doi.org/10.1177/1357034X07087531
Baert, P. and da Silva, F. C. (2010). *Social Theory in the Twentieth Century and Beyond*, 2nd edn. Cambridge: Policy Press.
Barry, C., Bresscall, V., Brownell, K. D. and Schlesinger, M. (2009). "Obesity Metaphors: How Beliefs about Obesity Affect Support for Public Policy". *The Milbank Quarterly*, 87: 7–47. https://doi.org/10.1111/j.1468-0009.2009.00546.x
Berger, P. L. and Luckmann, T. (1966). *The Social Construction of Reality: A Treatise in the Sociology of Knowledge.* Garden City, NY: Anchor Books.
Branicki, L. J. (2020). "COVID-19, Ethics of Care and Feminist Crisis Management". *Gender, Work and Organization*, 27 (5): 872–883. https://doi.org/10.1111/gwao.12491
Bryson, V. (2006). "Marxism and Feminism: Can the 'Unhappy Marriage' Be Saved?" *Journal of Political Ideologies*, 9 (1): 13–30. https://doi.org/10.1080/1356931032000167454
Burr, V. (2015). *Social Constructionism*, 3rd edn. London: Routledge.
Conrad, P. and Barker, K. K. (2010). "The Social Construction of Illness: Key Insights and Policy Implications". *Journal of Health and Social Behavior*, 51: 567–579. https://doi.org/10.1177/0022146510383495

Crenshaw, K. (1991). "Mapping the Margins: Intersectionality, Identity Politics, and Violence against Women of Color". *Stanford Law Review*, 43, (6): 1241–1299. https://doi.org/10.2307/1229039

Ehrenreich, B. and English, D. (2005). *For Her Own Good: Two Centuries of the Expert's Advice to Women*, 2nd edn. London: Anchor Books.

Epstein, S. (1996). *Impure Science: AIDS, Activism, and the Politics of Knowledge*. Berkeley: University of California Press.

Foucault, M. (1978–1979/2010). *The Birth of Biopolitics: Lectures at the Collège de France, 1978–1979: 5 (Lectures at the College de France)*. New York: St Martin's Press.

Giddens, A. (1984). *The Constitution of Society*. Cambridge: Polity Press.

Giddens, A. (1990a). *The Consequences of Modernity*. Cambridge: Polity Press.

Giddens, A. (1990b). "Structuration Theory and Sociological Analysis". In. J. Clark, C. Modgil and S. Modgil (eds.) *Anthony Giddens: Consensus and Controversy*. London: Falmer Press, 297–315.

Giddens, A. (1991). *Modernity and Self-Identity: Self and Society in the Late Modern Age*. Cambridge: Polity Press.

Greenhalgh, T. and Stones, R. (2010). "Theorising Big IT Programmes in Healthcare: Strong Structuration Theory Meets Actor-Network Theory". *Social Science and Medicine*, 70 (9): 1285–1294. https://doi.org/10.1016/j.socscimed.2009.12.034

Hempel, C. G. (1965). *Aspects of Scientific Explanation, and Other Essays in the Philosophy of Social Science*. New York: Free Press.

hooks, B. (2014). *Feminist Theory: From Margin to Center*. London: Routledge.

Horkheimer, M. (1947). *The Eclipse of Reason*. New York: Oxford University Press.

Inglis, D. and Thorpe, C. (2019). *An Invitation to Social Theory*, 2nd edn. Cambridge: Policy Press.

Kimmel, M. (2009). "Has a Man's World Become a Woman's Nation?" In. H. Boushey and A. O'Leary (eds.) *The Shriver Report: A Woman's Nation Changes Everything*. Washington, DC: Centre for American Progress, 323–357.

La Placa, V. G., McNaught, A. and Knight, A. (2013a). "Discourse of Wellbeing in Research and Practice". *International Journal of Wellbeing*, 3 (1): 116–125. doi:10.5502/ijw.v3i1.7

La Placa, V., McVey, D. MacGregor, E., Smith, A. and Scott, M. (2013b). "The Contribution of Qualitative Research to the Healthy Foundations Life-stage Segmentation". *Critical Public Health*, 24 (3): 266–282. https://doi.org/10.1080/09581596.2013.797068

La Placa, V. and Knight, A. (2017). "The Emergence of Wellbeing in Late Modern Capitalism: Theory, Research and Policy Responses". *International Journal of Social Science Studies*, 5 (3): 1–11. https://doi.org/10.11114/ijsss.v5i3.2207

Leavy, P. and Harris, A. (2019). *Contemporary Feminist Research from Theory to Practice*. London: Guildford Press.

Lester, D., Gunn, J. F. and Quinnett, P. (2014). *Suicide in Men: How Men Differ from Women in Expressing Their Distress*. Springfield: Charles C Thomas.

Marcuse, H. (1941). "Some Implications of Modern Technology". *Studies in Philosophy and Social Science*, 9: 414–439.

Marx, K. (1848/1978). "Manifesto of the Communist Party". In. R. Tucker (ed.) *The Marx/Engels Reader*. New York: Norton, 465–501.

McIntosh, M. (1968). The Homosexual Role. *Social Problems*, 16 (2): 182–192. https//doi.org/10.2307/800003

Montgomery, C., Hosegood, V., Busza, J. and Timaeus, I. (2006). "Men's Involvement in the South African Family: Engendering Change in the AIDs Era". *Social Science and Medicine,* 10: 2411–2419. https://doi.org/10.1016/j.socscimed.2005.10.026

Narayan, D. (2000). *Voices of the Poor: Can Anyone Hear Us?* Oxford: Oxford University Press.

Oakley, A. (1974/2018). *The Sociology of Housework (Reissue).* Bristol: Bristol University Press.

Office for National Statistics (ONS). (2021). "Coronavirus (COVID-19) and the Different Effects on Men and Women in the UK, March 2020 to February 2021". Available at: https://www.ons.gov.uk/peoplepopulationandcommunity/healthandsocialcare/conditionsanddiseases/articles/coronaviruscovid19andthedifferenteffectsonmenandwomenintheukmarch2020tofebruary2021/2021-03-10 (Accessed: 11 March 2021).

Renault, E. (2017). *Social Suffering: Sociology, Psychology, Politics.* London: Rowman and Littlefield International.

Rich, A. C. (1980/2003). "Compulsory Heterosexuality and Lesbian Existence". *Journal of Women's History,* 15 (3): 11–48. doi:10.1353/jowh.2003.0079

Stein, E. (1992). *Forms of Desire: Sexual Orientation and the Social Constructionist Controversy.* London: Routledge.

Stones, R. (2005). *Structuration Theory.* Basingstoke: Palgrave MacMillan.

Thompson, J. B. (1989). "The Theory of Structuration". In. D. Held and J. B. Thompson (eds.) *Social Theories of Modern Societies: Anthony Giddens and His Critics.* Cambridge: Cambridge University Press, 56–76.

UN Women UK. (2021). "Almost All Young Women in the UK have been Sexually Harassed, Survey Finds", The Guardian, 10 March. Available at: https://www.theguardian.com/world/2021/mar/10/almost-all-young-women-in-the-uk-have-been-sexually-harassed-survey-finds (Accessed: 16 March 2021).

Walby, S. (1990). *Theorizing Patriarchy.* Oxford: Blackwell.

Wallerstein, I. (1979). *The Capitalist World Economy.* Cambridge: Cambridge University Press.

Weitz, R. (1990). "Living With the Stigma of AIDS". *Qualitative Sociology,* 13: 23–38. https://doi.org/10.1007/BF00988594

World Health Organization. (2021). "Violence Against Women", World Health Organization, 9 March. Available at: https://www.who.int/news-room/fact-sheets/detail/violence-against-women (Accessed: 16 March 2021).

3

GLOBALISATION AND GLOBAL PUBLIC HEALTH

Vincent La Placa and Anneyce Knight

Introduction

This chapter will explore the concept of globalisation and its impact on global health and wellbeing, particularly in the light of COVID 19, as well as concepts of de-globalisation, and the future of conceptualising health and wellbeing on this level. It will contend against over reliance upon structural theories and foundationalism to locate discussions around globalisation, arguing for rich, detailed, and contextualised research to bridge the gap between theory and research. This places emphasis upon individual volition, action, agency, and standpoints, to build more in-depth contextualised knowledge around health, wellbeing, and global issues, and bridge the gap between practice, theory, and research.

Globalisation and Global Health

Over the past 30 years, an array of literature on globalisation, health, and wellbeing has emerged, although there is no agreed definition or agreement as to its consequences. Tomlinson (1999) defines it as a rapid development and ever deepening of a network of inter-links and independencies that characterise modern life, across politics, economics, culture, technology, and medicine. Modern life compresses and shrinks as geographical, social, and economic linkages are compounded, and information, people, products, and knowledge spread across boundaries, with less constraint, minimising spaces between people and countries (Ritzer, 2003; Chirico, 2014). For instance, enhanced technology and communications lessen geographical distances between people. Furthermore, increased trade between countries makes them more inter-dependent upon each other for prosperity. Greater movement of people entails a diminishing view of borders and 'separation', and recognition that what occurs in one part of the

DOI: 10.4324/9781003128373-3

globe assumes relevance for the rest, as COVID-19 has highlighted, and which is discussed later in this chapter.

Theorists differ precisely as to when globalisation began and its causes, although there is greater agreement, that it is connected, but not exclusively, to the development of modern capitalism in the Twentieth Century (Giddens, 2002). For instance, the rapid spread of free markets, production specialisation, technology, and consumerism homogenises the global economic system and legitimates free markets and their consequences (negative and positive) across the globe. This generates a global culture around 'neoliberal' ideologies and practices, as producers and consumers move knowledge and products unhindered across borders. This has prompted debate around whether the process homogenises global culture (in the interests of Western hegemony, but to the detriment of others in terms of, for instance, health inequalities) or whether heterogeneity is the result. Heterogeneity is the consequence of local fragmentation, engendered by communities and localities to resist universal culture, particularly Western colonial ones, and asserts difference and independence. This is captured in 'post-colonial' perspectives, which emphasise resistance to usually Western dominance and resultant inequalities (Ashcroft et al., 2006).

Globalisation is significant in studies of public health and wellbeing, especially in relation to healthcare systems, health inequalities, social justice, and equity, as well as relations between developed and developing nations, and global concepts of wellbeing. For example, in terms of health, diet, and lifestyle, it is argued that cognitive changes, precipitated by advertising and marketing of Western consumer goods, have facilitated the global spread and homogenisation of so-called 'lifestyle' diseases (such as obesity and tobacco-related illnesses) in specific populations within low- and middle-income countries, like those in the West. This then forces the low- and middle-income countries to adopt analogous Western methods of economic and healthcare reform and interventions, thereby enforcing further homogeneity. In terms of relations between low- and middle-income and high-income countries, greater population mobility means high-income countries formulate policies to deter high levels of immigration and so-called 'health tourism' (heterogenisation). However, the migration of health professionals from low- and middle-income countries offers benefits to understaffed health systems in high-income countries, but potentially at the expense of capacity in other countries (homogenisation). Globalisation has also precipitated developments in the concept of global wellbeing (La Placa and Knight, 2014), which have often been ignored in global public health studies.

Global Wellbeing

The term wellbeing is progressively important in social and behavioural science orientated public health, indicated by its correlation with health in the World Health Organization's 1948 constitution, 'Health is a state of complete physical, mental and social wellbeing and not merely the absence of disease or infirmity'

(WHO, 2021). Furthermore, the third goal of the 17 United Nations' Sustainable Development Goals (UNSDGs) specifically relates to 'Good Health and Wellbeing', and ensuring healthy lives, and promoting wellbeing for all at all ages (United Nations Development of Economic and Social Affairs, 2021). Nevertheless, although it is still entwined with health, wellbeing is increasingly perceived in social sciences, as a separate construct associated with, for instance, the development and complexity of late modern global capitalist society and firmly embedded within emergent public health discourses (La Placa and Knight, 2014).

As a term, wellbeing does not have one definitive globally understood definition, although historically, it is perceived from a positivist standpoint based purely on economics (consumerism), psychological (happiness and quality of life), and biomedical science, rather than as an all-encompassing concept (La Placa and Knight, 2014; Moreno-Leguizamon, 2014). Indeed, since the Second World War, material and measurable factors such as employment, income, economic growth, and Gross Domestic Product (GDP) were perceived as essentially equating to wellbeing (La Placa and Knight, 2014). However, as society has become progressively more individualistic in terms of individual lifestyle choices, increased consumerism, and developments in science and technology, wellbeing has emerged beyond a traditional reductionist lens, to a more multi-faceted concept. As the World Health Organization (2021) has proposed, wellbeing exists in two dimensions, subjective and objective. It comprises an 'individual's experience of their life as well as a comparison of life circumstances with social norms and values' (WHO Regional Office for Europe 2012: 1).

McNaught's (2011) definitional framework for wellbeing reflects this wider viewpoint as it includes the intricacies of an individual's lived reality, wherever they are situated globally, and provides for a more comprehensive approach. His structured framework identifies four domains of wellbeing: individual, family, community, and society, which includes a range of complex sub-categories, of both processes and relations, viewed from objective and subjective perspectives (McNaught, 2011). As an inclusive and holistic model, it also moves beyond the micro notion of individual and personal responsibility for wellbeing to the macro understanding of wellbeing, which is contingent on social, economic, geographic, and environmental dimensions, as these provide the fundamental resources and circumstances for wellbeing for society. It is important to remember, however, as McNaught (2011) ascertains, individuals are not merely passive recipients of wellbeing, based on external factors, as their unique actions, and choices, are also influential. The domains and inter-relationship of factors are illustrated within the framework in Figure 3.1.

When considering an exploration of wellbeing and global public health, the multi-dimensional nature of wellbeing should be considered beyond the lens of traditional public health, positive psychology, and quality of life. Although not explicitly referencing globalisation, McNaught's (2011) domains currently provide the most adaptable framework, which seeks to remove 'silo' and fragmented approaches to policy making, research, and public health interventions,

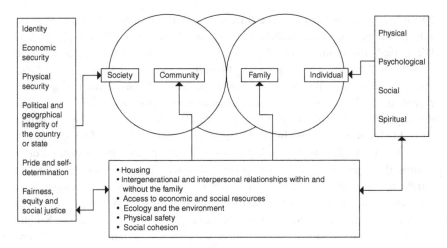

FIGURE 3.1   A structured framework for defining wellbeing. Figure 3.1 is reproduced from Knight and McNaught (eds) (2011) Understanding Wellbeing: An Introduction for Students and Practitioners of Health and Social Care, with permission from Lantern Publishing.

to improve both health and wellbeing at a local, national, and global level (the latter which requires more detailed knowledge and research). Indeed, the authors have previously proposed that McNaught's (2011) multi-levelled framework is helpful 'to enhance theoretical frameworks and to guide the design and development of both health and wellbeing interventions…[and] provides the philosophical underpinnings for wellbeing policy development' (La Placa et al., 2013: 116).

Undeniably, in the twenty-first century, the notion of promoting wellbeing throughout a population's lifespan should guide and be embedded within long-term global policy development and public health practice. This is to ensure that the impact of decision making is considered in relation to, not only their respective culture and society, but also to the individual, their family, communities, and decisions altered, if they are found to be detrimental. The aim is to broadly promote reflexivity, as well as self-actualisation, and ensure global social justice, rather than seeking a utilitarian approach, which may deny marginalisation, potential negative impacts on individual, family, community, and societal wellbeing, which heighten inequalities.

COVID-19 and Health and Wellbeing

Most recently, the continuing global COVID-19 pandemic, which began in 2019, with its global spread and search for solutions to it, has dominated debates around globalisation, global health, and wellbeing. The rapidity of modern transportation systems and population mobility has accentuated how infections can shift across the globe within a few hours (as illustrated by the SARS outbreak in 2002–2003 as well as COVID-19). Cash and Patel (2020) argue that global responses to COVID-19 have often been biased towards high-income countries and grounded within Western discourses of universal medicine. For instance, low-income countries were encouraged to lockdown, like high-income ones, but they question whether this was the appropriate response, given their younger population profiles, and lesser numbers of older people in care homes (Cash and Patel, 2020).

As a result, this may have increased deaths due to non-COVID 19 diseases, and increased the burden on lower-income people, than might otherwise have been the case. Poorer people, for instance, living in densely crowded urban slums, are subject to stringent lockdowns, even though social and physical distancing is much harder. This enforces greater hardships on those earning a living through the informal economy. Instead, policies focused on the unique demographics of a country, its different social conditions and cultures, precarious livelihoods, and constrained conditions and resources (particularly health resources) are necessary. As a result, the pandemic has illuminated issues around, not only health inequalities but also the failure of the global community, to ensure that the 'Global South' is adequately resourced and protected, similarly to the West.

The global pandemic has led theorists to address issues such as whether globalisation, and its gravitation towards intensified dependence and relations, is necessary, or has exceeded its benefits. For example, the pandemic caused a significant decline in international flows such as trade, foreign direct investment (FDI), consumption of health and non-health products, and international travel. Supply chain policies, particularly medical and health-related ones, have come to the forefront of global health debates and may reshape trade and FDI flows. The production, coordination, and transport of medicines, and pharmaceuticals, through to availability of life-saving personal protective equipment (PPE) for healthcare workers, have become delicate health, wellbeing, and security issues. Governments and healthcare systems have felt vulnerable to unexpected shortages of medical and health-related products, and this has led to a tendency towards protectionism. This is especially the case where production is over concentrated in specific parts of the globe, and the ability to produce many basic medicines has been foregone, as most global active pharmaceutical ingredients (APIs) are sourced globally.

Questions also emerge around the adequacy of reliance upon companies and other countries to produce and supply them when more diversification and national control and self-sufficiency are necessary in health emergencies. This, among many other factors, has precipitated debates around 'de-globalisation' whereby, for example, healthcare and economic systems become less connected and integrated and more regionalised. Thus, not only do nations assume more control over production and supplies of medicines and pharmaceuticals, but also over their responses to health emergencies, and resulting social and economic implications. Donald Trump's 'America First' and Joe Biden's 'Buy American' may not only appear to emanate from politically different perspectives but also represent a similar de-globalisation trend or, what the authors prefer to term, 'globalisation through equilibrium'. Concepts of de-globalisation emerged more strongly with Russia's invasion of Ukraine in early 2022. This has precipitated debates, especially in the West, and among its allies, about significant disentangling from reliance upon Russian oil and gas supplies and a shift to domestic supply instead (Peston, 2022). An invigorated emphasis on energy security will speed up the process and may enhance use of fossil fuels, which can have significant impacts on global health, and climate change. It may also mean the reconstruction of economies, where manufacturing and food production will occur closer to home, if not directly on the domestic level. The passing of the multi-billion-dollar bill, by the US House of Representatives in February 2022, aimed at increasing American competitiveness with China, and enhancing US semiconductor manufacturing, is another example of de-globalisation.

As a result, concepts of homogeneity then are replaced by ones such as 'competition', 'managed re-configuration', and 're-localisation', depending on context, and the perceived interest of a country/regional bloc. This may already be apparent in the often-failed attempt of the global community to mount an effective response to a global pandemic, reflected in its retreat into potential vaccine nationalism and protectionism, and ideological competition in terms of national responses, for instance, lockdowns and vaccination processes. Globalisation through equilibrium accentuates the contingent, agent lead, and contextual nature of global processes. It does not assume a one-dimensional trajectory, or an inevitable development of capitalism/s, beyond the control of healthcare professionals, policy makers, agents, patients, or, indeed, theoreticians.

Globalisation, Theory, and Public Health and Wellbeing Research

Discussions and uses of globalisation are increasingly important in global public health and wellbeing research and policy. However, definitions, causes, and solutions are also increasingly complex, as discussions are often framed within structural theoretical frameworks. Critical Public Health, Marxism, Feminism, Functionalism, and even Postmodernism tend to constitute the dominant frameworks, articulating distinct structural approaches as to, for example, its role in increasing/decreasing health inequalities, its distinctiveness from capitalism, and its impact upon responses to the pandemic (although, of course, postmodernists would achieve this with a pinch of scepticism). Often, these theories have paid scant attention to wellbeing, with an emphasis on physical health and illness.

Globalisation is also often approached through the lens of structures, systems, and how it interacts with other and wider dominant structures/systems. For example, critical theorists, often in conjunction with Marxists, have attempted to frame and articulate how health inequalities are caused by extensive globalisation and capitalism, but compounded in interaction with wider systems of, for instance, racism, heterosexism, and social exclusion, as the dominant narrative (Bhattacharyya, 2018; Chitty, 2020; Sell and Williams, 2020; Harvey, 2021).

However, whilst these issues are very important, and indispensable, if one perceives global public health as concerned with global equity and justice, there remains, as Stones (1996) asserts, the problem of building a bridge between theory and the complex evidence required to demonstrate its reality. There is also the issue of 'foundationalism', where one accepts abstract systems theory as reality itself, with very little empirical data to support it. Discussions of globalisation, the authors think, are often theorised with more than a little bias towards foundationalism.

Globalisation, capitalism, and forms of marginalisation may be intertwined. However, it would be impossible for a researcher to empirically confirm, once and for all, that global capitalism, in whatever historical shape, or definition, is primarily responsible for, or linked to other institutions/systems of oppression, or all health and economic inequalities, given the complexities involved. Empirically explaining how structural systems inter-link across time and space adequately is also a minefield. Neither should any attempt at this be taken lightly, given the implications for ensuring fairness, transparency, and equity in health policy. However, such an undertaking would entail the study of millions of market transactions, conducted by literally millions of individuals, potentially across hundreds of years of time and space, and continents. It would entail studying their interactions, motivations, reasons, opinions, and attitudes (either negative or positive) between the buyer and seller (was the buyer explicitly prejudiced against some aspect of the seller and did the seller experience the interaction as a form of marginalisation/oppression or racism, why, and in what sense?) and vice versa between the modern building developer and property buyer in contemporary economics. Clearly, this is impossible on an empirical level, whatever the ontological assumptions. It might be that innovative technology and knowledge, the higher qualifications required for it, and the higher rewards warranted for possessing them, may explain health and economic inequalities more effectively in some contexts. However, this is not accounted for through such analyses.

The transformation of China from communism to capitalism has been achieved through a series of discovery processes and interaction between individuals, ideology, historical interpretation, and cultural aspects, not all from a Western perspective (Coase and Wang, 2012). Attempting to empirically discover once and for all, unalterable connections between Chinese state capitalism (which is not a mirror image of Western capitalism), and Western notions of racism and colonialism, would surely somehow necessitate empirically asking and verifying whether Chinese traders, businesspeople, and consumers, across the second largest economy in the world, experience, and to what extent, the transformation has been racist, colonial, or anti-Chinese (it may or may not be or to different degrees). This might need to be attained through coverage of the last 40 years of economic development, across different regions, including Hong Kong, and across a whole array of agents, consumers, and actors, operating within, and externally to the current model. Clearly again, this is challenging, empirically, as well as theoretically, to confirm, once and for all. Failure to achieve empirical evidence has led to development of concepts, for instance, around 'post-colonial' studies (Ashcroft et al., 2006; Bakshi et al., 2016). However, this is not an adequate theoretical framework, but more a one-size-fits-all perspective, on knowledge interpretation (often comprising internal contradictions and arguments and one-sided opinions about who does and does not possess freedom and agency). The idea, for instance, that non-Western lesbians, gays, bisexuals, or transgendered people passively (consciously or unconsciously) accept Western discourses of sexuality and sexual practices and need to be 'de-colonised' as a result might produce a form of colonialism, eventually. It theoretically and empirically ignores the rich interplay of both Western and non-Western ideas, and the national and cultural-political interests of specific groups and institutions within countries to either retain or revise laws and practices, inherited from Empire, or across current or previous periods of Indigenous history, time and space, and specific contexts. Neither does it adequately address that non-Western discourses and cultural practices can marginalise or oppress others, independently of economic systems.

Rather, we argue that there is a durable place for systems theorising (from all standpoints), but one where ontological reality is grounded within more complex empirical analyses of globalisation on, for example, the local, contextual, and relational level, in terms of economics, health, and wellbeing. This may, for instance, assume the form of research into relations between health, wellbeing, and religious beliefs in rural India; or studies of the complex web of knowledge and relations that the local General Practitioner builds up as she or he attends to patients and hospitals between regional towns in Alabama; or it may focus upon how young people perceive and use social media, and its impact upon mental health and wellbeing, as they negotiate social media circuits across websites, social groups, and countries, and the contiguousness between events, across place and time.

We would encourage qualitative, hermeneutical, and Weberian social-action-orientated methodologies, as well as more traditional quantitative methods, aimed at discovery of structural realities. For instance, rich and detailed qualitative interviews and/or anthropological research with women in Sub-Saharan Africa around, for example, the social construction of perceptions and uses of contraception, Female Genital Mutilation (FGM), and sexual health and wellbeing, might shed light upon local or otherwise patriarchal attitudes towards women and their origins. It might also illuminate how they creatively organise resource to empower themselves in all women spaces, enabling other researchers to compare with similar studies, and build up global perspectives from women's points of view, and grounded within Feminist frameworks. Similarly, if one were to conduct contextualised research with Vietnamese garment/factory workers about their experiences of working for multinational companies, one could develop a range of perspectives, upon how they may or may not benefit from current economic contexts and impacts on health and wellbeing. The focus might be on potential forms of resistance, perceptions of work through the life-course, and organisation for workers' rights, as well as strategies to transmit changes, if any, in outlook and experience to their children. This continues to construct critical depictions of how social action in specific structural conditions actuates further resources, contexts, and consequences for further action (Bauman, 1992; Stones, 1996), like research strategies bracketed, but not exclusively, around Structuration theory and hermeneutics, considered in the previous chapter.

This we believe builds a bridge between theory, evidence, and action, whilst also refining and illustrating current frameworks in global public health and rendering a multi-layered perspective to empower people, and ensure voices are articulated by means of global perspectives. This is especially important given the complex emergence of wellbeing as distinct from other definitions and studies of health. The focus is on agency, consciousness, and empowerment from individuals' perspectives, as well as systems-orientated explanations, potential linkages, empirical confirmations, and contiguities between them. This, we believe, for instance, is an alternative to Kumar's (2020) interesting, if unlikely, discussion that the agency and actions of global garment workers are determined by structural systems of buyer and supplier chains within 'monopsony' capitalism.

Conclusion

This chapter has outlined key definitions of globalisation in public health and wellbeing and applied them to issues within global public health and the social sciences. It has argued against over reliance upon structural theories, to locate discussions around globalisation, but argued for rich, detailed, and contextualised research, to bridge the gap between theory and research; and place emphasis on individual, community, and contiguous realities to build knowledge.

Research Points and Reflective Exercise

With reference to the discussions in this chapter, begin to reflect upon the following:

- What do you understand by the term Globalisation, and what may explain its causes?
- How would you define global wellbeing?
- Do you agree with the authors' views as regards explanations of globalisation through reference to foundationalism? If not, why not?

Further Resources and Reading

McNaught, A. (2011). "Defining Wellbeing." In A. Knight and McNaught, A. (eds.) *Understanding Wellbeing: An Introduction for Students and Practitioners of Health and Social Care*. Banbury: Lantern Publishing, 7–22.

References

Ashcroft, B., Griffiths, G. and Tiffin, H. (2006). *The Post-Colonial Studies Reader*, 2nd edn. Abingdon: Routledge.

Bakshi, S., Jivraj, S. and Posocco, S. (2016). *Decolonizing Sexualities: Transnational Perspectives, Critical Interventions*. Oxford: Counterpress.

Bauman, Z. (1992). *Imitations of Postmodernity*. London: Routledge.

Bhattacharyya, G. (2018). *Rethinking Racial Capitalism: Questions of Reproduction and Survival*. London: Rowman and Littlefield International.

Cash, R. and Patel, V. (2020). "Has COVID-19 Subverted Global Health?" *The Lancet*, 395 (10238): 1669–1738. https://doi.org/10.1016/S0140-6736(20)31089-8

Chirico, J. (2014). *Globalization: Prospects and Problems*. London: Sage.

Chitty, C. (2020). *Sexual Hegemony: Statecraft, Sodomy, and Capital in the Rise of the World System*. London: Duke University Press.

Coase, R. and Wang, N. (2012). *How China Became Capitalist*. Basingstoke: Palgrave MacMillan.

Giddens, A. (2002). "The Globalization of Modernity". In. D. Held and A. McGrew (eds.) *The Global Transformations Reader: An Introduction to the Globalization Debate*. Cambridge: Polity, 60–66.

Harvey, M. (2021). "The Political Economy of Health: Revisiting Its Marxian Origins to Address 21st-Century Health Inequalities". *American Journal of Public Health*, 111 (2): 293–300. https://doi.org/10.2105/AJPH.2020.305996

Kumar, A. (2020). *Monopsony Capitalism: Power and Production in the Twilight of the Sweatshop Age*. Cambridge: Cambridge University Press.

La Placa, V., McNaught, A. and Knight, A. (2013). "Discourse on Wellbeing in Research and Practice". *International Journal of Wellbeing*, 3 (1): 116–125. https://doi.org/10.5502/ijw.v3i1.7

La Placa, V. and Knight, A. (2014). "Wellbeing: A New Policy Phenomenon?" In A. Knight, V. La Placa and A. McNaught (eds.) *Wellbeing: Policy and Practice*. Banbury: Lantern Publishing, 17–27.

McNaught, A. (2011). "Defining Wellbeing". In A. Knight and McNaught, A. (eds.) *Understanding Wellbeing: An Introduction for Students and Practitioners of Health and Social Care*. Banbury: Lantern Publishing, 7–22.

Moreno-Leguizamon, C. (2014). "Wellbeing in Economics, Psychology, and Health Sciences: A Contested Category". In A. Knight, V. La Placa and A. McNaught (eds.) *Wellbeing: Policy and Practice*. Banbury: Lantern Publishing, 7–16.

Peston, R. (2022). "The Invasion of Ukraine and the Death of Globalization, 3 March 2022". Available at: https://www.spectator.co.uk/article/the-invasion-of-ukraine-and-the-death-of-globalisation (Accessed: 8 March 2022).

Ritzer, G. (2003). "Rethinking Globalization: Glocalization/Grobalization and Something/Nothing". *Sociological Theory*, 21 (3): 193–209. https//doi.org/10.1111/1467-9558.00185

Sell, S. K. and Williams, O. D. (2020). "Health under Capitalism: A Global Political Economy of Structural Pathogenesis". *Review of International Political Economy*, 27 (1): 1–25. https://doi.org/10.1080/09692290.2019.1659842

Stones, R. (1996). *Sociological Reasoning: Towards a Past-Modern Sociology*. Basingstoke: MacMillan Press.

Tomlinson, J. (1999). *Globalization and Culture*. Chicago, IL: University of Chicago Press.

United Nations Development of Economic and Social Affairs. (2021). "Sustainable Development: The 17 Goals". Available at: https://sdgs.un.org/goals (Accessed: 2 August 2021).

World Health Organization. Regional Office for Europe. (2012). "Measurement of and Target Setting for Well-Being: An Initiative by the WHO Regional Office for Europe. Second Meeting of the Expert Group Paris, France, 25–26 June 2012". Available at: https://www.euro.who.int/__data/assets/pdf_file/0009/181449/e96732. pdf (Accessed: 2 April 2021).

World Health Organization. (2021). "WHO Remains Firmly Committed to the Principles Set Out in the Preamble to the Constitution". Available at: https://www.who. int/about/who-we-are/constitution (Accessed: 18 April 2021).

4

ECONOMICS AND GLOBAL HEALTH

Julia Ngozi Chukwuma and Kevin Deane

Introduction

Economics primarily appears in global health programmes in the guise of Health Economics. Broadly speaking, Health Economics involves two distinct strands. One strand focuses on the application of core neoclassical economic theories of the firm, the consumer, and the market to health-behaviour, and other health issues. It suggests a role for government intervention, only in the case of specific market failures (for example externalities, asymmetric information, moral hazard, and public goods) that distort market outcomes. Health Economics also promotes economic evaluation techniques that are used to assess the cost-effectiveness of competing interventions. However, what is rarely made clear to global public health students is that Health Economics, as a subfield of economics, applies only one version of economics (neoclassical economics), to health.

This chapter does not focus on traditional Health Economics – numerous textbooks exist that promote this way of thinking about the economics of health. Instead, this chapter discusses four alternative, non-neoclassical perspectives which are relevant to global health, namely, Keynesian, Political Economy, Feminist, and Ecological perspectives. We use the COVID-19 pandemic as a lens through which to introduce these perspectives and highlight the insights that they provide, for health inequalities, and planetary health.

Keynesian Economics and Health

While neoclassical economics promotes the notion of a perfectly functioning, free market, and sees an only limited role for state intervention, Keynesian economics accords a more active role to the government in steering the economy – especially in times of crisis. Indeed, neoclassical economics had very little to say

DOI: 10.4324/9781003128373-4

about either the causes of or solutions to the Global Financial Crisis (GFC) of 2007/08 and has been blamed by some economists for having caused the crisis, due to its attachment to free-market capitalism, and deregulation of the financial sector (Skidelsky, 2010a; 2010b).

While the GFC revealed the inherent flaws of unfettered capitalism and neoclassical economic theory championing it, the crisis which emerged in 2020 significantly exceeded the economic fallout of the GFC. What followed the declaration of the COVID-19 outbreak as a pandemic in March 2020 was a contraction of global economic output by 5.8 % – compared to 'only' 3.5 % in the aftermath of the GFC (UNCTAD, 2021). Within just a few weeks, the health crisis turned into a full-blown economic and social crisis. Across the globe, governments imposed movement restrictions on their citizens, ordering them to work from home to curb the spread of the COVID-19 virus, and shut down factories. Furthermore, like the measures adopted in reaction to the GFC, yet much greater in volume, national governments resorted once more to the 'Keynesian toolbox'.

Returning to 2008, the neoclassical economist Robert Lucas, known as one of the harshest critics of Keynesian macroeconomics, made headlines during the GFC when he proclaimed that 'everyone is a Keynesian in a foxhole' (Bello, 2017). Lucas' statement referred to the (non-neoclassical) economic theory behind the fiscal policy measures adopted by governments in response to the GFC: Keynesian economics owes its name to the British economist John Maynard Keynes (1883–1946). Keynes, observing an increasing number of unemployed workers, fewer firms engaging in manufacturing activity, and people buying fewer consumer goods during the years of the Great Depression of the 1930s, was of the view that the market would remain stuck in crisis, without the government stimulating demand. He was sceptical of the prevalent assumption of the time that, if left alone, the market mechanism would self-correct and ensure that the supply of products is met by the required demand (Heilbroner, 2011). Keynes argued that, in a world characterised by uncertainty about what the future may bring, investors do not automatically re-invest their savings but may want to wait for (pre-supposedly) better times (Keynes, 1936). Such lack of investment results in workers' disposable income and, consequently, their incentive to buy consumables decrease (Chang, 2014). Reduced consumption pushes investments even further down, and results in an additional loss of jobs, and so it continues. To halt the downward spiral, Keynes advocated that governments should 'manage' and intervene in the market by using public resources to boost the aggregate demand for goods and services and to create employment opportunities (Skidelsky, 2010a).

Having adopted a Keynesian's logic, the policy response of governments to the global economy's freefall in the wake of the GFC was unprecedented. For instance, 'fiscal policy measures' taken by the US Government included tax cuts and transfers to households, costing the taxpayer about 5.5 % of the country's entire 2008 Gross Domestic Product (GDP) (Guellec and Wunsch-Vincent, 2009).

Yet, the resources mobilised to stabilise the economy amidst the crisis prompted by COVID-19 far outweigh the money spent in response to the GFC. Within weeks of the on-set of the crisis, governments around the world – including conservative and libertarian regimes such as in the UK and the USA – de-emphasised their 'laissez-faire' philosophies. In the USA, a (first) fiscal stimulus package of an estimated US$ 2.3 trillion (around 11 % of GDP) was adopted as early as June 2020 (International Monetary Fund, 2021). In a similar vein, also UK politicians once again became Keynesians. The government introduced tax breaks for homeowners and entrepreneurs and a furlough scheme, providing financial support to companies, facing difficulties paying their workers' salaries, worth close to GB£ 70 billion (Francis-Devine et al., 2021) In other words, contrary to the pro-austerity narrative, rooted in neoclassical economics, which dominated policymaking for over a decade, governments and central banks, committed to heavily intervene in the market, to cushion the negative economic impact of the pandemic, and found their 'magic money tree' (BBC, 2018). This demonstrates that, in times of crisis, even the most committed free-market proponents turn to Keynesian economics.

Applying a Political Economy Lens to Health

Whilst Keynesian economics, in contrast to neoclassical economics, advocates for increased government expenditure and investment in times of crisis, political economy approaches go yet another step further and centre their analysis on the structural problems inherent to the capitalist economic system. Markedly, the COVID-19 pandemic has highlighted some of the systemic deficiencies of capitalism.

In May 2020, a Guardian headline read '*Black people four times more likely to die from COVID-19, ONS finds*' (The Guardian, 2020). Indeed, the Office for National Statistics reports that during the first wave of the COVID-19 pandemic, the rate of death in the UK of the 'black African group' was 3.7 times higher compared to the 'white British group' (ONS, 2020). During the second wave, the COVID-19 mortality rate of black Africans remained high vis-à-vis white Britons but was exceeded by the 'Bangladeshi group', with Bangladeshi men being five times more likely to die of COVID-19 than white British men (ONS, 2020). Similarly, research conducted in the USA highlights such health inequities, identifying higher infection and death rates among people of underrepresented ethnic and racial groups (Moore et al., 2020).

Whilst a neoclassical health economist may suggest that an individual will evaluate the cost and benefits associated with, for instance, leaving the safe environment of their own walls, to go to work amidst a raging contagious disease, the reality of the on-going pandemic highlights the 'structural drivers of injustice'. Remarkably, most people in countries of the Global South, or people in the Global North of a lower socio-economic class, were left with no choice, but to continue their work outside the household, to secure their livelihoods. At the same time, international COVID-19 vaccine inequality means that in many parts of the world, people do not have access to life-saving vaccines (Tatar et al., 2021). Consequently, any discussion that variance in outcome may be solely the result of genetic differences fell off the table swiftly. Instead, researchers and policymakers focused their attention on understanding how racial bias, disparate working and living conditions, and inequitable social circumstances, put disadvantaged groups at a higher risk of contracting and dying of COVID-19 (Milner et al., 2020; Yaya et al., 2020). For example, in the UK, people of African descent make up a considerable share of workers in the service industry and the 'essential' workforce (UNGA, 2020). They operate e.g., as bus drivers, delivery personnel, or social carers and cannot do their (often low paid) face-to-face jobs from the safety of their homes, exposing themselves more regularly to the threat of COVID-19. Likewise, deprived persons, and people of minority groups, often intersect and are also more likely to live in poor-quality accommodation, which increases their risk of getting infected with COVID-19 (Whitehead et al., 2021). By and large, the pandemic exposed the prevalence of existing economic and social inequalities and the deficiencies of how the current capitalist world economy is organised (Stevano et al., 2021b). At the same time, the crisis continues to shine light on the multiple ways in which the economy and health are interconnected.

In contrast to neoclassical health economics, concerns of equity and social justice are at the heart of political economy approaches to understanding health. Political economists are critical of asymmetric power relations (such as between business owners and workers, landowners, and tenants), which characterise contemporary capitalism, and perceive unjust working, living, and environmental conditions, as the root cause of inequitable health outcomes (Birn et al., 2017). Up until today, the German philosopher Karl Marx (1818–1883) remains one of the world's most famous political economists, having inspired a generation of Marxist political economists. Their focus of interest includes to understand how value is generated and distributed, what determines the worth of a good or service, and who benefits from the production of value. Adopting a Marxist political economy lens could help us answer some of the important questions that COVID-19 has brought to the fore, such as the working conditions that forced some workers to continue to expose themselves to the risk of contracting COVID-19, due to insecure working conditions in the gig economy. This also includes the question as to whether the salaries, which essential workers such as nurses, garbage collectors, or grocery vendors have received during the COVID-19 pandemic, truly reflect the actual value to society they continue to create, by saving our lives, keeping our streets clean, and providing us with food.

Feminist Approaches to Economics and Health

Alongside the inequalities highlighted by political economy approaches, Feminist economists have highlighted the gendered dimensions of COVID-19. Indeed, the pandemic has drawn attention to the many issues that Feminist economists have been working on for decades. One crucial aspect of this relates to the 'distribution of unpaid labour within the household', which was affected by lockdowns, and related control measures, introduced in the wake of the pandemic. Evidence from across the globe suggests that increased caring responsibilities, which resulted from school closures, and reduced access to health facilities, have been unevenly distributed, with women assuming more of this additional labour than men (Kabeer et al., 2021). This has exacerbated existing gendered inequalities in work within the home. Neoclassical economists have previously attempted to explain the gendered division of labour through the lens of comparative advantage, arguing that the unequal division of labour within the household is utility maximising, and reflects an optimal distribution of labour that assumes women have accumulated more domestic human capital than men (Becker, 1981). However, Feminist economists emphasise that the roots of these inequalities are due to a range of factors, including the artificial distinction made between 'paid' and 'unpaid' work, and how gendered conceptualisations of the economy, undervalue the importance of labour within the home. Perspectives such as 'social reproduction' reject these dualisms, instead of focusing on an analysis of how all labour that contributes to the reproduction of human life is organised, and the dynamics of this social process (Stevano et al., 2021a; 2021b; 2021c).

Inequalities in the distribution of labour within the household also reflect embedded labour market inequalities, such as the gender pay-gap, which shape unequal intra-household power relations and potential bargaining power. The COVID-19 pandemic has had a significant impact on the labour market and associated outcomes. Firstly, women are often over-represented in sectors that have been temporarily shut down or severely impacted in terms of activity, such as retail, hospitality, and service sectors (Kabeer et al., 2021), leading to higher rates of unemployment and reduced incomes. Across the globe, in contexts where formal employment is not the norm, many informal activities, engaged in by women, have been significantly impacted by lockdowns and reduced demand in the local economy. Recessions in the Global North, and depressed demand for consumer goods, have also disrupted global supply chains in key industries, such as the garment industry, with firms from the Global North cancelling orders, confining many to unemployment (Stevano et al., 2021c). Secondly, women are also more present in frontline services, such as care work or healthcare, having risked infection, and experienced the pressures of responding to the pandemic (Kabeer et al., 2021). Global dimensions of women's participation in the labour market also reflect changes in access to domestic work, as (often migrant) domestic labourers lose access to employment or are confined to the homes in which they work (Kabeer et al., 2021). Moreover, Feminist economists have been at pains to emphasise that these gendered inequalities are also shaped by class, race, and a range of other dimensions (such as, for example in the case of COVID-19, how many children women have).

One potential way forward, derived from a Feminist economics perspective, is a 'care-led recovery' from COVID-19 (De Henau and Himmelweit, 2021).

Given that the pandemic has enabled a reconsideration of what constitutes 'essential' work (Stevano et al., 2021a), a care-led recovery involves investing in the care sector to create more and better-paid jobs. This will ultimately help address gender inequality within the economy by relieving women of the burden of unpaid care within the home, acknowledging their work as valued, and thus transforming 'unpaid' work into 'paid' work. Economists have calculated that investing in the care sector would, in comparison to the more traditional Keynesian response of investing in construction and physical infrastructure, create more jobs and reduce gender inequality (De Henau and Himmelweit, 2021).

Ecological Economics and the Environment: The Importance of Planetary Health

Another issue that economists have addressed in relation to COVID-19 is the environment. Whilst, traditionally, public health crises like COVID-19 have been viewed as an external shock by neoclassical economists, environmental concerns that include climate change, environmental destruction, intensive industrial production systems, and loss of biodiversity, have long been linked with the increased likelihood of global zoonotic pandemics (Caminade et al., 2019; Gibb et al., 2020; Barouki et al., 2021). Therefore, rather than being an external shock, unrelated to economics, the pandemic is intimately linked with local and global economic processes, which have both created the conditions for the initial transmission of COVID-19 to the human population, and the global spread and degree of impact. Outbreaks like COVID-19 have long been predicted by scientists working in this field (Gruetzmacher et al., 2021). This has added further urgency to the need to reduce environmental destruction and halt climate change and engage with issues related to planetary health.

To date, neoclassical economists have focused on the role of the market as the most efficient mechanism through which to address the degradation of the environment, either by constructing market-based interventions, such as the carbon permit trading scheme, that aim to limit emissions or through the lens of the market failure framework, in which positive and negative externalities are corrected through taxes or subsidies (Groom and Talevi, 2020). However, there is growing recognition that market forces, combined with a focus on individual actions, are simply not strong enough to deliver the necessary degree of economic and social change to enable the human population to live within its planetary boundaries (Raworth, 2018).

Economists from outside the neoclassical tradition have forwarded a range of perspectives on the environmental crisis. For example, drawing on Keynesian ideas concerning the need for state direction and intervention, there have been many calls for a 'Green New Deal' (Pettifor, 2019). Echoing the stimulus package put together to respond to the Great Depression of the 1930s, the Green New Deal would provide large-scale public investment to radically re-structure and reorient the economy away from a continued reliance on fossil fuels, towards an ecological and sustainable path. Government intervention and financing are viewed as necessary to promote the development of and transition to green technology, and green jobs, to foster economic security and prosperity, and to soften the blow of what is viewed to be a 'costly transition' (Pettifor, 2019).

Drawing on a similar critique of the economic system, other economists identify capitalism and its inbuilt need for endless economic growth, as the primary cause of environmental destruction (Kallis et al., 2012; Hickel, 2021). The 'degrowth perspective' highlights the need for fundamental social and economic change, which would involve the reorientation of the economy towards human and planetary needs, instead of the current imperative of limitless growth and corporate profits. This requires a significant reduction (hence, the term degrowth) of the use of energy and resources by countries of the Global North, as well as the redistribution of income and resources to the Global South, where they are most needed. This approach is sceptical about the power of green technology to solve environmental issues, given that most new green technology (for example, the production of electric cars and expansion of charging infrastructure) involves the use of a considerable amount of energy and resources, in a situation in which more immediate action is needed to reduce consumption, and limit global warming.

Conclusion

This chapter has introduced a range of economic perspectives and ideas that would not normally be covered in a traditional Health Economics module in a public or global health programme. In times of a challenging health crisis, which has deep social and economic implications, these perspectives offer alternative ways forward to Neoclassical Economics for understanding and addressing human and planetary health. In contrast to the world of 'perfect markets' and 'rational individuals' described by Neoclassical Economics, these perspectives shed light on social and economic inequalities, the limitations of the market as a force for social good, and the need to engage critically with capitalism as the dominant economic system.

Research Points and Reflective Exercise

With reference to the discussions in this chapter, begin to reflect upon the following:

1 Look up some of the economic terms from one of the four different perspectives in the chapter. To what extent are these applicable to a global public health issue that you are interested in?

2 Look at an online version of a well-respected national newspaper and think about how the ideas presented in this chapter relate to articles, opinion

pieces, and commentaries about health and the economy that are presented in that publication.

Further Resources and Reading

Bellamy Foster, J. (1999). *The Vulnerable Planet: A Short Economic History of the Environment.* New York: Monthly Review Press.

Deane, K. and Van Waeyenberge, E. (2020). *Recharting the History of Economic Thought.* London: Red Globe Press.

Feminist Economics Volume 27, Issues 1–2, A special issue on Feminist Economic Perspectives on the COVID-19 Pandemic. https://www.tandfonline.com/toc/rfec20/27/1-2

Keen, S. (2011). *Debunking Economics: The Naked Emperor Dethroned.* London: Zed Books.

Mooney, G. (2009). *Challenging Health Economics.* Oxford: Oxford University Press.

References

Barouki, R., Kogevinas, M., Audouze, K., Belesova, K., Bergman, A. et al. (2021). "The COVID-19 Pandemic and Global Environmental Change: Emerging Research Needs". *Environment International,* 146: 106272. doi: 10.1016/j.envint.2020.106272.

BBC. (2018). "No Magic Money Tree". BBC News, 18 June. Available at: https://www.bbc.co.uk/news/uk-politics-44524605 (Accessed: 2 April 2021).

Becker, G. S. (1981). *A Treatise on the Family.* Cambridge, MA: Harvard University Press.

Bello, W. (2017). *Keynesianism in the Great Recession: Right Diagnosis, Wrong Cure.* Amsterdam: Transnational Institute.

Birn, A. E., Pillay, Y. and Holtz, T. H. (2017). *Textbook of Global Health.* Oxford: Oxford University Press.

Caminade, C., McIntyre, K. M. and Jones, A. E. (2019). "Impact of Recent and Future Climate Change on Vector-Borne Diseases". *Annals of the New York Academy of Sciences,* 1436 (1): 157–173. https://doi.org/10.1111/nyas.13950

Chang, H. (2014) *Economics: The User's Guide.* New York: Bloomsbury Publishing.

De Henau, J. and Himmelweit, S. (2021). "A Care-Led Recovery From Covid-19: Investing in High-Quality Care to Stimulate and Rebalance the Economy". *Feminist Economics,* 27 (1–2): 453–469. https://doi.org/10.1080/13545701.2020.1845390

Francis-Devine, B., Powell, A. and Clark, H. (2021). *Coronavirus Job Retention Scheme: Statistics.* London: House of Commons Library.

Gibb, R., Redding, D. W., Chin, K. Q., Donnelly, C. A., Blackburn, T. M., Newbold, T. and Jones, K. E. (2020). "Zoonotic Host Diversity Increases in Human-Dominated Ecosystems". *Nature,* 584 (7821): 398–402. https://doi.org/10.1038/s41586-020-2562-8

Groom, B. and Talevi, M. (2020). "How Does Economics Address the Environment?". In K. Deane and E. Van Waeyenberge (eds.) *Recharting the History of Economic Thought.* London: Red Globe Press, 247–268.

Gruetzmacher, K., Karesh, W. B., Amuasi, J. H., Arshad, A., Farlow, A., Gabrysch, S., Jetzkowitz, J., Lieberman, S., Palmer, C. and Winkler, A. S. (2021). "The Berlin Principles on One Health–Bridging Global Health and Conservation". *Science of The Total Environment,* 764: 142919. https://doi.org/10.1016/j.scitotenv.2020.142919

Guellec, D. and Wunsch-Vincent, S. (2009). *Policy Responses to the Economic Crisis: Investing in Innovation for Long-Term Growth, OECD Digital Economy Papers, No. 159.* Paris: OECD Publishing. https://doi.org/10.1787/222138024482

Heilbroner, R. L. (2011). *The Worldly Philosophers: The Lives, Times and Ideas of the Great Economic Thinkers*. New York: Simon and Schuster.

Hickel, J. (2021). *Less Is More: How Degrowth Will Save the World*. London: Windmill.

International Monetary Fund. (2021). "Policy Responses to COVID-19". Available at: https://www.imf.org/en/Topics/imf-and-covid19/Policy-Responses-to-COVID-19#U (Accessed: 2 April 2021).

Kabeer, N., Razavi, S. and van der Meulen Rodgers, Y. (2021). "Feminist Economic Perspectives on the COVID-19 Pandemic". *Feminist Economics*, 27 (1–2): 1–29. https://doi.org/10.1080/13545701.2021.1876906

Kallis, G., Kerschner, C. and Martinez-Alier, J. (2012). "The Economics of Degrowth". *Ecological Economics*, 84: 172–180. https://doi.org/10.1016/j.ecolecon.2012.08.017

Keynes, J. M. (1936). *The General Theory of Employment, Interest and Money*. London: Macmillan.

Milner, A., Franz, B. and Braddock, J. H. (2020). "We Need to Talk About Racism—In All of Its Forms—To Understand COVID-19 Disparities". *Health Equity*, 4 (1): 397–402. https://doi.org/10.1089/heq.2020.0069

Moore, J. T., Ricaldi, J. N., Rose, C. E., Fuld, J., Parise, M., Kang, G. J., Driscoll, A. K., Norris, T., Wilson, N. and Rainisch, G. (2020). "Disparities in Incidence of COVID-19 among Underrepresented Racial/Ethnic Groups in Counties Identified as Hotspots during June 5–18, 2020–22 States, February–June 2020". *Morbidity and Mortality Weekly Report*, 69 (33): 1122.

ONS. (2020). "Updating ethnic contrasts in deaths involving the coronavirus (COVID-19), England and Wales: deaths occurring 2 March to 28 July 2020". *Office for National Statistics Report*.

Pettifor, A. (2019). *The Case for the Green New Deal*. London: Verso.

Raworth, K. (2018). *Doughnut Economics: Seven Ways to Think Like a 21st-Century Economist*. London: Random House Business.

Skidelsky, R. (2010a). *Keynes: A Very Short Introduction*. Oxford: Oxford University Press.

Skidelsky, R. (2010b). *Keynes: The Return of the Master*. London: Pengiun.

Stevano, S., Ali, R. and Jamieson, M. (2021a). "Essential for What? A Global Social Reproduction View on the Re-Organisation of Work during the COVID-19 Pandemic". *Canadian Journal of Development Studies/Revue Canadienne d'études du Développement*, 42 (1–2): 178–199. https://doi.org/10.1080/02255189.2020.1834362

Stevano, S., Franz, T., Dafermos, Y. and Van Waeyenberge, E. (2021b). "COVID-19 and Crises of Capitalism: Intensifying Inequalities and Global Responses". *Canadian Journal of Development Studies/Revue Canadienne d'études du Développement*, 42 (1–2): 1–17. https://doi.org/10.1080/02255189.2021.1892606

Stevano, S., Mezzadri, A., Lombardozzi, L. and Bargawi, H. (2021c). "Hidden Abodes in Plain Sight: The Social Reproduction of Households and Labor in the COVID-19 Pandemic". *Feminist Economics*, 27 (1–2): 271–287. https://doi.org/10.1080/13545701.2020.1854478

Tatar, M., Shoorekchali, J. M., Faraji, M. R. and Wilson, F. A. (2021). "International COVID-19 Vaccine Inequality Amid the Pandemic: Perpetuating a Global Crisis?". *Journal of Global Health*, 11: 03086. https://doi.org/10.7189/jogh.11.03086

The Guardian. (2020). "Black People Four Times More Likely to Die from Covid-19, ONS Finds". 7 May. Available at: https://www.theguardian.com/world/2020/may/07/black-people-four-times-more-likely-to-die-from-covid-19-ons-finds (Accessed: 11 November 2021).

UNCTAD. (2021). "Impact of the COVID-10 Pandemic on Trade and Development: Transitioning to a New Normal". United Nations. Available at: https://unctad.org/system/files/official-document/osg2020d1_en.pdf (Accessed: 2 April 2020).

UNGA. (2020). "COVID-19, Systemic Racism and Global Protests, United Nations General Assembly, Report of the Working Group of Experts on People of African Descent". Available at: https://www.ohchr.org/en/issues/racism/wgafricandescent/pages/wgepadindex.aspx; https://doi.org/10.1136/bmj.n376 (Accessed: 8 August 2020).

Whitehead, M., Taylor-Robinson, D. and Barr, B. (2021). "Poverty, health, and covid-19". *BMJ*, 372, n376.

Yaya, S., Yeboah, H., Charles, C. H., Otu, A. and Labonte, R. (2020). "Ethnic and Racial Disparities in COVID-19-Related Deaths: Counting the Trees, Hiding the Forest". *MJ Global Health*, 5 (6): e002913. https://doi.org/10.1136/bmjgh-2020-002913

5

GLOBAL INEQUALITIES

The Impact on Health

Kafui Adjaye-Gbewonyo and Ichiro Kawachi

Introduction

Differences in health and social outcomes by population group have been observed across a wide range of conditions and risk factors. This chapter discusses concepts of inequality and inequity in relation to health both within and between nations. It explores inequalities in health by characteristics, such as social class, gender, ethnicity, and the intersection of these. Moreover, it discusses the importance of the social gradient of health. The chapter also addresses competing explanations for health and social inequalities globally, including poverty and material deprivation, psychosocial factors, discrimination, and structural determinants of health. We illustrate these concepts using examples from the COVID-19 pandemic and other health issues.

Health and Social Inequalities

Health inequalities can be defined as differences between individuals or groups in health status or health determinants (McKee et al., 2011; Arcaya et al., 2015). Health inequalities have been observed globally across a wide range of diseases and conditions—from infectious diseases to malnutrition and maternal and child health outcomes, injuries, mental health outcomes, and chronic noncommunicable diseases (GBD 2019 Diseases and Injuries Collaborators, 2020; Marmot et al., 2020).

A distinction is often drawn between 'inequalities' and 'inequities', where the term 'inequalities' refers descriptively to the existence of differences, while the term 'inequities' is used to denote differences that are unjust, avoidable, and systematic (Kawachi et al., 2002; McKee et al., 2011; Arcaya et al., 2015). Hence, the identification of a health inequity involves making a normative judgment

DOI: 10.4324/9781003128373-5

that a health disparity between groups is based upon an unfair or unjust distribution of the determinants of health, such as education, income, and wealth, secure jobs, and safe neighbourhoods, as well as the social bases of self-respect (Kawachi et al., 2002; Arcaya et al., 2015). It is often tricky to make this normative judgment. For example, men were consistently more likely to have severe illness and die of COVID-19 than women in China, in European countries, and in the USA, even though infection rates were similar between sexes (Mukherjee and Pahan, 2021). Does this disparity represent an inequity, or does it represent an underlying difference in susceptibility to severe illness due to biological sex (e.g., immune response, etc.)? The higher mortality from COVID-19 among men is partially explained by health behaviours, including higher rates of smoking, less healthcare seeking/utilisation, and subsequent higher levels of comorbidity among men (e.g., cardiovascular and respiratory disease) (Mukherjee and Pahan, 2021). In turn, this raises questions of personal responsibility; namely, to what extent are people responsible for 'choosing' to engage in health-damaging behaviours and to what extent are these behaviours influenced by determinants beyond personal control?

Health inequalities can occur, not only by sex or gender but also along dimensions of race or ethnicity, social class or socioeconomic position (SEP), religion, sexual orientation, immigrant status, disability status, geography, and so on. When looking at race or ethnicity, for example, the mortality rate from COVID-19 among black Caribbean females in the UK, from March through July 2020, was twice that among white females. For males, those of black African background had 2.7 times the mortality of those of white ethnic background after adjusting for age, socio-demographic factors, and pre-existing health conditions (Office for National Statistics, 2020). In terms of geography, people living in more deprived neighbourhoods have lower life expectancies on average compared to those living in less deprived neighbourhoods of England (Marmot et al., 2020).

Social Gradients in Health

The 'social gradient in health' expresses the idea that health status is often patterned and that each successive increment in social position (e.g., years of education) confers additional advantage (Kawachi et al., 2002). These gradients frequently occur by 'social class', 'SEP', or 'socioeconomic status (SES)'. Lynch and Kaplan (2000) defined SEP as 'the social and economic factors that influence what position(s) individuals and groups hold within the structure of society' (2000: 14). SEP and SES are viewed as fundamental 'social determinants of health' and are assessed through income, wealth, education, and/or occupation. Sometimes, where these indicators are not available, area of residence (e.g., level of neighbourhood deprivation) has been used as a proxy for individuals' SEP/SES (Lynch and Kaplan, 2000; Glymour et al., 2014; Marmot and Allen, 2014).

Most health outcomes and risk factors, as well as overall life expectancy, are known to be socially patterned, with those having higher SES typically faring better health-wise than those with lower SES (Solar and Iwrin, 2010; Glymour et al., 2014). For example, social gradients have been observed in many countries during the COVID-19 pandemic. A seroprevalence study conducted in Ghana by the West African Centre for Cell Biology of Infectious Pathogens (WACCBIP) showed potential social gradients in exposure to the novel coronavirus, SARS-Cov-2, which causes COVID-19. In a sample of 1,305 individuals in the capital city of Accra and the town of Kasoa, exposure to SARS-CoV-2 was higher among those with no or basic education (26.2%) compared to those with tertiary education (13.1%) (Quashie et al., 2021). Looking at another indicator of SEP—occupation—the authors found exposure rates to be higher among those in the informal sector (24%) compared to those in formal employment (15%) (Quashie et al., 2021). These data demonstrate clear socioeconomic gradients in virus exposure.

Socioeconomic gradients in health have been observed, not only across space and for a range of health outcomes but also over time. In the 1820s, French physician Louis René Villermé published data showing that Parisians living in wealthier neighbourhoods had better indicators of mortality, life expectancy, and stature (Krieger, 2011). Similarly, in his 1845 book, 'The Condition of the Working Class in England', Friedrich Engels (1845/2009) found that mortality rates followed a socioeconomic gradient by neighbourhood and household social class in Manchester (Krieger, 2011).

Measuring and Addressing Inequalities

The way in which inequalities are measured, and the ethical priorities adopted for health interventions may impact our understanding, of whether inequalities are improving or worsening with time. Imagine a hypothetical country in which infant mortality is 8 deaths/100,000 for those with high SES and 16 deaths/100,000 for those with low SES (for simplicity, we will assume that the country is equally split into high/low SES groups). After a healthcare intervention, the infant mortality rates drop to four deaths/100,000 for those with high SES and 10 deaths/100,000 for those with low SES. In this case, the *absolute* difference in mortality rates between the two groups decreased from a gap of eight deaths/100,000 (16 minus eight) before the intervention to a gap of six deaths/100,000 (10 minus four) following the intervention. However, the *relative* gap between the two groups has increased. Before the intervention, those with low SES had twice the rate of maternal mortality as those with high SES (16 divided by eight). After the intervention, the low SES group had 2.5 times the rate of maternal mortality compared to the high SES group (ten divided by four). Therefore, the way in which inequalities are measured, in absolute versus relative term, can affect our interpretation of whether they are improving or worsening over time. For this reason, it is critical to report both absolute and relative differences in health status (Kawachi, 2012).

Furthermore, interventions designed to 'maximise' health by reducing morbidity or mortality for all may end up widening inequalities. If we compare the intervention above to one which reduces the infant mortality rate for the high SES and low SES groups to six deaths/100,000 and nine deaths/100,000, respectively, we would find that this second intervention has produced a more 'egalitarian' outcome, i.e., it reduced the gap between low and high SES by more than the first intervention by improving outcomes for the low SES group more. However, the first intervention 'saves more lives' (in the aggregate), even though the relative gap widened between the low versus high SES groups. The reason is because in the first intervention, mortality rates dropped even more rapidly for the high SES group, compared to the second intervention. Another way to think about this is that the second intervention promoted health equity, but at the expense of maximising the lives that could have been saved. In the real world, educational interventions have often been observed to widen health inequalities, if those with higher SES are more able to use health information, than those with lower SES (Kawachi, 2012).

Explaining Health Inequalities

Social Selection Versus Social Causation

Several competing hypotheses have been offered to explain health inequalities. At the core is the question of whether these inequalities reflect 'social causation' or 'social selection' (Ritsher et al., 2001). By social causation, we mean that the health differences and gradients we observe are caused by social inequalities. For instance, this would mean that people who are poor end up with poor health because they are poor. Social epidemiologists are typically interested in social causation, how social factors cause or lead to different health outcomes.

The alternative explanation for health inequalities is sometimes referred to as social selection (Solar and Iwrin, 2010; McKee et al., 2011). According to this hypothesis, people 'select' or drift into different social conditions and social classes because of their health status. For example, people with worse mental or physical health during their youth could end up attaining lower levels of education or earning less income because of their illnesses. Similarly, people with worse health may move to low-income neighbourhoods because of limited income due to their health conditions. From a social epidemiological perspective, this would be an example of 'reverse causation' (Bhopal, 2016), where low social status is not leading to or causing poor health, but low SES is the result of poor health. This explanation could be invoked to explain both within- and between-country gradients in health status. There is some evidence in support of social selection and reverse causation when it comes to education and health (Case et al., 2005). However, research shows that for measures of SES, such as education and income, 'social causation' instead is the more dominant causal mechanism (Kroger et al., 2015), making these health inequalities, not only unequal but also inequitable and modifiable.

Materialist Explanations, Social Determinants and Poverty

Acknowledging social causation as an explanation for health inequalities, several possible mechanisms have been explored to explain how social conditions affect health. One is the 'materialist' explanation. This argues that material circumstances, including poverty, lead to inequities in health (Lynch et al., 2000; Solar and Iwrin, 2010; McKee et al., 2011). Poverty is a special case of extreme deprivation in which individuals do not have the basic necessities for survival or those viewed as standard in their society. This can include housing and shelter or adequate food and clothing. Poverty is clearly linked to health through material pathways. Having inadequate housing, for instance, can lead to overcrowding, exposure to weather elements, and pathogens causing illness. Lack of clean water and sanitation increases susceptibility to infectious disease or environmental toxins (Lynch and Kaplan, 2000; Solar and Iwrin, 2010).

However, social epidemiological research has demonstrated that it is not just absolute deprivation through poverty which can adversely impact health; being relatively deprived compared to others in society has also been shown to have negative effects on health (Lynch et al., 2000). For example, a person can have access to all the necessities of life, including housing, clothing, food, and healthcare, and still be in a state of relative deprivation, compared to others in society. They may lack sufficient heating in their homes or sufficient income to purchase fresh produce. These subtle differences by SEP could account for the social gradient in health described earlier. That is, health inequities are not just a matter of deprivation in the absolute sense.

The circumstances in which people are born, grow, learn, live, and work represent the 'social determinants of health' (CSDH, 2008; Solar and Iwrin, 2010). They can influence health, not only directly, such as through harmful exposures, but also indirectly through the ability to perform healthy behaviours (e.g., access to the time and environment for exercise or healthy eating). Social determinants frameworks place emphasis on 'upstream' determinants of health, such as economic factors, institutions, and the social and physical environment, in addition individual-level determinants of health (Solar and Iwrin, 2010).

Many of the socioeconomic gradients observed in COVID-19 outcomes could be explained through material pathways. Early in the pandemic, in countries such as the USA, news media outlets reported on how several celebrities seemed to have easy access to COVID tests while average citizens struggled to get tested (Twohey et al., 2020). Similarly, in October 2020, the then US President, Donald Trump famously received care above and beyond the national standard, including an experimental antibody treatment, while he was hospitalised with COVID (Cohen, 2020). These examples illustrate how status, wealth, and power may buy greater access to material resources, such as elite healthcare services to improve health outcomes.

Some of the racial and ethnic inequalities observed in COVID outcomes have also been attributed to material pathways. Based on their models, the Office for

National Statistics concluded that ethnic differences in COVID mortality in the UK were most strongly associated with socio-demographic factors such as occupation and place of residence rather than pre-existing health conditions (Office for National Statistics, 2020). This finding supports the role of social determinants of health such as living and working conditions in COVID outcomes.

Psychosocial Mechanisms

Additionally, social inequities in health status have also been explained through 'psychosocial' mechanisms (Marmot and Wilkinson, 2001). For example, having a lower relative position in the social hierarchy could lead to higher levels of stress due to social comparisons with those who have more or due to lack of material resources to cope with life's demands. This chronic psychosocial stress can again have direct impacts on both mental health and physical health, through the sympathetic nervous system, as well as indirect impacts, such as through maladaptive coping behaviours to deal with stress (over-indulging, smoking, alcohol, substance use, etc.) (Solar and Iwrin, 2010).

Several studies have examined potential psychosocial effects of inequality on health. Notably, the Whitehall Studies demonstrated that there was a social gradient in health among British civil servants and that psychosocial factors, such as having low levels of control in the workplace, were linked to inequalities in cardiovascular disease among these civil servants (Marmot and Wilkinson, 2001).

Discrimination and Inequality

Discrimination, defined as the unjust treatment of individuals or a group based on their characteristics, such as class or race, has also been implicated in the pathway between social factors and health (Krieger, 2014). In particular, there is evidence to suggest a role for discrimination in partially explaining health disparities and inequities observed across ethnic and racial lines, gender, sexual orientation, disability, etc. Discrimination can occur 'interpersonally', such as when individuals stereotype other people or groups. Discrimination can also occur 'institutionally', such as when police and security forces disproportionately profile, search, arrest, or kill individuals belonging to marginalised groups. The types of discrimination can also overlap (Krieger, 2014).

During the COVID-19 pandemic, there have been some suggestions of racial and ethnic discrimination impacting health outcomes. Stories of ethnic minorities who had died of COVID after being refused treatment or being released home made news headlines (Laville, 2020; Marsh, 2021). Additionally, the fact that ethnic inequalities in COVID mortality in the UK remained after controlling for socio-demographic variables and pre-existing health conditions may be indirectly suggestive of the potential role of factors such as unconscious bias, differences in quality of care, and institutional discrimination in the healthcare system (Apea et al., 2021).

Studies explicitly examining treatment differences by race and ethnicity have had mixed results, however. An American Heart Association study of patients across several US hospitals found that non-Hispanic black patients were least likely to be enrolled on COVID-19 trials for treatments such as Remdesivir compared to non-Hispanic white, Hispanic, and Asian/Pacific Islander patients; however, ethnic differences in mortality were no longer significant after adjusting for age (Rodriquez et al., 2021). A study in a New York City health system found that once hospitalised with COVID-19, black and Hispanic patients were less likely to die compared to white patients. Greater likelihood of testing positive for COVID-19, and higher rates of out-of-hospital mortality for COVID-19, may therefore have accounted for the higher rates of COVID-19 mortality among black and Hispanic populations generally (Ogedegbe et al., 2020). Nevertheless, given research highlighting potential ethnic differences in healthcare generally (Institute of Medicine, 2003), further systematic research into this issue may be warranted.

Intersectionality

In addition, health inequities due to discrimination and other factors can occur across the *intersection* of multiple characteristics of a single individual (Krieger, 2014). For example, an ethnic minority woman who identifies as 'queer', lives in a deprived area, and has less than secondary school education, may be disadvantaged by ethnicity, gender, sexual orientation, and social class, all at once. Intersectionality theory argues that the level of disadvantage a person experiences, due to the combination of factors, may be greater than the sum of each form of disadvantage separately (Krieger, 2014). The theory was first described by Crenshaw (1989) to illustrate the compounded experiences of discrimination faced by black women in the USA, experiences that were not adequately addressed by focussing on gender discrimination, racial/ethnic discrimination, and class discrimination separately (Crenshaw, 1989).

Structural Determinants and Socio-Political Frameworks

Our discussion so far has centred primarily on inequalities occurring within countries. However, global health inequalities between nations present starker contrasts than within-country comparisons. For example, high-income countries generally enjoy higher life expectancies than low-income countries (Gapminder, 2015; Lima Barreto, 2017). In 2019, an individual could expect to live to 53.3 years on average at birth in the Central African Republic, while in Hong Kong, an individual could expect to live an average of 85.1 years (The World Bank, 2021). Socio-political frameworks such as the 'World-Systems' theory, Political Economy of Health and Social Production of Disease' perspectives, approach global health inequalities as the product of exploitative relationships, operating through a system of global capitalism, and neo-colonialism (Wallerstein, 2004;

Krieger, 2011). That is, the distribution of health and illness across the globe is viewed in terms of disparities in power. For instance, countries that are often referred to as the 'Global North' hold more political and economic power globally compared to the 'Global South'. Many of the countries of the Global South also have a history of being recently colonised by countries of the Global North. The lingering legacies of colonialism and enduring neo-colonial or exploitative structures of the global economic system could be said to determine some of the fundamental structural causes that contribute to global inequalities. Processes of globalisation and neo-liberalism and policies such as the structural adjustment programmes of the International Monetary Foundation and World Bank have often been implicated in widening global inequities (Solar and Iwrin, 2010; Thomson et al., 2017; Daoud and Reinsberg, 2019).

Applying a socio-political framework to examine health inequalities, one could look at the example of Haiti, which is considered the poorest country in the Western Hemisphere. When it comes to health outcomes, Haiti consistently ranks poorly compared to its neighbours in levels of maternal mortality, infant mortality, HIV/AIDS, tuberculosis, malnutrition, etc. Haiti's healthcare system is also noted to be under-resourced (Farmer, 2007; Jean Paul et al., 2020). From a political economy of health perspective, one might explain the health and social inequities between Haiti and its neighbours in terms of its history of colonisation, forced reparations to France for the independence of its former slaves, military occupation by the USA, International Monetary Fund policies reducing local tariffs, and other deliberate geopolitical and economic factors that have impoverished the country (Farmer, 2007; Oliver-Smith, 2010).

Turning again to the COVID-19 pandemic, there have been vast inequalities in vaccination rates across countries, and the issue of 'vaccine nationalism' has become prominent (Santos Rutschman, 2020; Jha et al., 2021; Katz et al., 2021). Again, socio-political frameworks can be used to explain the unequal distribution of health resources such as vaccines globally (Richardson and Farmer, 2020). What are the political and economic situations that have led to the financial enrichment of countries in the Global North and at whose expense? By the same token, what are the factors that have led to the relative impoverishment of countries in the Global South and how has this affected scientific research and healthcare infrastructures? How has the current structure of the global health system evolved and who holds the power to determine agendas? How has access to resources for vaccine production been socially produced over time? How do commercial interests influence the situation? These are questions we can consider when examining global inequalities in the response to COVID-19 and many other health issues.

Conclusion

This chapter has introduced concepts of health inequalities and inequities. Social gradients in health are observed across a wide range of health outcomes and risk factors and have become highly visible during the recent COVID-19 pandemic. While there are some circumstances, where the mechanism linking social inequalities to health may be one of social selection, there is evidence that social causation explains more of the gradients in health, observed across education levels and income. Social inequities can affect health through material and psychosocial pathways, either directly or indirectly, through health behaviours. Further attention may need to be paid to the role that discrimination plays in creating health inequities, and to the structural and political factors, that contribute to national and global inequities in health. In addition, when addressing health inequalities and inequities through policy or other interventions, it is important to consider how inequalities are being measured and whether the ultimate goal is to maximise health or reduce inequalities.

Research Points and Reflective Exercise

Reflect on the pressing social and health inequalities in your country:

- Do you observe social gradients in health? In which direction?
- Have these inequalities improved or worsened with time?
- How might social selection and social causation explain the major health inequalities in your country?
- What structural, political, and economic factors do you feel have influenced the overall health status in your country compared to other countries?

Further Resources and Reading

Agenor, M. (2020). "Future Directions for Incorporating Intersectionality into Quantitative Population Health Research". *AJPH Perspectives*, 110 (6): 803–806. https://doi.org/10.2105/AJPH.2020.305610.

Bukhman, G. et al. (2020). "The Lancet NCDI Poverty Commission: Bridging a Gap in Universal Health Coverage for the Poorest Billion". *Lancet*, 396: 991–1044. https://doi.org/10.1016/S0140-6736(20)31907-3

Kawachi, I. and Kennedy, B. P. (2002) *The Health of Nations: Why Inequality Is Harmful to Your Health*. New York: The New Press.

Treloar, N. and Begum, H. (2021). *One Working Class: Race, Class and Inequalities. Facts Don't Lie (Runnymede Perspectives)*. London: Runnymede.

References

Apea, V. J., Wan, Y. I., Dhairyawan, R., Puthucheary, Z. A., Pearse, R. M., Orkin, C. H. and Prowle, J. R. (2021). "Ethnicity and Outcomes in Patients Hospitalised with COVID-19 Infection in East London: An Observational Cohort Study". *BMJ*, 11 (1): e042140. https://doi.org/10.1136/bmjopen-2020-042140.

Arcaya, M. C., Arcaya, A. L. and Subramanian, S. V. (2015). "Inequalities in Health: Definitions, Concepts, and Theories". *Global Health Action*, 8: 27106. https://doi.org/10.3402/gha.v8.27106

Bhopal, R. (2016). *Concepts of Epidemiology: Integrating the Ideas, Theories, Principles, and Methods of Epidemiology*, 3rd edn. Oxford: Oxford University Press.

Case, A., Fertig, A. and Paxson, C. (2005). "The Lasting Impact of Childhood Health and Circumstance". *Journal of Health Economics*, 24 (2): 365–389. https://doi.org/10.1016/j.jhealeco.2004.09.008

Cohen, J. (2020). "Update: Here's What is Known About Trump's COVID-19 Treatment", Science, 5 October. Available at: https://www.sciencemag.org/news/2020/10/-heres-what known-about-president-donald-trump-s-covid-19-treatment (Accessed: August 26 2020).

CSDH. (2008). *Closing the Gap in a Generation: Health Equity through Action on the Social Determinants of Health. Final Report of the Commission on Social Determinants of Health.* Geneva: World Health Organization.

Crenshaw, K. (1989). "Demarginalizing the Intersection of Race and Sex: A Black Feminist Critique of Antidiscrimination Doctrine, Feminist Theory and Antiracist Politics". *The University of Chicago Legal Forum*, 1989: 139–167.

Daoud, A. and Reinsberg, B. (2019). "Structural Adjustment, State Capacity and Child Health: Evidence from IMF Programmes". *International Journal of Epidemiology*, 48 (2): 445–454. https://doi.org/10.1093/ije/dyy251

Engels, F. (1845/2009). *The Condition of the Working Class in England*. Oxford: Oxford University Press.

Farmer, P. (2007). Whither Equity in Health? The state of the poor in Latin America. *Escola Nacional de Saude Publica*, 23 (Suppl. 1): S7–S12.

Gapminder. (2015). "How Does Income Relate to Life Expectancy?" Available at: https://www.gapminder.org/answers/how-does-income-relate-to-life-expectancy/ (Accessed: January 31 2022).

GBD. (2019). Diseases and Injuries Collaborators. (2020). "Global Burden of 369 Diseases and Injuries in 204 Countries and Territories, 1990–2019: A Systematic Analysis for the Global Burden of Disease Study 2019". *The Lancet*, 396 (10258): 17–23. https://doi.org/10.1016/S01406736(20)30925-9

Glymour, M. M., Avendano, M. And Kawachi, I. (2014). "Socieoeconomic Status and Health". In L. F. Berkman, I. Kawachi and M. M. Glymour (eds.) *Social Epidemiology.* Oxford: Oxford University Press, 17–62.

Institute of Medicine. 2003. *Unequal Treatment: Confronting Racial and Ethnic Disparities in Health Care.* Washington, DC: The National Academies Press. https://doi.org/10.17226/12875.

Jean Paul, A., Petit, M. and Archer, L. E. (2020). "Main Health Issues in Haiti: A Brief Review". *ScienceOpen Preprints.* https://doi.org/10.14293/S2199-1006.1.SOR-.PP7CWXJ.v1

Jha, P., Jamison, D. T., Watkins, D. A. and Bell, J. (2021). "A Global Compact to Counter Vaccine Nationalism". *The Lancet*, 397 (10289): 2046–2047. https://doi.org/10.1016/S01406736(21)01105-3

Katz, I. T., Weintraub, R., Bekker, L.-G. and Brandt, A. M. (2021). "From Vaccine Nationalism to Vaccine Equity – Finding a Path Forward". *The New England Journal of Medicine*, 384 (14): 1281–1283. https://doi.org/10.1056/NEJMp2103614

Kawachi, I. (2012). Lecture: Reducing and Eliminating Health Inequalities: A Policy Perspective. SHH 201, Society and Health, Boston, Massachusetts, delivered 20 October 2012.

Kawachi, I., Subramanian, S. V. and Almeida-Filho, N. (2002). "A Glossary for Health Inequalities". *Journal of Epidemiology and Community Health,* 56: 647–652. https://doi.org/10.1136/jech.56.9.647

Krieger, N. (2011). *Epidemiology and the People's Health: Theory and Context*. Oxford: Oxford University Press.

Krieger, N. (2014). "Discrimination and Health Inequities". In L. F. Berkman and I. G. Kawachi (eds.) *Social Epidemiology*. Oxford: Oxford University Press, 63–125.

Kroger, H., Pakpahan, E. and Hoffman, R. (2015). "What Causes Health Inequality? A Systematic Review on the Relative Importance of Social Causation and Health Selection". *European Journal of Public Health*, 25: (6): 951–960. https://doi.org/10.1093/eurpub/ckv111

Laville, S. (2020). "London Woman Dies of Suspected Covid-19 after Being told She Was 'Not Priority'", The Guardian, 25 March. Available at: https://www.theguardian.com/world/2020/mar/25/london-woman-36-dies-of-suspected covid-19-after-being-told-she-is-not-priority (Accessed: 26 Auguts 2021).

Lima Barreto, M. (2017). "Health Inequalities: A Global Perspective". *Ciencia & Saude Colletiva*, 22 (7): 2097–2108. https://doi.org/10.1590/1413-81232017227.02742017

Lynch, J. W., Davey Smith, G., Kaplan, G. A. and House, J. S. (2000). "Income Inequality and Mortality: Importance to Health of Individual Income, Psychosocial Environment, or Material Conditions". *British Medical Journal*, 320: 1200-1204. https://doi.org/10.1136/bmj.320.7243.1200

Lynch, J. and Kaplan, G. (2000). "Socioeconomic Position". In L. F. Berkman and I. Kawachi (eds.) *Social Epidemiology*. Oxford: Oxford University Press, 13-35.

Marmot, M. and Allen, J. (2014). "From Science to Policy". In L. F. Berkman and I. G. Kawachi (eds.) *Social Epidemiology*. Oxford: Oxford University Press, 562-576.

Marmot, M. and Wilkinson, R. G. (2001). Psychosocial and Material Pathways in the Relation between Income and Health: A Response to Lynch et al." *British Medical Journal*, 322: 1233-1236. https://doi.org/10.1136/bmj.322.7296.1233

Marmot, M., Allen, J., Boyce, T., Goldblatt, P. and Morrison, J. (2020). *Health Equity in England: The Marmot Review 10 Years On*. London: Institute of Health Equity.

Marsh, S. (2021). "Pregnant Nurse Who Died of COVID 'Unhappy' to be Sent Home from A&E". The Guardian, 23 March. Available at: https://www.theguardian.com/world/2021/mar/23/pregnant-nurse-who-died-of-covidunhappy-to-be-sent-home-from-er (Accessed: 26 August 2021).

McKee, M., Sim, F. and Pomerleau, J. (2011). "Inequalities in Health". In F. Sim and M. McKee (eds.) *Issues in Public Health*. Berkshire: Open University Press, 78-106.

Mukherjee, S. and Pahan, K. (2021). "Is COVID-19 Gender-Sensitive?" *Journal of Neuroimmune Pharmacology*, 38-42. https://doi.org/10.1007/s11481-020-09974-z

Office for National Statistics. (2020). Updating Ethnic Contrasts in Deaths Involving the Coronavirus (COVID-19), England and Wales: Deaths Occurring 2 March to 28 July 2020.

Ogedegbe, G., Ravenell, J., Adhikari, S., Butler, M., Cook, T., Francois, F. et al. (2020). "Assessment of Racial/Ethnic Disparities in Hospitalization and Mortality in Patients With COVID-19 in New York City". *JAMA Network Open*, 3 (12): e2026881. https://doi.org/10.1001/jamanetworkopen.2020.26881

Oliver-Smith, A. (2010). "Haiti and the Historical Construction of Disasters". *NACLA Report on the Americas*, 43 (4): 32-36. https://doi.org/10.1080/10714839.2010.11725505

Quashie, P. K., Mutungi, J. K., Dzabeng, F., Odura-Mensah, D., Opurum, P. C. et al. (2021) "Trends of SARS-CoV-2 Antibody Prevalence in Selected Regions across Ghana. *MedRxiv*. https://doi.org/10.1101/2021.04.25.21256067

Richardson, E. and Farmer, P. (2020). *Epidemic Illusions: On the Coloniality of Global Public Health*. Cambridge: The MIT Press.

Ritsher, J. E., Warner, V., Johnson, J. G. and Dohrenwend, B. P. (2001). "Inter-Generational Longitudinal Study of Social Class and Depression: A Test of Social Causation and Social Selection Models". *British Journal of Psychiatry*, 178 (S40): S84-S90. https://doi.org/10.1192/bjp.178.40.s84

Rodriquez, F., Solomon, N., de Lemos, J. A., Das, S., Morrow, D. A., Bradley, S. M. and Elkind, M. S. (2021). "Racial and Ethnic Differences in Presentation and Outcomes for Patients Hospitalized With COVID-19: Findings From the American Heart Association's COVID-19 Cardiovascular Disease Registry". *Circulation*, 143 (24): 2332-2342. https://doi.org/10.1161/CIRCULATIONAHA.120.052278

Santos Rutschman, A. (2020). "The Reemergence of Vaccine Nationalism". *Georgetown Journal of International Affairs, Forthcoming, Saint Louis U. Legal Studies Research Paper No. 2020-16*. https://doi.org/10.2139/ssrn.3642858

Solar, O. and Iwrin, A. (2010). "A Conceptual Framework for Action on the Social Determinants of Health. Social Determinants of Health Discussion Paper 2 (Policy and Practice)", World Health Organization. Available at: https://www.who.int/sdhconference/resources/ConceptualframeworkforactiononSDH_eng.pdf (Accessed: 25 January 2021).

The World Bank. (2021). "World Development Indicators", July 30. Available at: https://datacatalog.worldbank.org/dataset/world-development-indicators (Accessed: 2 September 2021).

Thomson, M., Kentikelenis, A. and Stubbs, T. (2017). "Structural Adjustment Programmes Adversely Affect Vulnerable Populations: A Systematic-Narrative Review of Their Effect on Child and Maternal Health". *Public Health Reviews*, 38 (13). https://doi.org/10.1186/s40985-017-0059-2

Twohey, M., Eder, S. And Stein, M. (2020). "Need a COVID Test? Being Rich and Famous May Help", New York Times, 18 March. Available at: https://www.nytimes.com/2020/03/18/us/coronavirus-testing-elite.html (Accessed: 6 November 2021).

Wallerstein, I. (2004). "World-Systems Analysis, in World System History" In G. Modelski (ed.) *Encyclopedia of Life Support Systems (EOLSS), UNESCO*. Oxford: Eolss Publishers, 1-14. http://www.eolss.net/ebooks/Sample%20Chapters/C04/E6- 94-01.pdf

6

ETHICS AND GLOBAL PUBLIC HEALTH

Nevin Mehmet

Introduction

This chapter argues for the location of ethics to be at the heart of global public health. It will discuss the definition of ethics, public health ethics, and global public health ethics. It will continue by exploring the core ethical theories of 'Utilitarianism', 'Deontology', and 'Virtue Ethics' and distinguish ethical principles of 'Autonomy', 'Beneficence', 'Non maleficence', and 'Justice' and how they generate ethical frameworks. Lastly, this chapter will focus on key global ethical challenges by exploring responses to global health inequalities and the COVID-19 pandemic in relation to lockdowns and liberty. Through this, it seeks to illustrate and apply some of the core theories and issues used throughout the chapter and increase their relevance to application in global public health practice and social sciences.

Ethics, Public Health Ethics, and Global Public Health Ethics

Ethics, from a philosophical perspective, is a branch of moral philosophy that addresses questions about morality; it attempts to appraise, define, and determine what is 'good', 'evil', 'right', and 'wrong', as well as what is justice and virtue to justify decision making and judgements (Mehmet, 2011). There are three key aspects that support our understanding of what we mean by ethics: 'Meta-ethics', 'Normative Ethics', and 'Applied Ethics'.

- Meta-ethics provide analytical thinking about the source of the meaning of words or concepts; it can be considered as a theoretical side of ethics and it aims to understand what we mean by 'morals' or the sources of 'morality'

DOI: 10.4324/9781003128373-6

and includes questioning the meaning of terms such as 'right' or 'wrong', within the context of morals;

- Normative Ethics attempts to give answers to moral questions and problems in relation to what the accepted morally right thing might be to do in each situation or whether someone is a morally good person;
- Applied Ethics attempts to answer difficult moral questions that people face in their lives, such as whether fluoride should be applied to national/ international water supplies, or whether all children should be compulsory vaccinated prior to starting school.

The combination of all three of these elements, Meta-ethics, Normative Ethics, and Applied Ethics, enables ethics to be at the centre of different contexts and issues from provision of equitable services through to reductions in health inequalities. Meta-ethics enables us to question terms, concepts, and definitions, to obtain greater understandings. Normative ethics enables us to place these concepts into 'real-life' situations and apply their meanings; for example, if we consider healthcare as a moral right, and this is a moral social norm, then the application of this norm precipitates the question, 'Should everyone have basic free healthcare?' or 'Should people who pay for private medical care get quicker or more advanced care, compared to those who do not?' Applied ethics provides a platform to apply ethics to specialised areas, such as public health and global public health within broader structural and relational contexts (World Health Organization, 2017), increasingly significant in applying social sciences perspectives to global public health.

Dawson (2011) states that public health ethics is a systematic process, which aims to clarify, prioritise, and justify possible practical courses of action and decisions within 'public health' at the population or community health level in line with accepted standards of ethics and morality. 'Global public health' ethics is a relatively new term which is used to conceptualise the process of applying moral values to issues within global public health (Stapleton et al., 2014) across nations and assumes an international perspective of globalised and inter-dependent communities and countries. Hunter and Dawson (2021) state that global public health ethics is often conceptualised in different ways within the literature. For example, the word 'public' is often missing, with the focus on global health ethics, and thus the ethical challenges associated with collective and global action may be overlooked (Stapleton et al., 2014). Ethical issues such as climate change, global pandemics, poverty, or issues, which can only be solved through worldwide collaboration, such as infectious disease control, are important components of global public health ethics, transcending national public health. Hunter and Dawson (2021) propose that the most widely and commonly accepted approach is to view global public health ethics as a 'normative project', one that seeks to establish common values in identifying global wrongs such as injustices in public health, global and structural inequalities, and imbalances of power and transcends the emphasis upon individuals, and nation states only, to generate truly global solutions.

Ethical Theories and Global Public Health

An understanding of the differences between ethical theories (Utilitarianism, Deontology and Virtue Ethics) and ethical principles (Autonomy, Beneficence, Non maleficence, and Justice) are important to consider action in any given situation, especially within the context of global public health. Ethical theories within global public health provide broad concepts, and understandings of moral reasoning and defensible abstract normative accounts and explanations around individuals and social systems, as well as effects on ethical principles. Ethical principles constitute general judgements to justify ethical prescriptions and evaluations of public health activities, which are often embedded within codes of conduct, and incorporated into broader 'Ethical Frameworks', discussed below.

Utilitarianism, proposed by Jeremy Bentham, and later John Stuart Mill, asserts that an action is morally good if it produces the 'greatest of good/welfare' for the greatest amount of people (greater good for the greater number) (Warnock, 1962; Upsur et al., 2013). There are many variations of utilitarianism. However, the idea always lies within maximising the overall wellbeing or net benefit. As the premise of public health is to promote health and wellbeing, improve public health services, and reduce inequalities on a population or global level, utilitarian ethics would therefore be viewed to be inherent or well suited as a theory for evaluating and justifying the morality of public health interventions and programs. By extension, it would be effective for determining what we should and should not do in the arena of public health internationally (Roberts and Reich, 2002; Holland, 2014).

The ethical theory of Deontology, also known as Kantian ethics, from the Greek word, *deontos*, meaning duty, obliges us to obey the rules that govern actions or conduct and considers whether an action is inherently right or wrong. Deontology ignores the issue of harmful or beneficial consequences, and relies on the rules of duty, to serve as the standard of judgement. For example, if we consider the rules of social norms, such as treating people fairly, the public health obligation here would be to ensure the right of health to all (the duty), so that everyone has an opportunity to maintain health.

Alternatively, virtue ethics stems from the work of Aristotle and focuses on virtues such as kindness, courage, respect for persons, honesty, and compassion. Habitual practice is necessary for developing these virtues, whose possession we equate with good character, and which equip a person to be effective in society or an organisation. Mackay (2021) argues that global public health can be viewed as a global arena to exercise core virtues such as honesty, courage, and justice. The application of these virtues can support, maintain, and defend the integrity of global public health. Mackay (2021) proposes that even though virtue ethics focuses on the individual, whilst public health is centred on the community or population level, there is a role for ethics in global public health in producing structures of virtues within societies (i.e., at the community or population and global level). This can be implemented within global public policy, and codes of practice, within global public health organisations. An example is the World Forum, developed by the World Health Organisation (WHO) (2015), which supports the development of policy to support global challenges, with the aim to assist policy makers, healthcare providers, and researchers to understand core public health values and virtues (such as justice, honesty, and compassion) by applying ethical principles to global public health issues.

Ethical Principles and Formations of Ethical Frameworks

The ethical principles proposed by Beauchamp and Childress (2012) are often used within global public health studies and decision making; these are Autonomy, Beneficence, Non maleficence, and Justice. Autonomy refers to issues around enhancing respect, confidentiality, and freedom. Beneficence focuses upon moral obligation to act for the benefit of others such as risk reduction and protection from harm. Non maleficence refers to the concept of doing no harm to others whilst Justice is grounded within obligations to equitably distribute benefits, risks, costs, and resources.

These principles determine a course of action and are often linked to broader moral theoretical frameworks, outlined above, to encompass given principles. When specific principles are combined or omitted to determine a structured course of action, this can be referred to as an 'Ethical Framework', which aims to provide structured guidance on how decisions ought to be made around ethical issues or dilemmas. Bernheim et al. (2007) suggest ethical frameworks should be considered as analytical tools that guide decision makers through reasoning and deliberation, without presuming that any one moral norm has greater weight than another. The four principles need to be taken to be 'prima facia', rather than absolute duties, meaning it is permissible to break or diminish one or more ethical principles if it is ethically justifiable. Ethical frameworks also enable us to find a balance between individuals and social determinants/societies, and the roles of both, when planning decisions.

Within global public health the development of a robust ethical framework is a complex process as decision makers are dealing with issues at global/population level, and not only, the individual or national level (e.g., the shift from public to global public health). Afolabi (2018) argues that a key feature of a global public health ethical framework is that it must have the capacity to resolve ethical concerns from a global perspective and internationally orientated ethics. Kass (2001) argues that ethics analysis should be conducted when planning and implementing all public and global health policy to enhance truth, fairness, and respect and because, from a more utilitarian perspective, public health work will be more effective if it produces benefits for the majority. This entails, for example, focusing on how benefits to participants can be balanced fairly; how approaches can minimise harm and burdens; and increase effectiveness in achieving goals of equity and equality.

The Ethics of Global Health Inequalities

A leading ethical global public health challenge is health inequalities. For example, public health in low-income countries is often compromised by social determinants, such as poverty, malnutrition, poor education, unhealthy living conditions, and a lack of access to healthcare (WHO, 2015). These social determinants impact on health outcomes in low-income countries. For example, in relation to maternal mortality, the rate in South Sudan is 1,150 maternal deaths per 100,000 live births compared to two maternal deaths per 100,000 live births in Norway (WHO et al., 2019). As discussed, the principle of justice highlights fairness, equal rights, and opportunities for all, including a right to good healthcare, irrespective of social determinants. Using a Kantian approach, which stipulates that access to basic healthcare can be considered a moral right, then the unavailability of healthcare to many people across the globe, and the ensuring increases in poorer health outcomes, would be considered morally wrong. This injustice has led to calls for collective ethical commitments and moral frameworks, which guide practice and policy, in reducing global health inequalities (Ruger, 2006).

Principles of justice furthermore enable consideration on how benefits and burdens ought to be distributed among individuals or communities as a matter of right and entitlement (Rawls, 1971). However, the principle of justice can be an unrealistic premise in achieving complete fairness and equality, as it presupposes someone is able to distribute money and resources fairly and efficiently. The inequitable distributions of resources of primary goods, for example, water, food, housing, health system financing, and income, are sensitive to a range of phenomena (migration, economic crisis, demographic changes), which can significantly impact any social justice resolutions. However, action around the ethical issue of global health inequalities puts emphasis on 'global solidarity' and thus implicates high-income countries in promoting global health equity as a moral obligation. Adopting this global solidarity approach to social justice, and to reducing global health inequalities, puts emphasis on global distributive justice, which is egalitarian (based on the principle that all people are equal and deserve equal rights and opportunities) as all 'global' citizens deserve a decent minimum of health for a decent human life (Pogge, 2008). Moreover, it could be argued that high-income countries, which have benefitted from colonial, and imperialist endeavours within low-income countries, have a moral duty in relation to distributive justice.

Hunter and Dawson (2021) consider whether geographical political boundaries have a 'moral significance', especially given their lesser significance in a globalised world. They propose that every person is a 'world citizen', therefore placing a universal and impartial moral duty to aid those in need, regardless of their nationality or proximity. This has been viewed as unrealistic, in that national boundaries do limit ethical considerations on a global scale, and prioritisation should be placed nationally, and not globally. Protection of national interests and the shift to potential de-globalisation, discussed in Chapter 3, may compound this, and impact the production of ethical frameworks. The debate that international aid itself is problematic and critiqued as contributing to global inequality and poverty (Moyo, 2009) illustrates this more broadly. The conditions on loans and aid, for example, through structural adjustment policies, as well as poverty reduction, have ethical implications, including questions about whose interests aid and loans serve (Standing, 2011; Sepúlveda Carmona, 2014).

Exploitation of low- and middle-income countries by high-income countries should be perceived as unjust; with the continued manipulation of global social structures privileging high-income counties at the expense of low- and middle-income countries, perpetuating global inequality. Rather, the global extension of economic and cultural relationships which transcend national borders (intensified through globalisation) requires the acknowledgement of global solidarity, or at the very least, a global 'social contract' as well as an understanding of the exploitative relationships which can occur between higher-income and low- and middle-income countries, and impacts upon generation of ethical frameworks to reduce this. Whilst adopting an egalitarian moralistic view may pose challenges within fair distribution of resources, as well as placing a moral obligation or duty on high-income countries to support low-income countries, it is contentious. However, Murphy (2000) argues that if we continue to develop these relationships between countries, we need to adopt the collective duty to maximise beneficence to those in need, through shared global responsibility. By doing so, we can have an impact on global health inequalities and inequalities in general.

COVID-19, Individual Liberty, and Lockdowns

Global pandemics, for example COVID-19, raise significant and novel ethical challenges to countries, healthcare systems, organisations, and the global practice of public health. These span from resource allocation, priority setting, quarantine, and isolation measures, obligations to conduct clinical trials, vaccination, and public health surveillance; these are exacerbated by the complexity of diverse health systems, unique cultures, and socio-economic context of different countries (MacGregor, 2019).

Pandemics cross national boundaries, and necessitate local national and international cooperation, to prevent, prepare, and respond to global pandemics. The recent COVID-19 global pandemic presented ethical challenges, which were demonstrable in how countries adopted differing approaches in their response to the virus. Public health strategies for timely outbreak response are important, and many high-income countries can provide rapid public health advice, and emergency response (MacGregor, 2019). The complexity of large-scale containment measures raises concerns about the impact of this disease in low- and middle-income countries, where unstable health systems, armed conflicts, competing priorities, poverty, and crowding may affect the capacity to manage rapid response to a global pandemic (Agyeman et al., 2020). However, as Tanveer et al. (2020) argue, there is a global moral responsibility for all countries to coalesce and support each other, in relation to emergency response and preparation.

Moreover, countries that impose containment strategies, such as lockdowns, pose ethical tensions, as they may breach ideas of 'freedom' or 'liberty', which are considered a human right in terms of Kantian ethics, so may be perceived as wrong; on the other hand, in relation to utilitarianism, lockdowns could be perceived as acceptable, as their aim is to bring about benefit i.e., the reduction of infection and the protection of the vulnerable (Savulescu et al., 2020). Within a global pandemic, such as COVID-19, Savulescu et al. (2020) state that the utilitarian approach is not simple or easy. It requires choosing the course of action that benefits most people to the greatest degree, however difficult or counterintuitive, that may appear. For utilitarianism, wellbeing is all that matters. Liberty and rights are only important as far as they secure wellbeing. Thus, a utilitarian approach to lockdown may be prepared to override the right to privacy or liberty to protect global wellbeing. However, Tanveer et al. (2020:3) suggest that lockdowns must be both 'proportionate' and 'non-discriminatory', and effective public engagement is key to developing public trust. Coercive measures in low-income countries, exhibiting low levels of literacy and social, religious, and cultural complexities, as well as populations without access to information channels, may be problematic in a pandemic. Therefore, the global community has a moral duty to ensure that access to information and resources, which embody the values of respectfulness and cultural appropriateness, are available.

A unified response to a global pandemic can be considered a moral obligation by all countries to curb the spread of the pandemic through isolation (restricting the movement of infected and symptomatic individuals) and quarantine (restricting the movement of otherwise healthy individuals exposed to an infectious disease) (Henning, 2021). However, there are variations in how this is adopted. Countries that radically curtail liberty, and protect health and security, are often criticised for being overly authoritarian, whereas more 'liberal countries' which assume a 'softer' form of quarantine and isolation and aim to protect liberty and incur greater infection risks are criticised for failing to protect the vulnerable and secure public health. Savulescu et al. (2020) assert that regardless of the varying ways that are adopted, curtailing autonomy, liberty, or factoring in cultural relativism, utilitarianism provides a clear framework, as it takes an impartial approach to everyone's health and wellbeing.

The global response to COVID-19 witnessed a threat to the lives, health, and welfare of others and provided the legitimacy in restricting individual liberty to protect the population and community. This universal approach, such as restricting travel, implementing national and global quarantine measures, may signify a sign of global solidarity through principles of universality and equity, so that a global pandemic could be contained.

Conclusion

This chapter has provided a critical understanding of ethics and theories of ethics. It then proceeded to discuss ethical principles and how they combine to produce ethical frameworks, keeping in mind the distinction between balancing, for example, individuals and populations and public health and global public health. The chapter used issues around health inequalities, COVID-19, liberty, and lockdowns to illustrate ethical issues, and the need to consider the ethics of global public health.

Research Points and Reflective Exercises

With reference to the discussions in this chapter, begin to reflect upon the following:

- What do you understand by the term 'global solidarity' in relation to global public health?
- Reflect upon what you consider to be a global public health issue and think about which interventions/strategies can be applied globally and consider what ethical issues this may present.

Further Resources and Reading

Harris, D. (2011). *Ethics in Health Services and Policy: A Global Approach*. San Francisco, CA: Jossey-Bass.

Landrigan, P. J. and Vicini A. (2021). *Ethical Challenges in Global Public Health: Climate Change, Pollution, and Health of the Poor*. Eugene, OR: Pickwick Publications.

References

Afolabi, M. O. (2018). *Public Health Disasters: A Global Ethical Framework*. Pittsburgh, PA: Springer.

Agyeman, A. A., Laar, A. and Ofori-Asenso, R. (2020). "Will COVID-19 be a Litmus for Post Ebola Sub-Saharan Africa?". *Journal of Medical Virology*, 10: 1-3. https://doi.org/10.1002/jmv.25780

Beauchamp, T. L. and Childress, J. F. (2012). *Principles of Biomedical Ethics*, 7th edn. New York: Oxford University Press.

Bernheim, R. G., Nieburg, P. and Bonnie, R. J. (2007). "Ethics and the Practice of Public Health". In R. A. Goodman (ed.) *Law in Public Health Practice*, 2nd edn. New York: Oxford University Press.

Dawson, A. (2011). *Public Health Ethics: Key Concepts and Issues in Policy and Practice*. Cambridge: Cambridge University Press.

Henning, N. (2021). "Humanitarian Aid, Infectious Diseases and Global Public Health". In. P. J. Landrigan and S. J. Vicini (eds.) *Ethical Challenges in Global Public Health: Climate Change, Pollution, and Health of the Poor*. Eugene, OR: Pickwick Publications, 181-193.

Holland, S. (2014). *Public Health Ethics*, 2nd edn. Cambridge: Polity Press.

Hunter, D. and Dawson, A. (2021). "Is There a Need for Global Health Ethics? For and Against". In. S. Benatar and G. Brock (eds.) *Global Health Ethical Challenges*, 2nd edn. Cambridge: Cambridge University Press, 98-157.

Kass, N. E. (2001). "An Ethics Framework for Public Health". *American Journal of Public Health*, 91 (11): 1776–1782. https://doi.org/10.2105/ajph.91.11.1776

MacGregor, H. (2019). "Global Public Health, Noncommunicable Diseases, and Ethics". In. A. C. Mastroianni, J. P. Kahn, and N. E. Kass (eds.) The *Oxford Handbook of Public Health Ethics*. Oxford: Oxford University Press, 524-536.

Mackay, K. (2021). "Public Health Virtue Ethics". *Public Health Ethics*. phab027: 23-32. https://doi.org/10.1093/phe/phab027

Mehmet, N. (2011). "Ethics and Wellbeing". In. A. Knight and A. McNaught (eds.) *Understanding Wellbeing: An Introduction for Students and Practitioners of Health and Social Care*. Banbury: Lantern Press, 37-50.

Moyo, D. (2009). *Dead Aid: Why Aid Is Not Working and How There Is Another Way for Africa*. London: Penguin.

Murphy, L. B. (2000). *Moral Demands in Non-Ideal Theory*. Oxford: Oxford University Press.

Pogge, T. (2008). *World Poverty and Human Rights Cosmopolitan Responsibilities and Reforms*. Cambridge: Cambridge Polity Press.

Rawls, J. (1971). *A Theory of Justice*. Cambridge, MA: Harvard University Press.

Roberts, M. J. and Reich, M. R. (2002). "Ethical Analysis in Public Health". *Lancet*, 359 (9311): 1055-1059. https://doi.org/10.1016/S0140-6736(02)08097-2

Ruger, J. P. (2006). "Ethics and Governance of Global Health Inequalities". *Journal of Epidemiology and Community Health*, 60 (11): 998–1003. https://doi.org/10.1136/jech. 2005.041947

Savulescu, J., Persson, I. and Wilkinson, D. (2020). "Utilitarianism and the Pandemic". *Bioethics*, 34: 620-632. https://doi.org/10.1111/bioe.12771

Sepúlveda Carmona, M. (2014). *From Undeserving Poor to Rights Holder: A Human Rights Perspective on Social Protection Systems*, Kent, MI: Development Pathways.

Standing, G. (2011). "Behavioural Conditionality: Why the Nudges Must be Stopped – An Opinion Piece". *Journal of Poverty and Social Justice*, 19 (1): 27-38.

Stapleton, G., Schroder-Black, P., Laaser, U., Meershoek, A. and Popa, D. (2014). "Global Health Ethics: An Introduction to Prominent Theories and Relevant Topics". *Global Health Action*, 7: 23569. https://doi.org/10.3402/gha.v7.23569

Tanveer, F., Khalil, A. T., Ali, M. and Shinwari, Z. K. (2020). "Ethics, Pandemic and Environment: Looking at the Future of Low Middle Income Countries". *International Journal Equity Health*, 19 (182): 1-12. https://doi.org/10.1186/s12939-020-01296-z

Upsur, R. E. G., Benatar, S. and Pinto, A. D. (2013). "Ethics and Global Health". In. A. D. Pinto and R. E. G. Upshur (eds.) *An Introduction to Global Health Ethics*. Oxon: Routledge, 16-36.

Warnock, M. (1962). *Utilitarianism: John Stuart Mill*. London: Fontana Press.

World Health Organisation. (2015). *Global Health Ethics Key Issues: Global Network of WHO Collaborating Centres for Bioethics*. Available at: https://www.who.int/publications/i/item/9789241549110 (Accessed: 10 January 2022).

World Health Organisation. (2017). *Code of Ethics and Professional Conduct*. Available at: https://www.who.int/about/ethics/code_of_ethics_full_version.pdf (Accessed: 10 January 2022).

WHO, UNICEF, UNFPA, World Bank Group, and the United Nations Population Division. (2019). *Trends in Maternal Mortality: 2000 to 2017*. Geneva: World Health Organization.

7

ENGAGING CRITICAL PEDAGOGY WITHIN GLOBAL HEALTH TEACHING AND LEARNING

Jennifer Randall

Introduction

As hooks (1994: 14) states 'the classroom remains the most radical space of possibility in the academy'. Times of 'radical' social and ecological change require 'radical thinking' and perhaps a 'radically minded pedagogy'. This chapter discusses perspectives within educational philosophy and focuses on three dimensions of radicality for a teaching practice, for global public health, that these times require. The terms radical and radicality are engaged provocatively, and in the spirit imbued within the writing, of hooks (1994). A radical pedagogy engenders a safe, supported, and challenging space, for conscientisation or raising of critical consciousness. Drawing on an anthropological sensibility and critical pedagogy through the voices of, for example, hooks 1994), Freire (1968), Palmer (1997), and Giroux (2014), this work does not propose a methodology. Instead, it poses a series of questions, and a new concept for learners and teachers of global health, to consider when creating education spaces. This is a learning and teaching practice that engages with emotion, intimacy, and identity transformation, rather than information transmission. This chapter discusses three key concepts: 'identity', 'risk', and 'power'.

Critical Pedagogy and Global Health

Global health, as Arthur Kleinman asserts, 'is more a bunch of problems than a discipline' (Kleinman 2010). Often, global health teachers originate from a range of disciplinary backgrounds. As economists, clinicians, or anthropologists, we approach research and teaching, with a particular set of tools and ways of understanding problems and designing solutions. Those disciplines draw from different ontological and epistemological perspectives, which are advantageous

DOI: 10.4324/9781003128373-7

for students, who can then access a plurality of ideas and methods. But this multi-disciplinarity poses challenges in helping students synthesise their own practice amongst a range of approaches.

In addition to the range of disciplines, learners must also deal with the emotions that accompany studying these problems. Global health topics can be upsetting, traumatising, and can sometimes lead to nihilism and hopelessness. Within 'critical' programmes, we often situate our understanding of global health within a deep historical context. The roots of colonialism, resource extraction, and neoliberal ideology and destroy natural environments. Structural violence, and the reflexivity that can accompany it, leaves students uncomfortable with an acknowledgement of their own complicity (Farmer, 2004). In this multidisciplinary and emotive study, is there a pedagogy that can help us reach students that engages their intellect and empowers their actions? Are there particular techniques to help students to find the skills and the will to analyse and tackle problems, as well as develop solutions?

Critical pedagogy, and adaptations of it (often subsumed under Critical Public Health theory), can facilitate transformative education by which global health practitioners, come to not only critique problems, but actively engage in their solutions. Noted as the father of critical pedagogy, Paulo Freire was a Brazilian educator who worked as an English teacher with peasant communities (Freire, 1968). Coming from the intellectual and political tradition of liberation theology, he argued for an education that served the purpose of transforming the social world. Regardless of experience, everyone who enters a learning space or classroom brings with them wisdom and a valid understanding of the world. Furthermore, all participants gain insights from these varied worldviews. The role of the educator is to leverage those understandings in the service of a bigger social concern. Learning is transformative, reflective, and critical for individuals and society alike. His most famous writing, 'Pedagogy of the Oppressed' (1968) argued that education's purpose was to dismantle systems of oppression, and who better to lead that structural change, than those who experience its oppression. Education is a political endeavour, and he knew this better than many as he was forced to live in exile for several years.

Many people critique, discuss, and adapt his intellectual insights, most notably, hooks (1994) and Henry Giroux (2014). Furthermore, Freire's ideas also hold prominence with a range of participatory research methodologies. Photovoice and other participatory techniques are grounded in the belief that those living within environments in need of 'development' should be the leaders and directors of the research process (Wang, 1996). These methods are less extractive and are positioned, so that participants' voices, with the support of researchers, can raise everyone's critical consciousness of the complex actors and processes, that create and maintain global health and development problems (Reynolds and Sarolio, 2018). Disrupting the traditional paradigms that define education practice is key to a radical global health pedagogy. This chapter outlines three dimensions, that each learner and teacher can consider, to enhance the ability to learn and change, and offers probing questions, to help teachers and learners define critical aspects of their own pedagogical practice.

Identity

To begin, it is crucial to disrupt the hegemonic idea that education is about information. Instead, let us see it as a space for radical imagination in the transformation of new identities. All participants within learning experiences should work to reframe learning as a 'transformation of identity', not a transmission of information. Education is an intimate connection in which humans come together to learn something new and expand their thinking: and these processes, therefore, change who they 'are', not only what they 'know'. For example, one does not learn medicine; they 'become' a doctor. Being a doctor is an embodied knowledge practice that ultimately works in the service of others. But medical education is not just a knowledge transmission system, but a transformation of people, in which they have internalised its rules, concepts, and critical structures (Palmer, 2007). As such, this is a deeply personal endeavour. It is fragmentation and rebuilding of their identity. Understanding how this process affects students is key, and it should also be mirrored in the educator.

When teachers are 'self-actualised' (hooks, 1994), they disarm their students. As educators demonstrate a revelation of their own predispositions, this serves as an invitation for students to engage in a more profound experience of learning. Working alongside teachers, students can experience an education that sees, listens, invites, and supports. If educators make their own journeys of learning available to students, those learners can then see why and how these transformations of identity can materialise. This integrated identity, which is shared with students, will serve as a model for other students to follow. For only when people are seen, heard, guided, and held, can they begin to challenge their own assumptions, privileges, and vulnerabilities and ultimately question the structures which facilitate and maintain the suffering, which is often the object of their learning. Any change of identity requires a willingness to risk personal revelations.

Risk

Even seasoned educators and researchers can feel vulnerable when they make ideas permanent, whether in pixel or print. Regardless of how well-evidenced, passionately articulated, or perfectly printed in poetic prose, anxiety might always lie beneath the surface when analyses are publicly presented. 'Someone will read this and react'. Surely, at least one person will do so with critique or negativity. In today's social media climate, that can feel particularly vulnerable, when our lives are lived in an environment of global reach. Our students suffer a similar anxiety, and it is our first responsibility to help people feel comfortable in taking risks. Learning means changing; changing feels scary, and when we are scared, we need to feel safe, so that we can take 'risks', not just to learn something new, but become something different. When viewed as an object, and not attending to the subjective experiences of our students, we diminish the capacity of our classrooms to become safe spaces for taking risks.

Teaching global health is not about wearing social justice as a cloak or observing the material suffering and analytical structures of power from afar; it is about engaging a practice of embodied learning for teacher and learner alike. Thus, this becomes a practice that serves, not only to engage the minds and intellect, but attends to the emotional response, so natural to the learning occurring in the classrooms we inhabit (hooks, 1994); an environment where students and teachers feel safe in saying 'I want to take the risk of becoming something new'.

Learning how to take risks and change one's identity within a classroom is an important experience for future global health work. The experience of reframing or unlearning serves as a model by which those who have been stirred and nurtured by such practice can then model this work in their re-engagement within their 'rhizomal' and 'tentacular' connections (Haraway, 2016). For example, students may be invited to confront hegemonic stories about certain groups, e.g., all drug users are personally responsible for their misuse. While this statement may seem axiomatic within certain contexts, it is not underpinned by much of the literature on this issue (Singer and Page, 2014; Hart, 2021). When educators provide the time and 'safe' space to articulate these problematic ideas, and gently work to reframe the students' views on these challenging topics, they undergo personal change and start to perceive the world differently. They are then able to create safe spaces for risk-taking in their networks. Education is at the heart of global health work. When built on the philosophy that learning is about feeling safe to change one's thinking and become something different, powerful sustainable transformations can be nurtured.

Power

Within classrooms, we all aim to 'empower' our students (a working definition inspired by Collins (2000) is discussed below). We hope to engage them in critical analysis of how this work of empowerment can be carried out within and beyond the classroom and in the context of their future global health work. Hence, when teaching a module, it can be helpful if the educator can articulate their perspective on this process. Educators can clearly address how they theoretically and practically engage in empowering work, both within the context of classrooms, but then in all the spaces where health education, public health, and behaviour change work is achieved. How students experience empowerment within classrooms defines how they will do this work with others in the future.

The neoliberal university and learning spaces, which many of us occupy, present new challenges and barriers to an engaged, radical pedagogy (Cowden and Singh, 2013; Collini, 2017). It is increasingly difficult to nurture a sense of responsibility to one's learning and creating a safe space for the unlearning and reframing of internalised oppressive structures. Students are positioned as consumers, as objects upon which information is foisted. While this chapter cannot address this ecosystem with the needed detail, neoliberal learning settings view students as both simultaneous objects to receive information, but also as active, powerful consumers within the micro and macro environments. Subjective experiences of customer satisfaction become the goal of a … 'quality-controlled' operation driven by standardisation and a banking pedagogy (Darder, 2018: 142–143). This paradox creates a tension that must be properly addressed. Power is thus consistently in tension within higher education spaces.

When combining the ideas of critical pedagogy, as described by hooks (1994) and Freire (1968), with the matrix of oppression, as it is outlined by Collins (2000), we can identify a theory of power and a potential intervention, by which learning can disrupt or reframe power (Collins, 2000). Collins provides four domains of the matrix of power: structural, disciplinary, hegemonic, and interpersonal. Briefly, structural power resides within institutions and organisations within society, and they 'organise' power. Disciplinary power is the bureaucracy within those organisations, and it is the force that 'manages' communities oppressed by this power. Hegemonic power includes the invisible and reinforced stories (Mkhwanazi, 2016) articulated about the communities or groups of people that are managed by the disciplinary power and organised by those structures. Hegemonic power thus 'justifies' the entire system. And the final domain is interpersonal power, which is the collection of intimate, daily interactions, between groups of people, by which intersectional identities can result in power 'over' another individual, e.g., a white lecturer with her racially minoritised students.

Empowerment within this matrix is therefore derived from this matrix by creating empowering learning environments for disempowered groups. It is argued here that these spaces must be guided by a critical pedagogy approach. This is not about information transmission. These spaces must offer an opportunity for reflection and demystification of these domains of power. Students and teachers create a learning space to identify and reflect upon how those structures define their lives. Students are introduced to a vocabulary to describe those structures and the numerous ways in which it impacts their lives. Most importantly, this must be a space to tell new stories, to reframe, and change the hegemonic power, which justifies maintaining the system as it is. For example, in the case of disproportionate policing of BAME communities, peer to peer programmes like YStop in the UK serve to provide a space where young people experiencing over policing can share stories and reframe those experiences (Shiner et al., 2018).

A Radical Pedagogical Practice

Critical pedagogy becomes the philosophy and methodologically influenced mechanism by which empowering environments can be made for marginalised groups to acknowledge, speak, and redefine the stories, told about them, to maintain their oppression. This framework can potentially dismantle a dualism often observed in community engagement. Participants or targeted communities can be seen either as a group completely stripped of its agency or having full responsibility placed upon their shoulders to fracture sclerotic systems of oppression. The teacher or educator thus becomes the architect of a space for careful reflection, connection with innovative ideas, and a demystification of the structures, by which oppression of self and others is manifested. Learners and students can come to identify the role that individuals play within those structures and then they can find resources and support, by which they can have their voices, and so challenge hegemonic narratives and power to shift other structural, disciplinary, and interpersonal domains of the power matrix.

Various social movements have deployed these mechanisms to change the narrative and structural barriers to their protection and respect of inalienable human rights. Sex workers, drug users, disability activists, and trans activists, all use these methods in their work to reframe and challenge the 'single stories' of who they are and can thus facilitate their reclamation of power. One prominent example comes from the work of VANDU, the Vancouver Network of Drug Users. Kerr (2006) and Hari (2015) narrate the role of the presence of drug users in political spaces. Using direct action, activists initiated the telling of a different story, of who they are and how many were needlessly dying. These actions ultimately changed the hearts, minds, and eventually the structural political system in the form of the Mayor, Philip Owens, unlearning and being open to a transformation of who he was (Osborn and Small, 2006). VANDU activists changed the mayor, so that he became an advocate of the drug users' rehumanising demands. These powerful examples of the willingness to take risks, to shift identities, and use their power in the service of others, are profoundly inspiring and are key examples of how this transformative work is done.

Our students enter our classrooms with the intention of studying global health. This collection of problems (Kleinman, 2010) can overwhelm students as they wrestle with the details of the material and corporeal suffering they witness in academic literature and media outlets. As students work with lecturers to discover and expose histories that feel calcified, hegemonic, and mystified, apathy extinguishes optimism. The revelation of these ideas and the connections students have to the personal, as well as the political, can often leave students feeling lost, overwhelmed, or nihilistic. These are all perfectly 'reasonable' responses to what is often seen as an 'unreasonable' world.

The power of this approach is evidenced by work conducted by the author in a programme entitled 'Reflections for Change' (Randall, 2020) and a project in preparation for publication, 'Sowing Empowering and Engaging Discussions on Substances' (SEEDS). In these projects, students worked alongside the educator to start with a reflection on the varied lives of the people in those classrooms. Building conversations around those stories, and introducing new vocabulary, connected students with tools and concepts, to describe and analyse their past and present. Threading those conversations together built new stories about who these students are and what they mean to the institutions of higher education that host their learning experiences. Working collectively to create new knowledge, both projects designed, developed, and disseminated the stories and ideas of students, as tools for critical conversations outside of formal learning spaces. As educators leverage their institutional power, students were provided opportunities to speak 'truth to power' in formal dissemination events. SEEDS was a 50-day social media, and in person campaign, designed by students for their 'communities' to seed conversations on harm reduction and drug policy reform. Over 40 students from more than ten countries produced 50 videos and materials in English, Somali and Bengali, to help shift the dialogue locally and globally. Public health outreach in the form of formal and informal conversations was carried out in person and online and these 'rhizomal' connections continue to grow and mature.

Navigating learning that asks its students and teachers to reframe ideas that may be entrenched or hegemonic requires a transformative learning and un-learning process for all. The COVID pandemic revealed structural inequities and polarised political proclivities, but that does not mean we give up on learning and unlearning. The work needed for us to address global health problems feels overwhelming. At the heart is the need for 'conversations'. It is important to consider who, why, and what frames these conversations. A capacity to change behaviour and thinking is possible for us all (Berg and Seeber, 2016). Learning and education become a process for a radical reflection on why we live the life we lead. It builds connections to people and ideas. It also facilitates a personal reckoning with empathy and power. Finally, it can engender an ability and a willingness to act. For the purpose of memorable wordplay and social science cultural practices, let us call this RECONEMPACT: a portmanteau of REflection, CONnection, EMPathy/EMPower, and ACTion.

RECONEMPACT can be enacted by asking a series of questions to catalyse these courageous conversations. Why do I experience privilege or vulnerability within certain spaces? Where are the silent or invisible privileges, and where are the noisy and omnipresent vulnerabilities, created by intersecting characteristics of who I am? With what disciplines and paradigms can I connect my understanding of the world? With whom do I connect and find inspiration? How can I leverage my capacity for empathy, and the power within my reach, to engage in conscientious change?

Conclusion

To address issues of power and inequalities, more effective critical pedagogies are required for global public health learning and teaching. We need to embody the roles of student and teacher in all the spaces we occupy in our various 'communities'. Working alongside people from a range of backgrounds, we can all learn to reflect, connect, find power, nurture critical empathy, and act. The work of social justice is not just political protests on the streets, but also slow, continuous, critical, and empathetic conversations in our communities. Dialogue between students and teachers connect the lives of others, and entwine knowledge and insights, not just about the object of study within our literal gaze, but with the interpretation of others, from various worldviews and lives lived. We must envision education as a process of transformations of identity, rather than information transmission. It encourages the creation of safe learning spaces for risking a change in that identity and is a way for us to identify individual and collective power, for effective change within global public health.

Research Points and Reflective Exercise

With reference to the discussions in this chapter, begin to reflect upon the following:

1 What is the role of critical pedagogy in teaching global public health and enabling students to see and provide solutions to health inequalities?
2 What is the role of educators and learners in ensuring that global public health solutions and interventions transform the health and wellbeing of marginalised communities?

Further Resources and Reading

hooks, b. (2003) *Teaching Community: A Pedagogy of Hope.* New York: Routledge.

References

Berg, M. and Seeber, B. (2016). *The Slow Professor: Challenging the Culture of Speed in the Academy.* Toronto: University of Toronto Press.

Collini, S., (2017). *Speaking of Universities.* London: Verso Books.

Collins, P. H. (2000). *Black Feminist Thought: Knowledge, Consciousness, and the Politics of Empowerment,* 10th Anniversary edn. New York: Routledge.

Cowden, S. and Singh, G. S. (2013). *Acts of Knowing: Critical Pedagogy in, Against and Beyond the University.* London: Bloomsbury Publishing.

Darder, A. (2018). *Radical Imagine-Nation: Public Pedagogy and Praxis.* New York: Peter Lang Publishing.

Farmer, P. (2004). "An Anthropology of Structural Violence". *Current Anthropology,* 45 (3): 305–325. http://doi.org/10.1086/382250

Freire, P. (1968). *Pedagogy of the Oppressed,* 6th edn. New York: Herder and Herder.

Giroux, H. (2014). *Neoliberalism's War on Higher Education.* Toronto: Between the Lines.

Haraway, D. (2016). *Staying With the Trouble: Making Kin in the Chthulucene.* Durham: Duke University Press.

Hari, J. (2015). *Chasing the Scream: The First and Last Days of the War on Drugs.* London: Bloomsbury.

Hart, C. (2021). *Drug Use for Grown-Ups: Chasing Liberty in the Land of the Free.* New York: Penguin Random House.

hooks, b. (1994). *Teaching to Transgress: Education as the Practice of Freedom.* New York: Routledge.

Kerr, T. E. A. (2006). "Harm Reduction By A 'User-Run' Organization: A Case Study of the Vancouver Area Network of Drug Users (VANDU)". *International Journal of Drug Policy*, 17: 61–69. http://doi.org/10.1016/j.drugpo.2006.01.003

Kleinman, A. (2010). "The Art of Medicine: Four Social Theories for Global Health". *The Lancet*, 375: 1518–1520. http://doi.org/10.1016/S0140-6736(10)60646-0

Mkhwanazi, N. (2016). "Medical Anthropology in Africa: The Trouble with a Single Story". *Medical Anthropology: Cross-Cultural Studies in Health and Illness*, 35 (2): 193–202. http://doi.org/10.1080/01459740.2015.1100612

Osborn, B. and Small, W., (2006). "'Speaking Truth to Power': The Role of Drug Users in Influencing Municipal Drug Policy. *International Journal of Drug Policy*, 17: 70–72. http://doi.org/10.1016/j.drugpo.2005.09.001

Palmer, P. (1997). *The Courage to Teach*. San Francisco, CA: Jossey-Bass Publishers.

Palmer, P. (2007). "A New Professional: The Aims of Education Revisited. Change". *The Magazine of Higher Learning*, 39 (6): 6–13. http://doi.org/10.3200/CHNG.39.6.6-13

Randall, J. (2020). "Transformative Identities: Journeys through the Neoliberal University in Search of Social Justice". *Practicing Anthropology*, 42 (1): 52–55. http://doi.org/10.17730/0888-4552.42.1.52

Reynolds, L. and Sarolio, S. (2018). "The Ethics and Politics of Community Engagement in Global Health Research". *Critical Public Health*, 28 (3): 257–268. http://doi.org/10.1080/09581596.2018.1449598

Shiner, M., Carre, Z., Delsol, R. and Eastwood, N. (2018). *The Colour of Injustice: 'Race'. Drugs, and Law Enforcement in England and Wales*. London: StopWatch.

Singer, M. and Page, B. (2014). *The Social Value of Drug Addicts: Use of the Useless*. New York: Routledge.

Wang, C. E. A. (1996). "Chinese Village Women as Visual Anthropologists: A Participatory Approach to Reaching Policymakers". *Social Science and Medicine*, 42 (10): 1391–1400. http://doi.org/10.1016/0277-9536(95)00287-1

8

ISSUES IN DESIGN, IMPLEMENTATION, AND EVALUATION OF MATERNAL HEALTH INTERVENTIONS IN LOW- AND MIDDLE-INCOME COUNTRIES

Aduragbemi Banke-Thomas and Ejemai Eboreime

Introduction

Despite diverse efforts invested in strengthening health systems and improving health outcomes, many global public health challenges remain unresolved, as new ones emerge. Many maternal health interventions have been implemented with several failing to achieve their intended results. As has been established, failure in achieving desired outcomes may be related to how the intervention was designed (design failure) or how it was implemented (implementation failure) (Allen and Gunderson, 2011). No other domain of global public health highlights these failures better than maternal health. Within the maternal health domain, despite a 38% reduction in global maternal deaths since 2000, 295,000 women still die annually due to pregnancy and childbirth complications. Almost all maternal deaths occur in low- and middle-income countries (LMICs) with Nigeria accounting for over two-fifths of the global burden. A key target of the 'Sustainable Development Goals' is to reduce the global maternal mortality ratio to less than 70 per 100,000 live births by 2030 (United Nations, 2016). This chapter will use case studies of two maternal health interventions, implemented in Nigeria, to highlight and discuss issues in design, implementation, and evaluation of maternal health interventions and policies in LMICs.

Maternal Health Interventions

Nyamtema et al. (2011) found that various supply- and demand-side and evidence-based interventions, with the aim of improving maternal outcomes, have been implemented. Generally, more supply-side interventions have been implemented due to the evidence which suggests that about two-thirds of maternal deaths can be prevented with good quality obstetric care. These interventions

DOI: 10.4324/9781003128373-8

include training of health workers, improving supply of medicines, establishing, and strengthening blood banks, strengthening referral systems, construction of comprehensive emergency obstetric care facilities, establishing maternal waiting homes, and mobile maternal health services. Conversely, demand-side interventions, that have been implemented, include community-based health education, voucher schemes, community-based funds to fund ambulances or loans for obstetric complications, training, and/or linking traditional birth attendants to the health system (Nyamtema et al., 2011). In addition to recognising the maternal health interventions to implement, the other critical consideration is establishing if and how the interventions work in specific contexts.

Two large-scale maternal health interventions that have been implemented in Nigeria, Midwives Service Scheme (MSS) and Àbíyè (Safe Motherhood) programme, are described below and used as case studies to discuss issues in design, implementation, and evaluation of maternal health interventions and policies in LMICs.

The Midwives Service Scheme

Recognising the marked variation in maternal health access and outcomes across geopolitical zones, and between rural and urban areas, the Federal Ministry of Health (FMOH) continues to deploy interventions to foster equity. Nigeria launched the MSS in December 2009 as a response to the shortage of skilled health personnel in rural areas, which is thought to be an important supply-side constraint, linked to poor utilisation of health services, and poor health outcomes in these areas (Abimbola et al., 2012). The scheme was largely funded by the Paris Club debt relief agreements awarded to Nigeria in 2005. The MSS was designed as a collaborative intervention between the three tiers of government (local, state, and federal) and was formalised through a memorandum of understanding. The expected theory of change was that an increased supply of midwives would translate to improved access, perceived quality utilisation of services, satisfaction with care, and ultimately, reduction in maternal mortality (Abimbola et al., 2012; Okeke et al., 2015).

The midwives were recruited and deployed from the federal level to selected Primary Health Centres (PHCs) where they worked for one year. They received basic health insurance, as well as a monthly stipend from the Federal (N30,000) (US$200) and state government (N20,000) (US$133), while local government provided the midwives with free accommodation and additional stipend (N10,000) (US$66). Through the MSS, the FMOH employed new graduates, unemployed, and retired midwives, to fill human resource gaps in rural areas. A cluster model was utilised to select four eligible rural PHC facilities which have basic infrastructure and minimum equipment, and are in proximity to a selected General Hospital, which could provide comprehensive emergency obstetric care. Distribution of MSS facilities was mostly determined by estimated maternal mortality for the different geopolitical zones in the country. The north-eastern and north-western states, which were deemed to exhibit very high mortality zones, were allocated 24 facilities each. The north central and south-south states, with their supposed high mortality zones, were allocated 16 facilities each, while the southwest and southeast states, categorised as moderate mortality zones, were allocated 12 facilities each (Okeke et al., 2015).

Using a difference-in-difference approach, results showed that there was about a seven-percent increase in antenatal care (ANC) utilisation after the first year, with no programme effect evidenced afterwards. In addition, minimal evidence of an increase in the number of four or more ANC visits, as recommended by the World Health Organization, was recorded. The scheme also had a negligible impact on skilled birth attendance (Okeke et al., 2015). In a separate study, overall institutional MMR dropped from 789 per 100,000 live births for July-December 2009 to 572 per 100,000 live births for the same period in 2010. When disaggregated by zones, the north central zone had the greatest reduction in institutional MMR while the ratio about doubled, during the same period, in the north-eastern and south-eastern zones (Abimbola et al., 2012). As per available evidence, it is clear that the scaling up of the supply of midwives is necessary but is in no way a 'magic bullet' for improving maternal health outcomes in Nigeria.

The Àbíyè (Safe Motherhood) Programme

In October 2009, the Government of Ondo state, southwest Nigeria, under the leadership of a newly elected Governor launched the Àbíyè (Safe Motherhood) programme. This was designed as a response to the evidence from the 2008 Nigeria Demographic and Health survey (NDHS), which showed that Ondo state had the worst maternal outcomes in southwest Nigeria with MMR of 765 per 100,000 live births (Ajayi and Akpan, 2020). The programme aimed to ensure every pregnant woman received quality health care, to expand universal access to quality maternity care by removing barriers to care in a sustainable fashion, and implement an equitable allocation of the state's limited resources, based on identified needs and performance-driven principles.

As part of design, the state conducted a needs assessment to identify technical and sociocultural drivers of poor health outcomes in the state. This assessment identified delays in access to care across four phases of care, which predispose women to maternal deaths in the state, and sought home-grown solutions to each phase (Mimiko et al., 2013). The delays identified and strategies deployed in the programme were:

- Delay in seeking care: The state mobilised 'health rangers', which were trained community workers, assigned to 25 pregnant women in their community, who they monitored and counselled during pregnancy. Women were also given mobile phones with which they communicated with their assigned health ranger;

- Delay in reaching care: Health rangers were provided with transportation (including motorcycles, tricycle ambulances, and four-wheeled ambulances) to help transport their assigned women to health facilities;
- Delay in accessing care: The state government employed and trained health workers, renovated five PHCs, and built 11 new ones. The state also deployed strategies to ensure the supply of essential drugs and consumables, following findings from the needs assessment;
- Delay in referring care: It strengthened the existing two-way referral system and constructed an apex referral centre.

These interventions were initially piloted in one of the 18 local government areas (LGAs) of the state. Lessons learnt, while piloting, helped to identify what worked and what did not work. For example, it helped policy makers to realise that procuring tricycles to serve as ambulances to transport pregnant women in emergency situations would not be an effective use of resources, as the poor terrain and road network minimised their efficiency and effectiveness. The pilot also led to the exclusion of the plan to distribute mobile phones to all pregnant women in the full scale-up (Ajayi and Akpan, 2020).

In a study that compared maternal health indices pre- and post-programme, using the 2013 and 2018 NDHS, the authors reported that ANC utilisation increased from 80% in the 2013 NDHS to 98% in the 2016 survey. The authors also reported a 29.1% increase in births occurring in health facilities from 56.5% in the 2013 NDHS to 85.6% in the 2016 survey (Ajayi and Akpan, 2020). In a case-control study that compared the pilot LGA with a control LGA, the provision of mobile phones to pregnant women, and improvement of maternal health services, was deemed to have significantly improved service utilisation, though no effect was observed on pregnancy outcomes (Oyeyemi and Wynn, 2014).

Reviewing Design and Implementation of Maternal Health Interventions

Every public health intervention consists of core and adaptable elements. Both elements may be viewed as answering two key questions. Core elements respond to 'what is being delivered to cause change?' and adaptable elements respond to 'how is the intervention delivered to cause change within context?' Core elements are responsible for the impact of an intervention (Fixsen et al., 2009) while adaptable elements make them suitable for contexts such as local culture, language, or socio-political considerations. Adaptable elements can therefore be modified to align with contextual nuances, optimising effectiveness. However, compromising the core elements, during the design or implementation phases, may result in failure. The field of implementation science has evolved theories, models, and methods, aimed at improving the quality of implementation and the effectiveness of interventions (Nilsen, 2015). Specifically, for global health, the Theory-Design-Implementation (TyDI) framework is a useful tool

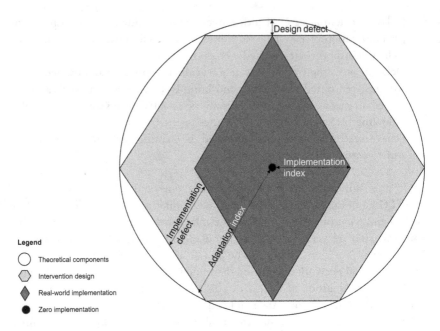

FIGURE 8.1 An illustration of the TyDI concepts and parameters.

for supporting programme managers and policy makers in designing and implementing interventions successfully (Eboreime et al., 2020).

The TyDI framework comprises three main elements, a rhomboid (representing 'real-world' programme implementation), a hexagon (representing the intervention design), and a circle (the underpinning theory of the intervention) (Figure 8.1). Interaction between these elements can be assessed by two indices (implementation index and adaptation index) and two defects (design and implementation). The implementation index measures the extent to which the intervention was implemented in the real world. Conversely, the adaptation index measures the extent to which the adapted programme aligned with the core components of the intervention. Ideally, an intervention should align optimally with core components, both in design and implementation. But in the real world, design and implementation defects occur. The implementation defect is the component of the design that was not implemented, reflecting the gap between intervention-as-delivered in comparison to the intervention-as-designed or planned. The two case studies described depict how interventions are commonly challenged either in the design, implementation, or both.

Using the TyDI framework, the MSS had a key design defect. Whereas the intervention theory accounted for the decentralised (federal) governance system of Nigeria, the adapted design at initiation assumed a strong centralised approach. Programme funding, recruitment, and deployment of human resources (midwives), monitoring and evaluation systems, were all managed by the National Primary Health Care Development Agency (a parastatal of the federal government), rather than the state (subnational) governments (Okpani and Abimbola, 2016; Eboreime et al., 2017). During an evaluation of the MSS, programme stakeholders opined that a consequence of this design defect was that the homogenous design of the MSS (with the attendant top-down approach to management), created critical challenges in implementation at the subnational level. The stakeholders believed that contextual issues were not considered during the design of the programme; rather, the defective adaptation was subsequently 'forced' on them for implementation (Okeke et al., 2015). There are other questions with design. Was it enough to allocate facilities, based on burden of disease, as was done on the MSS? What about access, travel time, and geographical barriers, that need to be overcome to reach health facilities? Evidence suggests that women face significant challenges in accessing facilities, even in urban settings, which are meant to have the so-called 'urban advantage'. These challenges include traffic congestion, poor road conditions, and disruption by security forces (Banke-Thomas et al., 2020). In addition, women are known to bypass nearby facilities for assorted reasons (Kruk et al., 2009; Banke-Thomas et al., 2020). In many settings, these design effects are context specific.

The other critical design consideration for the MSS is the incentive package given to the skilled health personnel (described above). As per WHO guidelines, an effective incentive scheme for health workers should have clear objectives, be realistic and deliverable, and reflect the needs and preferences of health workers. It should also be effectively designed, strategic, and fit-for-purpose, contextually appropriate, fair, equitable and transparent, measurable, and incorporate financial and non-financial elements. While the MSS incentive package had some of these characteristics, some were not addressed. Questions remain on the sufficiency of the package in meeting the needs of the health workers, many of whom still needed to borrow money from relatives to make ends meet (Ibeh, 2015). The other key design issue relates to the sufficiency of a one-year initial contract renewable dependent on performance. Was a one-year contract sufficient for health workers who had to relocate to start jobs in a rural environment? We argue that this short-term contract does not provide health workers with the stability for a major career shift.

Another key issue relates to the adequacy of the additional midwives added to the health workforce pool. In all, 2,488 midwives were deployed, with each clinic receiving four midwives to enable them to run shifts providing 24-hour coverage (Okeke et al., 2015). At baseline, Nigeria, despite having one of the highest maternal deaths, has only 12 nurses and midwives per 10,000 population, which is one of the lowest density of nurses and midwives per population ratios globally. Countries with fewer than 23 physicians, nurses, and midwives per 10,000 population, generally fail to achieve adequate coverage rates for selected primary healthcare interventions. Available data shows that though Africa carries 25% of the world's disease burden, it has only 3% of the world's health workers (World Health Organization, 2006). Another consideration is that some shifts may be busier than others, as will some rural areas and health facilities. These are crucial factors in allocating midwives to the facilities, especially as health workers in Nigeria, who are part of similar incentive-based schemes, led to corollary increased clinical workload and record keeping (Bhatnagar and George, 2016). Even for those health workers who were on the scheme, many were not paid for as long as nine months, with Government blaming budget delays (Ibeh, 2015).

In addition, varying financial barriers in accessing care across the various states have been reasons provided by MSS stakeholders to explain the differential achievement of programme outcomes (Okpani and Abimbola, 2016). Critically, there were other issues that influenced effectiveness of the programme which were not the focus of the programme; for example, sociocultural factors, which encourage women to opt for home deliveries, despite proximity to MSS facilities in some parts of the country (Abimbola et al., 2012; Okeke et al., 2015).

The success of the Abiye programme was attributed to strong political commitment, stakeholder goodwill, evidence-based and technically sound programme design, implementation fidelity, and dynamics, significant grassroot mobilisation, and monitoring, as well as removal of user fees (Mimiko et al., 2013). As the initiating Governor's tenure ended, there were concerns about its continuity with the transition of power to a new Governor in 2017. The new Governor promised to sustain and improve the achievements of the previous regime and has proceeded to attract over $US6.5 million additional investment from the World Bank and MedShare, an American non-profit organisation (Johnson, 2020). The new Governor, in response to the funding gap and drive to ensure sustainability, launched the Abiyamo Maternal and Child Health Insurance Scheme (ODCHC, 2019). A critical point is that programme design was based on a robust needs assessment that identified the multiple points of delay that women experienced in accessing care and generated 'home grown' strategies to address them.

These two case studies underscore the importance of appropriate intervention design. They also demonstrate that a poorly designed intervention will result in poor outcomes, irrespective of how well it is implemented. Also important is that addressing implementation challenges cannot correct the design defects. Design failure can only be addressed by de-implementation and redesign of the defective intervention (Eboreime et al., 2020).

Reviewing Evaluation of Maternal Health Interventions

With evaluation, there are two questions that are important for programme implementers and researchers. These relate to efficiency and effectiveness. Efficiency relates to outputs and can be reported if robust data systems are incorporated as part of the programme design. With effectiveness, this relates to outcomes, and is for the most part, out of the control of implementers, but an important question. The evaluation of whether an intervention was effective or not should be based on data that demonstrates the attributable gains of the intervention itself. This typically requires specific data collection, as part of the evaluation process, or secondary data from existing surveys or health information management systems.

For the Àbíyè programme, while improvements were noted based on data from the NDHS conducted before and after the intervention (Ajayi and Akpan, 2020), it is not clear how much of the improvements could be specifically attributed to the intervention. For programmes that have specific data collection processes, study designs, such as randomised controlled trials (RCTs), and quasi-experimental studies, will be ideal. However, for ethical reasons, it is difficult to conduct RCTs regarding interventions to reduce maternal mortality. The challenge with demonstrating programme impact in LMICs, including those related to the rarity of the event, inadequacy of health management information systems, and the quality of the available data, has long been recognised (Graham et al., 1996). The difference-in-difference approach used by Okeke et al. (2015) in the MSS evaluation is gaining popularity. However, specific data collection processes attract additional cost. In recent years, and with the increasing donor funding of maternal health interventions, there has been demand, to demonstrate cost-effectiveness, and more broadly value for money (Banke-Thomas et al., 2017). This requires clear lines of attribution of costs to outcomes achieved because of the intervention. There is also the need for greater transparency and accountability with costs disbursed on implementing the interventions.

Conclusions

The challenges faced by pregnant women in accessing and utilising maternal health services are multi-faceted and multi-tiered. As such, integrated programmes with multiple interventions are needed and have been shown to have more significant impact on pregnancy outcomes of mothers (Nyamtema et al., 2011). Where there are gaps in adaptation and implementation, these have important implications for maternal health, especially in LMICs. Through the integration of several supply and demand-side interventions and innovations, it is possible to make considerable progress in maternal health, like in the Abiye programme. The TyDI framework helps to identify and evaluate gaps or defects in core and adaptable elements in the design and implementation of health programmes. For evaluation, more robust, integrated, and agile data systems are needed. In the end, we want to answer what works? How well did it work? And why did it work? Comprehensive answers will contribute to improved outcomes for maternal health interventions.

Research Points and Reflective Exercise

With reference to the discussions in this chapter, begin to reflect upon the following:

• Reflecting on a specific maternal health intervention to be implemented in your setting or country, what are some of the key adaptable elements that require consideration?

- How will you engage end users of intervention during design and implementation of maternal health implementation?
- Why is it a challenge to demonstrate value-for-money of maternal health interventions?

Further Resources and Reading

Banke-Thomas, A., Nieuwenhuis, S., Ologun, A., Mortimore, G. and Mpakateni, M. (2019). "Embedding Value-for-Money in Practice: A Case Study of a Health Pooled Fund Programme Implemented in Conflict-Affected South Sudan". *Evaluation and Program Planning*, 77: 101725. https://doi.org/10.1016/J.EVALPROGPLAN.2019.101725
Eboreime, E. A., Eyles, J., Nxumalo, N., Eboreime, O. L. and Ramaswamy, R. (2019). "Implementation Process and Quality of a Primary Health Care System Improvement Initiative in a Decentralized Context: A Retrospective Appraisal Using the Quality Implementation Framework". *The International Journal of Health Planning and Management*, 34 (1): e369–e386. https://doi.org/10.1002/HPM.2655

References

Abimbola, S., Okoli, U., Olubajo, O., Abdullahi. J. and Pate, M. A. (2012). "The Midwives Service Scheme in Nigeria". *PLOS (Public Library of Science) Medicine*, 9 (5): e1001211. https://doi.org/10.1371/journal.pmed.1001211
Ajayi, A. I. and Akpan, W. (2020). "Maternal Health Care Services Utilisation in the Context of 'Abiye' (Safe Motherhood) Programme in Ondo State, Nigeria". *BMC Public Health*, 20: 362. https://doi.org/10.1186/s12889-020-08512-z
Allen, C. R. and Gunderson, L. H. (2011). "Pathology and Failure in the Design and Implementation of Adaptive Management". *Journal of Environmental Management*, 92 (5): 1379–1384. https://doi.org/10.1016/j.jenvman.2010.10.063
Banke-Thomas, A., Balogun, M., Wright, O., Ajayi, B., Abejirinde, I. O. O. et al. (2020). "Reaching Health Facilities in Situations of Emergency: Qualitative Study Capturing Experiences of Pregnant Women in Africa's Largest Megacity". *Reproductive Health*, 17 (1): 145. https://doi.org/10.1186/s12978-020-00996-7
Banke-Thomas, A., Madaj, B., Kumar, S., Ameh, C., and van den Broek, N. (2017). "Assessing Value-for-Money in Maternal and Newborn Health". *BMJ Global Health*, 2: e000310. https://doi.org/10.1136/ bmjgh-2017-000310
Bhatnagar, A. and George, A. S. (2016). "Motivating Health Workers Up to a Limit: Partial Effects of Performance-Based Financing on Working Environments in Nigeria". *Health Policy and Planning*, 31 (7): 868–877. https://doi.org/10.1093/HEAPOL/CZW002
Eboreime, E. A., Abimbola, S., Obi, F. A., Ebirim, O., Olubajo, O. et al. (2017). "Evaluating the Sub-National Fidelity of National Initiatives in Decentralized Health Systems: Integrated Primary Health Care Governance in Nigeria". *BMC Health Services Research*, 17 (1): 227. https://doi.org/10.1186/s12913-017-2179-2
Eboreime, E. A., Olawepo, J. O., Banke-Thomas, A., Abejirinde, I.-O. O. and Abimbola, S. (2020). "Appraising and Addressing Design and Implementation Failure in Global Health: A Pragmatic Framework". *Global Public Health*, 16 (7): 1122–1130. https://doi.org/10.1080/17441692.2020.1814379
Fixsen, D. L., Blase, K. A., Naoom, S. F. and Wallace, F. (2009). "Core Implementation Components". *Research on Social Work Practice*, 19 (5): 531–540. https://doi.org/10.1177/1049731509335549

Graham, W. J., Filippi, V. G. A. and Ronsmans, C. (1996). "Demonstrating Programme Impact on Maternal Mortality". *Health Policy and Planning*, 11 (1): 16–20. https://doi.org/10.1093/HEAPOL/11.1.16

Ibeh, N. (2015). "How Nigerian Govt Ruins Midwives Scheme, Fails to Fight Maternal Deaths", Premium Times, 27 April. Available at: https://www.premiumtimesng.com/news/headlines/182131-how-nigerian-govt-ruins-midwives-scheme-fails-to-fight-maternal-deaths.html (Accessed: 1 November 2020).

Johnson, D. (2020). "Healthcare: The Slow Start in Ondo", Vanguard Newspaper, 31 May. Available at: https://www.vanguardngr.com/2020/05/healthcare-the-slow-start-in-ondo (Accessed: 1 November 2020).

Kruk, M. E., Mbaruku, G., McCord, C. W., Moran, M., Rockers, P. C. and Galea, S. (2009). "Bypassing Primary Care Facilities for Childbirth: A Population-Based Study in Rural Tanzania". *Health Policy and Planning*, 24 (4): 279–288. https://doi.org/10.1093/heapol/czp011

Mimiko, O., Nair, D., Mai, M. M. and Cooke, J. (2013). "Maternal Health in Nigeria: Progress is Possible". Available at: https://s3-eu-west-1.amazonaws.com/s3.sourceafrica.net/documents/120327/Expanding-the-Abiye-Model.pdf (Accessed 1: November 2021).

Nilsen, P. (2015). "Making Sense of Implementation Theories, Models and Frameworks". *Implementation Science*, 10: 53. https://doi.org/10.1186/S13012-015-0242-0

Nyamtema, A. S., Urassa, D. P., and Roosmalen, J. van. (2011). "Maternal Health Interventions in Resource Limited Countries: A Systematic Review of Packages, Impacts and Factors for Change". *BMC Pregnancy and Childbirth*, 11: 30. https://doi.org/10.1186/1471-2393-11-30

ODCHC. (2019). "Akeredolu Flags-off Abiyamo Maternal and Child Health Insurance Scheme", Health Insurance Scheme. Available at: https://odchc.on.gov.ng/akeredolu-flags-off-abiyamo-maternal-and-child-health-insurance-scheme/ (Accessed: 1 November 2020)

Okeke, E. N., Glick, P., Abubakar, I., Chari, A., Pitchforth, E. et al. (2015). *The Better Obstetrics in Rural Nigeria (BORN) Study: An Impact Evaluation of the Nigerian Midwives Service Scheme*. Rand Corporation. Santa Monica, Calif.: RAND Corporation, RR-1215-3ie, 2015. https://www.rand.org/pubs/research_reports/RR1215.html

Okpani, A. I. and Abimbola, S. (2016). "The Midwives Service Scheme: A Qualitative Comparison of Contextual Determinants of the Performance of Two States in Central Nigeria". *Global Health Research and Policy*, 1: 16. https://doi.org/10.1186/s41256-016-0017-4

Oyeyemi, S. O. and Wynn, R. (2014). "Giving Cell Phones to Pregnant Women and Improving Services May Increase Primary Health Facility Utilization: A Case–Control Study of a Nigerian Project". *Reproductive Health,* 11 (1): 1–8. https://doi.org/10.1186/1742-4755-11-8

United Nations. (2016). "Sustainable Development Goals: 17 Goals to Transform Our World". Available at: http://www.un.org/sustainabledevelopment/sustainable-development-goals/ (Accessed: 1 December 2022).

World Health Organization. (2006). "Working Together for Health: The 2006 World Health Report". Available at: https://www.who.int/whr/2006/whr06_en.pdf (Accessed: 1 November 2022).

9

SOCIAL ENTREPRENEURSHIP AND SOCIAL INNOVATION IN GLOBAL PUBLIC HEALTH PRACTICE

Charles Oham, Maurice Ekwugha and Gladius Kulothungan

Introduction

The values and principles of privately owned enterprises are perceived as more efficient in the delivery of public services. These results of social enterprises, and not-for-profit organisations, are often overlooked globally (Durkin and Oham, 2016; Kay et al., 2016; Macaulay et al., 2018). Yet, not-for-profit organisations, such as social enterprises, can improve the scale and effectiveness of public health interventions. Their value lays in the ability to be independent, innovative, flexible, and responsive (Dees, 2007; Department of Health, 2008), leading to systemic change, that addresses public health challenges. This chapter will define social entrepreneurship and enterprise and proceed to discuss the role of social entrepreneurship in global public health.

Social Entrepreneurs and Social Enterprise

A social entrepreneur is an individual who uses entrepreneurial principles, such as earned income strategies, to effect social change, because of a government, market, or societal failure (Boschee, 2006; Mair, 2010; Baggot, 2013). Governmental failure occurs when governments fail to provide the basic goods and services for their people, for example, hospitals. Market failure arises when businesses focus on profit at the expense of their social and ethical responsibility, for instance, oil companies polluting the environment in the Niger Delta area of Nigeria. Societal failure occurs when people ignore their basic responsibilities and accept as a norm, injustices, biases, and traditions, which deny others their rights, e.g., stigmatisation of children with special needs in Africa. Social entrepreneurs create hybrid organisations, that enable them to combine a plurality of social actions and economic principles, and form collective and democratic organisations,

DOI: 10.4324/9781003128373-9

aimed at producing positive effects on social outcomes (Kulothungan, 2010). Possessing an entrepreneurial and innovative orientation, social entrepreneurs, and social enterprises address a particular social need (e.g., health inequalities) to create social value (benefits to the community), which leads to social impact, and improved health outcomes (Beugre, 2017).

Social enterprises are, therefore, the vehicles which social entrepreneurs use to deliver social outcomes, through 'trading activity' centres. Trading activity, or an earned income strategy, is a critical function of social entrepreneurship, and this distinguishes it from charities and not-for-profit organisations, who rely mostly on donations (Boschee, 2006). The term 'trading' is broad and could mean retail, merchandising, wholesale, business-to-business trading, contracting, or commissioning from buyers, such as governments and institutions like the World Health Organization (WHO). For example, Bromley Healthcare in the UK is a social enterprise, commissioned by the Bromley Clinical Commissioning Group (CCG) to provide health and social care services to the population of Bromley in Southeast London. In the UK, the CCGs are responsible for health budgets at a local level and fund General Practitioners (GPs) and health providers to deliver health services to the community. Social enterprises include a spectrum of trading organisations, such as cooperative societies, charities involved in trading activity, civic enterprises, established by local government, credit unions, and microcredit organisations, and not-for-profit health and social care organisations (Galera and Borzaga, 2009).

Social enterprises and social entrepreneurs employ business models to address persistent social problems, such as social exclusion, health inequalities, environmental issues, injustice, and poverty (Hayday, 2016; Konsti-Laakso et al., 2016). As a result, social entrepreneurs and enterprises can add value to solving global public health challenges. In India, 'Glocal' has built ten fully functional, 100-bed multi-speciality hospitals in several states and initiated 250 digital dispensaries, which provide video consultations, examinations, investigations, and automated medicine dispensing. During the second wave of COVID-19 in 2021, Glocal launched a free telemedicine consultation for COVID-19 screenings (World Economic Forum, 2021).

Furthermore, the characteristics of social entrepreneurs and enterprises are grounded within 'Entrepreneurship' theory, covering three domains, namely, finding new products and services to satisfy needs (innovation), creating organisations using available resources (e.g., abundance of cocoa trees in Ghana), and creating wealth by adding value, e.g., creating employment (Mellor, 2009). Schumpeter (1950; 1954) noted that entrepreneurs actively create opportunity using innovative combinations, which often included creative destruction of passive or lethargic economic markets, making the entrepreneur, a lynchpin of economic development.

A subset of social enterprise, increasingly recognised, is 'faith-based' social enterprises. They are organisations initiated and run by faith institutions such as churches, synagogues, temples, and mosques, or their adherents (Dinham, 2007;

Oham, 2013). 'First Fruit Group', based in East London, UK, is a faith-based social enterprise, that provides refuge for women affected by domestic violence (Oham and Massa, 2022). In the USA, several types of faith-based organisations exist, providing a range of services, including public health interventions. However, these organisations are less understood and face a range of challenges, such as a lack of support. A study found that religious organisations providing microfinance (a form of social enterprise) to alleviate poverty had difficulties in obtaining funding (Zhao and Lounsbury, 2016). A lack of funding and support can impact the work of faith-based social enterprises. However, faith-based social enterprises present a plethora of opportunities for systemic change in global public health interventions, due to their ability to reach wide audiences. An exemplar of faith-based organisations operating in a social entrepreneurial and innovative way in Biafra (1967-1970) was 'Joint Church Aid', with a network of over 2,000 feeding centres. As a result, millions of people, especially children, were saved from starvation during the war (Oham, 2013).

Another form of social enterprise is 'Fair-Trade' organisations. They act as hybrids, comprising a strategy of generating revenue from trading activity, and the social advancement of farmers, as a social objective (Doherty et al., 2014). One example of a fair-trade organisation is 'Kuapa Kokoo Farmers' Cooperative', based in Ghana, and major shareholders of 'Devine Chocolate Ltd.' in the UK. They are a fair-trade farmers' cooperative that started in 1993 and supplies over 1,000 tons of cocoa to the European Union each year (Devine Chocolate, 2021). The profits realised from obtaining a higher premium for their cocoa beans have been used to provide public healthcare services that support the comprehensive healthcare delivery of their farmers. Clinic attendance stands at 3,293 registered attendants and there have been over 23,000 visits since its establishment. Kuapa Kokoo has also established a health insurance scheme for farmers to access health services in any government facility. Other programmes operated include the building and running of schools, Agro-Forestry, TeleAgric, campaigns against child labour, gender-based violence, and labour rights (Kuapa Kokoo, 2022).

Social entrepreneurship is situated within the broader theoretical context of the 'Political Economy Approach', with significant affiliations to 'Critical Public Health'. The concern is with issues of equity and social justice and challenges neoliberal and classical approaches to understanding health and the economy. As was mentioned in Chapter 4, political economists are critical of asymmetric power relations (such as between business owners and workers, landowner, and tenants) and seek alternatives to the current structures of capitalism, and resource distribution, to achieve more equitable economic and health outcomes (Doyal and Pennel, 1979; Karl; 2012; Birn et al., 2017). Social entrepreneurship is part of a tradition, which seeks to understand how value is produced and distributed, which processes impel the worth of a good or service, and who benefits from the production of value, and produce alternatives, where these processes produce inequality. Similarly, Galloway et al. (2015) argue, from a Feminist perspective, that normative constructs of entrepreneurialism and leadership are currently framed within masculinised discourses and frameworks, which valorise men, and masculinity only. Women's contributions to leadership and enterprise are often overlooked, and new Feminist frameworks, beyond classical approaches, are required to understand how the latter are often gendered, and the contributions women can make to economic life and entrepreneurship.

Social entrepreneurship and social enterprise continue the 'assets-based approach', deeply ingrained within the Political Economy and Critical Public Health theoretical frameworks. The assets-based approach to health and wellbeing seeks to empower communities to address the social determinants of health, which produce inequalities (Roy, 2017). It provides a framework to assist communities to drive economic and health development processes, through identifying and mobilising existing, and often unrecognised, assets, and in the process, produce more local economic opportunities, to drive community development (Roy, 2017). Its focus is upon challenge existing structures of enterprise and capitalism, and production of social value (Young, 2006).

Social Entrepreneurship and Social Innovation in Public Health

An assets-based approach requires that social innovation creates social value from innovative ideas, applications, and combinations of existing circumstances and resources (Young, 2006). Social innovation, which is the development of new ideas that work in solving problems, was found to have a close link with social entrepreneurship. When innovation, for example, the introduction of novel products and services, is used for social purposes, like improving the health and wellbeing of a population, it is classified as social innovation. Resource limitations can act as a push for social enterprises to be highly innovative and precipitate sustainability (Oham and Okeke, 2022). Social entrepreneurial philosophy proceeds beyond profit-making to innovation and resilience when challenges occur. 'Sustainable Health Enterprises' (SHE), based in Rwanda and East Africa, are involved in working with schools and stakeholders to address 'period' poverty amongst schoolgirls, who are unable to afford or access sanitary pads. Innovatively, SHE have also developed the use of banana tree fibres to manufacture high-quality sanitary pads (Beugre, 2017).

The contribution of social entrepreneurship to change, or strategic management initiatives, occurs when social entrepreneurs introduce, through social innovation, new management practices, new technologies, or new ways of labelling, or describing a problem ('rhetorical innovation') to arrive at a solution (Hartley, 2005). 'Wellbeing Enterprises CIC' is a UK public health social enterprise, working with GPs to provide person and community-centred health approaches, e.g., social prescribing, which recommends social activities for patients experiencing loneliness and isolation to address mental health and wellbeing challenges.

Social entrepreneurs use social innovation to develop simple and effective tools to address global public health challenges. 'One World Institute' is a social enterprise that is transforming global public health through innovation, funding new trials, and repurposing old medicines and vaccines, especially those relating to diseases of low- and middle-income countries (Beugre, 2017). These cases demonstrate the need for policy development and action, which includes all stakeholders (social enterprises) during strategic planning of public health programmes, leading to cost savings by leveraging existing resources, and strengthening the assets-based approach (Stewart and Cornish, 2009).

Human and Social Capital Development in Public Health Social Enterprises

Although a social entrepreneur's passion and desire for social change are high, gaps could exist in their skill sets. Regular auditing of skills, and the capacity of the social entrepreneur to carry out requisite roles and responsibilities, ensures that the social enterprise fulfils its mission. This is important because some social enterprises may not invariably operate efficiently in meeting objectives, due to a lack of competence (Royce, 2007; 2009). The acquisition of leadership, managerial, team building, and financial skills will improve performance (Peattie and Morley, 2008). The capability approach is one method, which is applied to improve social enterprise capabilities, focusing primarily on human development (Wongtschowski, 2015). Research on social enterprises by Martin and Novicei (2010) ascertained that the success of programmes may be attributed in part to individual and group cultural learning and the appropriateness of the 'servant leader' approach (a goal to serve others on the team). It suggests that leadership development assumes a salient position in social entrepreneurship growth and impact.

'Social capital' refers to the trust, bonds, and social networks, built up within a community and which encourage reciprocal behaviours, links between community groups, and community resilience (Oham et al., 2009). Social capital is a key resource, used by community health practitioners, to deliver on health promotion initiatives to marginalised groups. It has enabled practitioners to mobilise local communities, generate bottom-up activism against unfair policies, e.g., the 'Treatment Action Campaign' that emerged in South Africa, when millions of people were dying from AIDs, because of a lack of access to life-saving drugs (Campbell, 2020).

Social entrepreneurs consider social capital as a critical part of their input when initiating programmes and are integral to the assets-based approach within Political Economy and Critical Public Health theories. In 2001, 'Schwab Foundation for Social Entrepreneurship' established the 'Global Exchange for Social Investment' (GEXSI) to render the global social capital market more efficient and transparent. The idea for a social capital market was to accumulate and combine social capital with other forms of capital platforms, such as economic capital, so that social entrepreneurs, with replicable projects, can obtain the financial and in-kind support, required to scale up their projects and create systemic change.

Examples of systemic change include micro-credit lending to the world's poor from Bangladesh to Africa, enabling those on low incomes, to improve their standard of living. Replicating innovative ideas in low- to middle-income countries requires a range of capital (social, economic, symbolic, cultural, spiritual, and human). The 'Global Steering Group for Impact' (GSG) is an organisation with a mission to stimulate impact investing and entrepreneurship to benefit people across the globe. They aim to encourage investors to consider the environmental impact of their investment on societies, rather than a sole focus on profits. They have currently initiated national advisory boards in 33 countries to encourage impact investing, which addresses, for instance, climate change and poverty, both significant global public health challenges.

Effective monitoring and evaluation models are required to capture all types of benefits from public health social enterprises, to demonstrate social impact, and value for money, and resource use to stakeholders. 'Social impact' is defined as beneficiary outcomes from prosocial behaviour, which are enjoyed by intended targets of that behaviour within the community, and across organisations and environments (Rawhouser et al., 2019). The concept is an evolution in measuring performance in the non-profit sector, a critical tool which social entrepreneurs use to capture broader and longer-term outcomes (Oham and Okeke, 2022). Tools which can be used for monitoring and evaluations include the 'Theory of Change' and 'Social Return on Investment', enabling the social entrepreneur to measure social impact, and explain it to stakeholders. Social entrepreneurs must be strategic and intentional, possessing or outsourcing relevant monitoring and evaluation skills and tools, which capture extensive data on interventions. This is because stakeholders require this information to formulate policy and funding decisions. Stakeholders include health commissioning institutions, governments, user-led groups, the community, and philanthropic organisations, e.g., the Bill and Melinda Gates Foundation.

Further Research Opportunities

Social entrepreneurship is a growing area of study (Granados et al., 2011). Nonetheless, there is still a significant gap in knowledge of how, and to what extent, such activities can impact the social determinants of health, particularly concerning health-enhancing mechanisms and causal pathways (Macaulay et al., 2018). Further research is needed to understand the impact of social enterprises on long-term public health outcomes (Roy et al., 2014). Several systematic reviews, albeit with limited evidence, point to social enterprise activity impacting positively on mental health, self-reliance/esteem, health behaviours, reducing stigma, constructing social capital, and enhancing the health and wellbeing of a community (Roy et al., 2017). For example, 'Park Dale Green Thumb Enterprises' in Ontario, Canada, is a social enterprise, employing people with significant mental health challenges, to design green spaces, and provide horticultural services for clients (Roy et al., 2017). However, there is a need for more empirical research-based evidence upon the impact of social entrepreneurship on global public health, located within the traditions of Critical Public Health. Moreover, social enterprises, in turn, need access to public health and wellbeing research, which is essential to developing socially innovative solutions, based around lifestyle and health-related behaviour change (Macke et al., 2018; La Placa and Oham, 2019).

Conclusion

This chapter defined and discussed the roles of social enterprise and provided evidence on how they create social value, through social innovation and entrepreneurship to meet global public health agendas. It pointed to the need for policy development that engages with, and enables, social enterprises to become mainstream within global public health. This is because entrepreneurialism and social innovation, which foster solutions to health inequalities and health inequities, are key values of social entrepreneurship, and the Critical Public Health approach.

Reflective Questions and Further Research

With reference to the discussions in this chapter, begin to reflect upon the following:

1   What benefits can social enterprises bring to global public health?
2   What policy actions can health commissioners take to partner with social enterprises in addressing health inequalities and inequities?
3   How can public health practitioners in low- to middle-income countries actively engage in social entrepreneurship?

Further Reading

Oham C. A. and Okeke O. J. (2022) "Strategic Formulation and Implementation of Social Entrepreneurs". In C. A. Oham (ed.) *Cases of Survival and Sustainability Strategies of Social Entrepreneurs*. Hershey, PA: IGI Publishers.

Oham C. and Macdonald D. (2016) *Leading and Managing a Social Enterprise in Health and Social Care*. London: Community Training Partners.

Wei-Skillern, J., Austin, J. E., Leonard, H. and Stevenson, H. (2007). *Entrepreneurship in the Social Sector*. London: Sage.

Websites

Institute for Social Entrepreneurs: Www.socialent.org
Mercy Project Ghana: https://mercyproject.net/
One World: https://www.path.org
SHE Enterprises: https://sheinnovates.com/
Wellbeing Enterprises CIC: www.wellbeingenterprises.org.uk/

References

Baggot, R. (2013). *Partnership for Public Health and Well-being: Policy and Practice.* London: Palgrave Macmillan.

Beugre, C. (2017). *Social Entrepreneurship, Managing the Creation of Social Value.* New York: Routledge.

Birn, A. E., Pillay, Y. and Holtz, T. H. (2017). *Textbook of Global Health.* Oxford: Oxford University Press.

Boschee, J. (2006). "Social Entrepreneurship: The Promise and the Perils". In A. Nicholls (ed.) *Social Entrepreneurship: New Models of Sustainable Social Change.* Oxford: Oxford University Press, 356-391.

Campbell, C. (2020). "Social Capital, Social Movements and Global Public Health: Fighting for Health-Enabling Contexts in Marginalised Settings". *Social Science and Medicine,* 257: 112153. https://doi.org/10.1016/j.socscimed.2019.02.004

Dees, J. (2007). "Taking Social Entrepreneurship Seriously". *Transaction Social Science and Modern Society,* 44 (3): 24-31.

Department of Health. (2008). *Social Enterprise, Making a Difference: A Guide to the Right to Request.* London: The Stationery Office.

Devine Chocolate. (2021). "The Beginnings and Structure of Kuapa Kokoo | Blog - Divine Chocolate". Available at: http://www.Devinechocolate.com/devineworld (Accessed: 17 November 2021).

Dinham, A. (2007). "Faiths and Frontiers on the Starship: Boldly Going as Faith-Based Entrepreneurs?" Faith Based Regeneration Network. Available at: http://www.fbrn. org.uk/files/*STARSHIP*.pdf (Accessed: 16 March 2016).

Doherty, B., Huagh, H. and Lyon, F. (2014). "Social Enterprises as Hybrid Organisations: A Review and Research Agenda". *International Journal of Management Review,* 16: 417-436.

Doyal, L. and Pennel, I. (1979). *The Political Economy of Health.* London: Pluto Press.

Durkin, C. and Oham, C. (2016). "Social Innovation Management and Capital Literacy". In. C. Oham and D. MacDonald (eds.) *Leading and Managing a Social Enterprise in Health and Social Care.* London: Community Training Partners, 89-111.

Galloway, L., Kapasi, I. and Sang, K. (2015). "Entrepreneurship, Leadership, and the Value of Feminist Approaches to Understanding Them". *Journal of Small Business Management,* 53 (3): 683–692. https://doi.org/10.1111/jsbm.12178

Galera, G. and Borzaga, C. (2009). "Social Enterprise: An International Overview of its Conceptual Evolution and Legal Implementation". *Social Enterprise Journal,* 5 (3): 210-228. https://doi.org/10.1108/17508610911004313

Granados, M. L., Hlupic, V., Coakes, E. and Mohamed, S. (2011). "Social Enterprise and Social Entrepreneurship Research and Theory: A Bibliometric Analysis". *Social Enterprise Journal,* 7 (3): 198-218.

Hartley, J. (2005). "Innovation in Governance and Public Services: Past and Present". *Public Money and Management,* 25 (1): 27-34. https://doi.org/10.1111/j.1467-9302.2005.00447.x

Hayday, M. (2016). "Managing Trends in Finance and Social Finance for Social Enterprise". In. C. Oham and D. Macdonald (eds.) *Leading and Managing a Social Enterprise in Health and Social Care.* London: Community Training Partners, 233-253.

Karl, M. (2012). *A Critical Analysis of Capitalist Production.* Hertfordshire: Wordsworth.

Kay, A., Roy, M. J. and Donaldson C. (2016). "Re-Imagining Social Enterprise". *Social Enterprise Journal,* 12 (2): 217-234. https://doi.org/10.1108/SEJ-05-2016-0018

Konsti-Laakso, S., Koskela, V., Martikainen, S. J., Melkas H. and Mellanen, L. (2016). "Participatory Design of a Social Enterprise for Rehabilitees." *Work,* 55 (1): 145-153. https://doi.org/10.3233/WOR-162383. PMID: 27612064

Kuapa Kokoo. (2022). "Healthcare Services". Available at: https://kuapakokoo.com/programmes/health (Accessed: 19 January 2022).

Kulothungan, G. (2010). "What Do We Mean By 'Social Enterprise'? Defining Social Entrepreneurship". In. R. Gunn and C. Durkin (ed.) *Social Entrepreneurship: A Skills Approach*. Bristol: Policy Press, 23-33.

La Placa, V. and Oham, C. (2019). "Loneliness and Young People Experiencing Mental Health Difficulties: Evidence and Further Research". *PEOPLE: International Journal of Social Sciences*, 5 (2): 1024-1039. https://doi.org/10.20319/pijss.2019.52.10241039

Macaulay, B., Roy, M. J., Donaldson, C., Teasdale, S. and Kay, A. (2018). "Conceptualizing the Health and Well-Being Impacts of Social Enterprise: A UK-Based Study". *Health Promotion International*, 33 (5): 748-759. https://doi.org/10.1093/heapro/dax009

Macke, J., Sarate, J. A. R., Domeneghini, J. and Silva, K. A. (2018). "Where Do We Go From Now? Research Framework for Social Entrepreneurship". *Journal of Cleaner Production*, 183: 677-685. https://doi.org/10.1016/j.jclepro.2018.02.017

Mair, J. (2010). "Social Entrepreneurship: Taking Stock and Looking Ahead". In. A. Fayolle and H. Matlay (eds.) *Handbook of Research on Social Entrepreneurship*. Cheltenham: Edward Edgar Publishing, 15-29.

Martin, J. S. and Novicevic, M. (2010). "Social Entrepreneurship Among Kenyan Farmers: A Case Example of Acculturation Challenges and Program Successes". *International Journal of Intercultural Relations,* 34: 482-492. https://doi.org/10.1016/j.ijintrel.2010.05.007

Mellor, R. B. (2009). "The Economics of Entrepreneurship and Innovation". In. R. B. Mellor, G. Coulton, A. Chick, A. Bifulco, N. Mellor et al. (eds.) *Entrepreneurship for Everyone: A Student Textbook*. London: Sage, 18-31.

Oham, C., Stewart, J. and Cornish, Y. (2009). "Social Capital Social Enterprise and Community Development". In J. Stewart and Y. Cornish (eds.) *Professional Practice in Public Health*. Devon: Reflect Press, 191-206.

Oham, C. (2013). "Could there be Treasures in Our Faith? The Recognition and Utilisation of Spiritual Capital Values". In. D. Singleton (ed.) *Faith With Its Sleeves Rolled Up*. London: Faith Action.

Oham, C. A. and Massa, N. (2022). "Entrepreneurial Parenting Through Spiritual Capital: A Case Study on First Fruit Group Social Enterprise", IGI Global, Publisher of Timely Knowledge. Available at: https://www.igi-global.com/teaching-case/entrepreneurial-parenting-through-spiritual-capital/296028 (Accessed: 21 January 2022).

Oham C. A. and Okeke O. J. P. (2022). "Strategic Formulation and Implementation of Social Entrepreneurs". IGI Global, Publisher of Timely Knowledge. Available at: https://www.igi-global.com/teaching-case/strategic-formulation-and-implementation-of-social-entrepreneurs/296022 (Accessed: 21 January 2022).

Oham C. and Macdonald D. (2016) *Leading and Managing a Social Enterprise in Health and Social Care*. London: Community Training Partners.

Peattie, K. and Morley, A. S. (2008). *Social Enterprises: Diversity and Dynamics, Contexts and Contributions. (Discussion Paper)*. Cardiff: BRASS/ESRC/Social Enterprise Coalition.

Rawhouser, H., Cummings, M. and Newbert, S. L. (2019). "Social Impact Measurement: Current Approaches and Future Directions for Social Entrepreneurship Research". *Entrepreneurship Theory and Practice*, 43 (1): 82–115. https://doi.org/10.1177/1042258717727718

Roy, M. J., Donaldson, C., Baker, R. and Kerr S. (2014). "The Potential of Social Enterprise to Enhance Health and Well-Being: A Model and Systematic Review". *Social Science and Medicine*, 123: 182–193. https://doi.org/10.1016/j.socscimed.2014.07.031

Roy, M. J. (2017) "The Assets-Based Approach: Furthering a Neoliberal Agenda or Rediscovering the Old Public Health? A Critical Examination of Practitioner Discourses". *Critical Public Health*, 27 (4): 455–464. https://doi.org/10.1080/09581596.2016.1249826

Roy, M. J., Lysaght, R. and Krupa, T. M. (2017). "Action on the Social Determinants of Health Through Social Enterprise". *Canadian Medical Association Journal*, 189 (11): E440–E441. https://doi.org/10.1503/cmaj.160864

Royce, M. (2007). "Using Human Resource Management Tools to Support Social Enterprise: Emerging Themes from the Sector". *Social Enterprise Journal*, 3 (1): 10–19. https://doi.org/10.1108/17508610780000718

Royce, M. (2009) *Management for Social Enterprise*. London: Sage.

Schumpeter, J. A. (1950). *Capitalism, Socialism and Democracy, 3rd edn*. London: Allen and Unwin.

Schumpeter, J. A. (1954). *History of Economic Analysis*. New York: Oxford University Press.

Stewart, J. and Cornish, Y. (2009). *Professional Practice in Public Health*. Devon: Reflect Press.

Wongtschowski, A. (2015). *Social Enterprise Capabilities and Human Development DPU Working Paper No.174, Special Issue on Capability Approach in Development Planning and Urban Design*. London: Development Planning Unit/The Bartlett/University College London.

World Economic Forum. (2021). "6 Ways Social Entrepreneurs are Saving Lives During India's Covid-19 Crisis", 4 May 2021. Available at: https://www.weforum.org/agenda/2021/05/6-ways-social-entrepreneurs-are-saving-lives-in-india/ (Accessed: 18 January 2022).

Young, R. (2006). "For What It's Worth: Social Value and the Future of Social Entrepreneurship". In. A. Nicholls (ed.) *Social Entrepreneurship: New Models of Sustainable Social Change*. Oxford: Oxford University Press, 56–74.

Zhao, E. Y. and Lounsbury, M. (2016). "An Institutional Logics Approach to Social Entrepreneurship: Market Logic, Religious Diversity and Resource Acquisition by Microfinance Organizations". *Journal of Business Venturing*, 31: 643–662. https://doi.org/10.1016/j.jbusvent.2016.09.001

10

PLANETARY HEALTH AND THE ANTHROPOCENE

Stefi Barna, Sonali Sathaye and Vanita Gandhi

Introduction

Human societies exist in an ecological context upon which they are dependent on air, water, food, and health. In this chapter, we describe a framework for identifying types of environmental degradation, called the 'planetary boundaries', and their effects on human health. We then examine the causes of the degradation, from European colonialism to the industrial revolution and global capitalism. We also consider ways to safeguard the health of people, and of the planet simultaneously, from the United Nations Sustainable Development Goals (SDGs), to the re-framing of global public health as 'planetary' health. Finally, we describe an example of a grassroots initiative to ensure basic needs within ecological limits.

The Climate and Ecological Emergency

Agricultural human settlements emerged after the last glacial ice age, about 11,700 years ago, and developed because of predictable environmental conditions (Wiedmann et al., 2020). The stable climate and the abundant biodiversity of what is called the 'Holocene' (or 'present') epoch enabled urban settlements to increase across the world. Over time, ideas of health and illness, and practices of care and healing, came to assume relatively unchanging climatic and ecological cycles, and eventually to regard the individual human body, as the locus of health and illness, disregarding the role of the social and environmental determinants of health. Over the last few decades, it has become apparent that an industrialised and technologically complex, global society serves the interests of a small minority by over-extracting natural resources (Weinzettel et al., 2013; Wiedmann et al., 2020). Far from enabling the distribution of technological and

DOI: 10.4324/9781003128373-10

financial resources across the human population equally, the pursuit of economic development, separate from natural systems, has instead served to vitiate the resources, essential to the survival of humans, such as water, air, and food. Since 1980, global greenhouse gas emissions have doubled, and human activity has removed over half of the wild birds, mammals, fish, invertebrates, and insects on the planet (Grooten and Almond, 2018). Global consumption of materials and energy has increased dramatically, even during a time, when industrial production has been slowed by the COVID-19 pandemic (Dhara and Singh, 2021). The cutting, dredging, and in-filling of land for agriculture, the loading of soils with chemical fertilisers, the re-purposing of air, water, and land, as part of industrial practices, and the killing of biologically diverse organisms have driven exponential increases in non-communicable diseases, infectious, and vector-borne diseases, and malnutrition (Donohoe, 2003). Just as devastating, have been the psychological effects of injury, trauma, and displacement, which emerge in the wake of extreme weather events, climate-related migration, and conflict over access to natural resources, such as water, land, or oil.

A growing body of scientific evidence, called the 'planetary boundaries framework' (Rockström et al., 2009), identifies and quantifies the effects of human activities on the earth system processes, which are essential for the sustenance of human life. A planetary boundary is a limit to how much the Earth system can be disturbed, without proceeding into a new state, which would be unsafe for human societies. Staying within each of the nine earth-system boundaries provides human societies with a 'safe space' for functioning.

The nine planetary boundaries are (1) climate change, (2) ocean acidification, (3) stratospheric ozone depletion, (4) nitrogen and phosphorous cycle, (5) global freshwater, (6) land system change, (7) biodiversity loss, (8) atmospheric aerosol loading, and (9) chemical pollution. Alarmingly, four of these boundaries have already been transgressed. These are land-use change (the conversion of forest, grassland, wetland, and other ecosystems to agriculture), biodiversity loss (the collapse in the number and variety of species), nitrogen pollution (from chemical fertilisers and industrial waste), and climate change (the warming of the Earth caused by greenhouse gases from human activities). With regards to climate change especially, extreme weather events, such as storms, floods, droughts, and fires, lead to food and water shortages and the higher food costs, set the stage for malnutrition, homelessness, and the disruption of education, employment, and health services (Romanello et al., 2021). Extreme weather events can cause mental health challenges, such as post-traumatic stress disorder (PTSD). One in six people met the diagnostic criteria for PTSD in areas affected by Hurricane Katrina (Lowe et al., 2013), and 15.6% of a community affected by extreme bushfires had symptoms of PTSD several years after their experience (Bryant et al., 2014). There are also associations between extreme heat and violence (Cane et al., 2014), and even extreme heat and antibiotic resistance (MacFadden et al., 2018).

Burning fossil fuels also increases particulate matter air pollution and ground-level ozone (a key component of smog), which is associated with diminished lung function, increased hospital admissions, and emergency room visits for asthma, as well as increases in premature death and low birth weight or pre-term birth (Health Effects Institute, 2020), diabetes, dementia, and mental illness (Padhy et al., 2015). Coal combustion also produces mercury, a potent neurotoxin, which can affect cognitive ability, and motor function in the developing foetus (Wiedmann et al., 2020). Worldwide, climate-sensitive infections, such as dengue and malaria, are rising, due to spread of vectors, such as mosquitoes, beyond their original habitat (Thu et al., 1998). Finally, as climate refugees grow in number, mass migrations will affect social and demographic configurations and health services (Abubakar et al., 2018). This alarming list of the health effects of breaching the climate boundary continues to grow as new connections and feedback loops are discovered.

Colonisation, Industrialisation, and Globalisation

Who gets to consume what, how much, for how long, and at what cost? These are questions of history, of global and societal hierarchies, and of the power to determine what is fair. The overconsumption of natural resources, and the emphasis on financial profit, regardless of need or consequence, has been made possible by histories of inequity, fuelled by technological innovation. The Sixteenth-Century colonisation of the Americas gave birth to plantation economies and global trade, enabled by the enslavement of African people and the homogenisation of agriculture in the colonies of the Americas (Tsing, 2015; Moore, 2017). The industrial revolution of the Eighteenth Century drastically altered the cycles of resource extraction and consumption (McGregor et al., 2016), and the colonisation of Asia provided new materials and labour for the factories of the colonisers. Beliefs justifying the superiority of some humans over others, and of humans over animals, justified the exploitation of the planet's natural systems and paved the way for economic growth beyond limits (Lewis and Maslin, 2018). In other words, while environmental change accelerated after 1850, and even more so after 1945, the change was enabled by the patterns of power, profit, and production, established four centuries earlier (Moore, 2017).

The global ecological crisis has its roots in, and perpetuates, ecological and social injustice. It disproportionately impacts the most vulnerable groups in society (Thomas et al., 2019) and is therefore inextricable from struggles for human rights and equity. It is now understood that the climate and ecological emergencies cannot be solved without addressing the underlying economic system that produced them (Bullard, 2001). Geologists assert that there is now evidence of human activity in the geological record itself, from the radioactive isotopes of nuclear explosions to the layers of plastic and concrete, which now cover most parts of the Earth, and the sheer volume of domestic chicken bones buried near human settlements (Bennett et al., 2018). They suggest a new term for this epoch, 'the Anthropocene', from the Greek word 'anthropo' for human and 'cene' for new (Crutzen and Stoermer, 2000). Whilst the term Anthropocene helpfully identifies what has occurred, it does not explain the how: in other words, the change is not due to the behaviour of a species, but rather to a system in which the benefits and harms of extraction and development are not equally distributed. In this view, the term 'Capitalocene' is more apt than the term 'Anthropocene' (Moore, 2017).

From a social sciences perspective, such understandings of the role of social and economic systems, and their ecological impact, link to the theory of 'social suffering' within Critical Public perspectives. Social suffering focuses upon how, for instance, human consequences of war, poverty, inequality, and disease are often the result of a holistic assemblage of human problems and suffering, and which result from what political, economic, and institutional power imposes upon people (as well as the human responses to social problems as they are influenced by those forms of power) (Kleinman et al., 1997). Renault (2010) argues that social suffering theory is integral to any analyses of power and social injustice, and challenges disciplinary boundaries, traditionally established to demarcate individual and social phenomena. Combining health and social problems breaks down the boundaries between them and accentuates the interrelatedness of health and social factors. 'Structural violence', for example, is a type of social suffering which occurs due to social and institutional structures, such as racism, Patriarchy, and poverty, and which limits human agency and experience. Readers can refer to Chapter 12 for a more detailed focus on structural violence. The chapter now proceeds to a focus on the UN SDGs, which like Critical Public Health perspectives focuses on reductions in health inequalities and social inclusion.

The UN Sustainable Development Goals

The United Nations' Agenda for Sustainable Development (2015) was triumphantly adopted by all United Nations member states, with a blueprint for ending poverty and reducing inequality, whilst simultaneously addressing the climate crisis, and restoring degraded oceans and forests. Whereas the eight Millennium Development Goals (2000–2015) had applied only to low- and middle-income countries, the SDG's 17 goals were applied to all UN member states. This was a recognition that while countries of the global North might enjoy a higher Gross Domestic Product (GDP) per capita, they also embodied grotesque social and economic inequalities, with many of their citizens unable to meet their basic needs with dignity and opportunity. The SDGs draw on the definition of sustainability developed by the UN Brundtland Commission (1987), which emphasised that sustainable development meets the needs of the present, without compromising the ability of future generations to meet their own needs. They aim to balance economic growth, social inclusion, and environmental protection.

The SGDs have been criticised on conceptual and practical grounds. First, the breadth of the 17 goals and 169 targets were produced by inherently political processes; in other words, they were negotiated by a wide range of state, private sector, and not-for-profit stakeholders, and this renders them contradictory at times. For example, it has been argued that on a planet, which is reaching its resource limits, the aim of economic growth will never bring about environmental sustainability (Hickel, 2019).

To address this, some have argued that high-income countries, as the greatest contributors to the problem, should now focus on environmental protection policies, while low- and middle-income countries focus on socio-economic policies in the short term (Swain, 2018). Second, the SDGs are difficult to quantify and, therefore, also difficult to implement and monitor. Third, they are non-binding, with each nation responsible for creating and ratifying their national or regional plans. Fourth, they do not apply to financial resources and investments. Finally, the SDGs assume, as do most national and international policies, that our human experience will play themselves out in an unchanging ecological context. The COVID-19 pandemic, a small example of the effects of breaching planetary boundaries, has exposed the fragility of the SDGs' dependence on economic growth.

Another framework which usefully brings together the planetary boundaries with the SDGs has been proposed by the economist Kate Raworth (2018). Dubbed the 'Doughnut Model', it illustrates the need to stay within the planet's earth system boundaries (the 'ceiling') whilst also meeting the basic needs of all members of the human community (the 'floor'). This defines not only a 'safe' operating space for humanity within ecological limits but also a 'just' one that ensures fundamental social guarantees (see Figure 10.1). At present very few countries can meet the basic needs of their residents; none have done so without overconsuming their share of natural resources (Fanning et al., 2022).

One Health and Planetary Health

Indigenous people have long recognised the interconnectedness of all living things, including the impact of all elements of the natural world on wellbeing, health, and spirituality, and, as a result, acted as custodians of the environment (Romanelli et al., 2015). More recently, health professionals have begun to expand their understanding of illness, care, healing, and health to these broader socio-ecological determinants of health. The 'One World, One Health' concept was created in 2004 to address the health of humans, animals, and ecosystems simultaneously. It brought together veterinarians, doctors, and ecologists to consider the role of ecological, evolutionary, and environmental sciences in infectious and non-communicable diseases (Destoumieux-Garzón et al., 2018).

Building on this work, the 'Planetary Health' movement moved to include the social sciences, politics, ethics, and law, to the understanding of the different ways human societies interact with animals and ecosystems, and perceptions of risk. Planetary health urges us to (1) recognise the socio-ecological drivers of illness; (2) protect biological diversity and cultural diversity; (3) improve

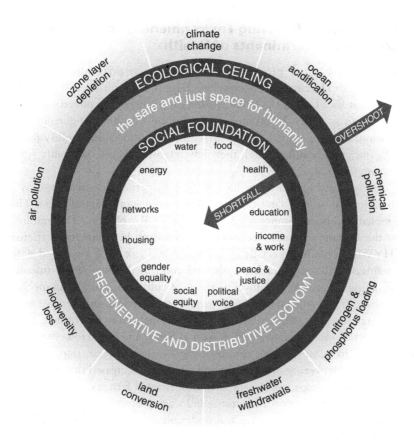

FIGURE 10.1 The Doughnut model for sustainable development within social and planetary boundaries (Creative Commons by SA4.0).

accountability and decision-making by calculating threats to ecosystem integrity; (4) redefine growth and prosperity away from GDP towards measures which enable better quality of life for all; and (5) develop research and governance structures and processes to respond to environmental threats to health and life (Whitmee et al., 2015). It argues that applying a planetary health lens to policy negotiations could bring together the fragmented agendas of health, environment, human rights, and security (de Paula, 2021). A multitude of policy and grassroots initiatives have emerged globally to meet basic needs whilst preserving and re-generating natural resources. The case study below is an effective example of thinking systemically in ways that address the principles underpinning planetary health, doughnut economics, and the SDGs.

Case Study: Addressing Environmental, Social, and Economic Determinants of Health

The United Nations' prestigious Equator Initiative prize was awarded to the 'Deccan Development Society' in 2020, in recognition of its work to address at least four of the SDGs: eliminating hunger and poverty in their communities (SDG 2), promoting gender equality and refiguring caste relations in more equitable ways (SDG 5), promoting sustainability (SDG 12), and good health through their low intensity-high food quality agriculture (SDG 3).

Hunger and malnutrition have at various periods loomed large over the arid, semi-desert landscape of Telangana in south-central India. The problem has been compounded by the 'Green Revolution'. This resulted in the initiation of new technologies, including high-yielding varieties (HYVs) of cereals, especially dwarf wheat and rice. It is associated with chemical fertilisers, agrochemicals, and controlled water-supply (usually involving irrigation) and novel methods of cultivation, including mechanisation. It also engendered a shift towards more irrigation-intensive agricultural practices, which allowed traditional staple crops like millets, to be replaced by more lucrative cereals such as wheat and rice. However, these practices have, in the long run, over-exploited freshwater, impoverished soils through overuse of pesticides and fertilisers, decreased the nutritional quality of the crops, and, eventually, immiserated farmers. Global warming, with its erratic rainfall patterns and searing summer heat, has further compounded water shortages and undermined crop yields (Shiva, 1991; Behal, 2020).

Millets are rain-fed crops that require no chemical intervention can withstand scorching temperatures and are traditionally co-cultivated with legumes to fix organic carbon into the soil. They contain high amounts of iron, calcium, and vitamins A and B, besides quantities of potassium, often lacking in the diets of the poor. In the 1980s, The Deccan Development Society worked with a group of women from the most marginalised castes, to form a cooperative, to harness the power of millets, to end hunger and malnutrition in the area. Today about 2,700 women cultivate their own fields, hold their own seed banks, feed themselves and their families, and set their prices through fair trade type agreements and markets, thus challenging patriarchal understandings of agriculture, including who counts as a 'farmer'. Their work has created a million person-days of employment, recharged fields with mulch and organic fertilisers, and produced three times as much food as when they started. The model acts on intertwined ecological, economic, social, and therefore health drivers, to demonstrate an equitable and sustainable solution. Disenfranchised and socially marginalised lower caste Dalit women have created climate-resilient, bi-odiverse farmlands, whilst managing their market and media presence. In doing so, they have challenged several systems of authority – from caste and gender hierarchies to those of the State and the market.

Conclusion

This chapter has focused on the relationship of the climate-and-ecological crisis to colonisation, industrialisation, and globalisation. In the Twenty-First Century, health cannot be viewed primarily through a scientific or medical lens. Instead, given the close links between environmental and human health, and the direct relationship between ecology and economic systems, any effective global public health intervention involves an urgent redressal of socio-economic and ecological inequity. The authors explored some theoretical models and perspectives which recognise the inseparable links between society, economy, and environment. The chapter ended with a case study, which demonstrated an example of hunger alleviation in the Indian sub-continent, by addressing social determinants of health (food and income) within the needs of the local ecosystem.

Research Points and Reflective Exercise

With reference to the discussions in this chapter, begin to reflect upon the following:

1   Do you feel that social hierarchies in your country, such as class, gender, or caste, have played a role in the environmental crisis? If yes, which one?
2   How would you reconcile the need for a better standard of living for the poor, with the urgent imperative to consume less globally?

Further Resources and Reading

Duff H., Faerron Guzmán, C., Almada, A., Golden, C., and Myers, S. (2020). "Planetary Health Case Studies: An Anthology of Solutions". https://doi.org/10.5822/phanth9678
Kothari, A. (2014). "Radical Ecological Democracy: A Path Forward for India and Beyond". *Development*, 57 (1): 36–45. https://doi.org/10.1057/dev.2014.43

References

Abubakar, I., Aldridge, R. W., Devakumar, D., Orcutt, M., Burns, R., Barreto, M. L., et al. (2018). "The UCL–Lancet Commission on Migration and Health: The Health of a World on the Move". *The Lancet*, 392 (10164): 2606–2654. https://doi.org/10.1016/S0140-6736(18)32114-7

Behal, A. (2020). "The Green Revolution and a Dark Punjab", Down to Earth, 16 July. Available at: https://www.downtoearth.org.in/blog/agriculture/the-green-revolution-and-a-dark-punjab-72318 (Accessed: 11 January 2022).

Bennett, C. E., Thomas, R., Williams, M., Zalasiewicz, J., Edgeworth, M., Miller, H., et al. (2018). "The Broiler Chicken as a Signal of a Human Reconfigured Biosphere". *Royal Society Open Science*, 5 (12): 180325. https://doi.org/10.1098/rsos.180325

Brundtland, G. H. (1987) *Our Common Future: Report of the World Commission on Environment and Development.* Geneva, UN-Dokument A/42/427.

Bryant, R., Waters, E., Gibbs, L., Gallagher, H. C., Pattison, P., Lusher, D., et al. (2014). "Psychological Outcomes Following the Victorian Black Saturday Bushfires". *Australian and New Zealand Journal of Psychiatry*, 48: 634–643. https://doi.org/10.1177/0004867414534476

Bullard, R. D. (2001). "Environmental Justice in the 21st Century: Race Still Matters". *Phylon*, 49 (3/4): 151–171.

Cane, M. A., Miguel, E., Burke, M., Hsiang, S. M., Lobell, D. B., Meng, K. C., et al. (2014). "Temperature and Violence". *Nature Climate Change*, 4 (4): 234–235.

Crutzen, P. J. and Stoermer, E. F. (2000). "The 'Anthropocene'". *IGBP Newsletter,* 41: 17–18.

de Paula, N. (2021). "Planetary Health Diplomacy: A Call to Action". *The Lancet Planetary Health*, 5 (1): e8–e9. https://doi.org/10.1016/S2542-5196(20)30300-4

Destoumieux-Garzon, D., Mavingui, P., Boetsch, G., Boissier, J., Darriet, F., Duboz, P., et al. (2018). "The One Health Concept: 10 Years Old and a Long Road Ahead". *Frontiers in Veterinary Science,* 5. https://doi.org/10.3389/fvets.2018.00014

Dhara, C. and Singh, V. (2021). 'The Elephant in the Room: Why Transformative Education Must Address the Problem of Endless Exponential Economic Growth". In R. Iyengar and C. T. Kwauk (eds.) *Curriculum and Learning for Climate Action Toward an SDG 4.7 Roadmap for Systems Change (E-Book (PDF)),* 120–143.

Donohoe, M., (2003). "Causes and Health Consequences of Environmental Degradation and Social Injustice". *Social Science and Medicine*, 56, (3): 573–587. https://doi.org/10.1016/S0277-9536(02)00055-2

Fanning, A. L., O'Neill, D. W., Hickel, J and Roux, N. (2022). "The Social Shortfall and Ecological Overshoot of Nations". *Nat Sustain*, 5: 26–36. https://doi.org/10.1038/s41893-021-00799-z

Grooten, M. and Almond, R. E. (2018). *Living Planet Report-2018: Aiming Higher: Living Planet Report-2018:* Aiming Higher.

Health Effects Institute. 2020. *State of Global Air 2020. Special Report.* Boston, MA: Health Effects Institute.

Hickel, J. (2019). "The Contradiction of the Sustainable Development Goals: Growth versus Ecology on a Finite Planet". *Sustainable Development.* 27, (5): 873–884. https://doi.org/10.1002/sd.1947

Kleinman, A, Das, V. and Lock, M. M. (1997). *Social Suffering.* Berkeley University of California Press.

Lewis, S. L and Maslin, M. A. (2018). *The Human Planet: How We Created the Anthropocene. New Haven.* London: Yale University Press.

Lowe, S. R., Manove, E. E. and Rhodes, J. E. (2013). "Posttraumatic Stress and Posttraumatic Growth Among Low-Income Mothers Who Survived Hurricane Katrina". *Journal of Consulting and Clinical Psychology.* 81 (5): 877–889. https://doi.org/10.1037/a0033252

MacFadden, D. R., McGough, S. F., Fisman, D., Santillana, M. and Brownstein, J. S. (2018). "Antibiotic Resistance Increases with Local Temperature". *Nature Climate Change*, 8 (6): 510–514. https://doi.org/10.1038/s41558-018-0161-6

McGregor, H., Gergis, J., Abram, N. and Phipps, S. (2016). "The Industrial Revolution Kick-Started Global Warming Much Earlier than When We Realized". The Conversion Blogsite.

Moore, J. W. (2017). "The Capitalocene, Part I: On the Nature and Origins of Our Ecological Crisis". *The Journal of Peasant Studies*, 44 (3): 594–630. https://doi.org/10.1080/03066150.2016.1235036

Padhy, S.K., Sarkar, S., Panigrahi, M. and Paul, S. (2015). "Mental Health Effects of Climate Change". *Indian Journal of Occupational and Environmental Medicine*, 19 (1): 3–7. https://doi.org/10.4103/0019-5278.156997

Renault, E. (2010) "A Critical Theory of Social Suffering". *Critical Horizons*, 11 (2): 221–241. https://doi.org/10.1558/crit.v11i2.221

Raworth, K. (2018). *Doughnut Economics: Seven Ways to Think Like a 21st-Century Economist*. London: Random House Business Books.

Rockström, J., Steffen, W., Noone, K., Persson, Å., Chapin, S., Lambin, E., et al. (2009). "Planetary Boundaries. Exploring the Safe Operating Space for Humanity". *Ecology and Society*, 14: (2): 32. (online). URL:http://www.ecologyandsociety.org/vol14/iss2/art32/.

Romanelli, C., Cooper, D., Campbell-Lendrum, D., Maiero, M., Karesh, W.B., Hunter, D., et al. (2015). *Connecting Global Priorities: Biodiversity and Human Health: A State of Knowledge Review*. WHO/CBD 344p. ISBN 978 92 4 150853 7.

Romanello, M., McGushin, A., Di Napoli, C., Drummond, P., Hughes, N., Jamart, L., et al. (2021). "The 2021 Report of the Lancet Countdown on Health and Climate Change: Code Red for a Healthy Future". *The Lancet*, 398 (10311): 1619–1662. https://doi.org/10.1016/S0140-6736(21)01787-6

Shiva, V. (1991). *The Violence of the Green Revolution*. London: Zed Books.

Swain R. B. (2018). "A Critical Analysis of the Sustainable Development Goals". In: Filho W. L. (ed.) *Handbook of Sustainability Science and Research*. Cham, Springer, 341–357.

Thomas, K., Hardy, R. D., Lazrus, H., Mendez, M., Orlove, B., Rivera-Collazo, I., et al. (2019). "Explaining Differential Vulnerability to Climate Change: A Social Science Review". *Wiley Interdisciplinary Reviews: Climate Change*, 10 (2):e565. https://doi.org/10.1002/wcc.565

Thu, H. M., Aye, K. M. and Thein, S. (1998). "The Effect of Temperature and Humidity on Dengue Virus Propagation in Aedes Aegypti Mosquitos". *The Southeast Asian Journal of Tropical Medicine and Public Health*, 29 (2): 280–284.

Tsing, A. (2015). *The Mushroom at the End of the World: On the Possibility of Life in Capitalist Ruins*. Princeton: Princeton University Press.

United Nations General Assembly. (2015). "Transforming Our World: The 2030 Agenda for Sustainable Development", 21 October, A/RES/70/1. Available at: https://www.refworld.org/docid/57b6e3e44.html (Accessed: 19 February 2022).

Whitmee, S., Haines, A., Beyrer, C., Boltz, F., Capon, A. G, de Souza Dias, B. F., et al. (2015). "Safeguarding Human Health in the Anthropocene Epoch: Report of The Rockefeller Foundation-Lancet Commission on Planetary Health". *The Lancet*, 14 386 (10007): 1973–2028. https://doi.org/10.1016/S0140-6736(15)60901-1.

Wiedmann,.T, Lenzen, M., Keyßer, L. T. and Steinberger, J. K. (2020). "'Scientists' Warning on Affluence". *Nature Communications*, 11 (1): 1–10. https://doi.org/10.1038/s41467-020-16941-y

Weinzettel, J., Hertwich, E. G., Peters, G. P., Steen-Olsen, K. and Galli, A. (2013). "Affluence Drives the Global Displacement of Land Use". *Global Environmental Change*, 23 (2): 433–438. https://doi.org/10.1016/j.gloenvcha.2012.12.010

11

THE CLIMATE EMERGENCY AND ZERO-CARBON HEALTHCARE

Vanita Gandhi and Stefi Barna

Introduction

Climate change is recognised as one of the Twenty-First Century's greatest threats to population health and health equity. It also offers an opportunity to make systemic changes that will improve the health of the public. This chapter explores how the healthcare sector contributes to the climate emergency and how it might instead contribute to a sustainable world. We will discuss the intersections between the social determinants of health, health inequities, and the effects of a warming climate. A framework for building a zero-carbon healthcare system will be considered. Finally, we will consider a public health intervention to improve the health of people and the planet.

An Unsustainable Health System

In 1987, the United Nations (UN) Brundtland Commission defined sustainability as that which 'meets the needs of the present generation without compromising the ability of future generations to meet their own needs' (UN, 1987). In healthcare, the term sustainability traditionally refers to financial challenges, i.e., how to fund the rising cost of healthcare from ageing populations, accelerating rates of chronic disease, and the increasing cost of technology. It generally does not consider the natural resources which supply healthcare or the quantity of pollution healthcare produces. To understand how healthcare is unsustainable in this definition, and potential ways to mitigate this, we will examine the example of the climate emergency. Climate change is caused by human activities which emit greenhouse gases, such as carbon dioxide and methane, which trap heat in the atmosphere, causing the Earth's temperature to rise. All countries will experience significant and growing health impacts from climate change. Ironically,

DOI: 10.4324/9781003128373-11

however, the health sector makes a significant contribution to the climate crisis and thus the evolving global health emergency. Healthcare produces 4.4% of the world's greenhouse gases; if it were a country, it would be the fifth largest emitter on the planet (Healthcare Without Harm, 2019). The top three emitters, the United States, China, and collectively the countries of the European Union (including the UK), comprise 56% of the world's total healthcare climate footprint. Direct emissions from healthcare facilities and vehicles make up 17% of the sector's footprint, indirect emissions from purchased energy sources such as electricity comprise 12%, and the remaining 71% is primarily derived from supply chains, through the production, transport, and disposal of goods and services, such as pharmaceuticals and equipment (Healthcare Without Harm, 2019).

Health systems will bear high costs resulting from extreme climate events and must become resilient to climate's impacts. In the 2015 Paris Agreement, all countries agreed to reduce emissions to keep global warming below two degrees Celsius (UN Framework Convention on Climate Change, 2015). Establishing the capacity for the health sector to understand, measure, and track its climate footprint is a fundamental step to alignment with the ambition of the Paris Agreement. The contribution of healthcare to the climate change emergency is also increasingly important to Critical Public Health theorists in understanding how the design and function of healthcare can produce and perpetuate health inequalities and the differential impacts of climate change on poorer and marginalised communities especially (La Placa et al., 2013).

A country-wide attempt to do this is underway in the UK. As the largest public sector carbon emitter, the English National Health Service (NHS) has pledged to reduce its directly controlled emissions to net zero by 2040, and the emissions it can influence (such as through supply chains) to net zero by 2045 (England NHS and Improvement NHS, 2020). In doing so, it became the first major national health system to commit to transition to a low carbon economy.

At the 2021 UN Climate Change Conference, called COP26, 52 countries (including Indonesia, Malawi, Morocco, Spain, and the USA) committed to building health systems which are low carbon, sustainable, and able to withstand the impacts of climate change (COP26 Health Team, 2021). These include 47 countries, representing over a third of global healthcare emissions, which have committed to develop a sustainable, low carbon health system. Fourteen of these 47 countries have set a deadline of 2050 to reach net zero (WHO, 2021). For example, the government of Fiji is responding to the increase in cyclones and rising sea levels by building more climate-resilient health infrastructures and providing healthcare facilities with sustainable energy services.

A Zero-Carbon Health System

A sustainable health system would operate with the available financial, social, and environmental resources to protect health for all, now, and in future generations. These three elements together are often referred to as the 'triple bottom line'

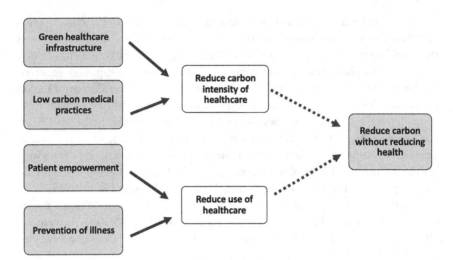

FIGURE 11.1 Components of a zero-carbon health system. Adapted with permission from Centre for Sustainable Healthcare's principles of sustainable clinical practice (Mortimer et al., 2018; Gandhi et al., 2020).

(Elkington, 1997). A zero-carbon health system must be based on low carbon infrastructure, less resource-intensive medical practices, the empowerment of patients to manage their own care, and, wherever possible, keeping people out of hospitals by preventing illness (Mortimer, 2010). Figure 11.1 illustrates the components of a zero-carbon health system, which reduces both wasteful activities and the environmental impact of necessary activities, whilst maintaining high standards of care.

Green Healthcare Infrastructure

When we think about reducing carbon emissions, we usually turn first to the infrastructure, buildings, energy, and appliances of hospitals and clinics. To decarbonise, the health system, like other sectors, must cease burning fossil fuels and make the most of existing renewable energy, by insulating buildings and using energy-efficient appliances (Rasheed et al., 2021). The UN Development Program's 'Solar for Health' Project (2018) installed solar panels on over 400 health centres in Zimbabwe, facilitating quality care, reducing costs, and building resiliency with zero emissions. In 2019, the Santa Izabel Hospital in Brazil implemented efficient lighting, solar water heating, and improvements to heating and ventilation, resulting in a 2% reduction in their greenhouse gas emissions (Healthcare Without Harm, 2019).

Low Carbon Medical Practices

Medical activities produce high levels of waste and pollution. One way to reduce the environmental footprint is switching to lower carbon treatments.

For example, in Kenya, anaesthetists and pharmacists collaborated with the government and pharmaceutical companies to negotiate substitutions to lower carbon anaesthetic gases and to make propellant-free inhalers cheaper respectively, and encouraged their use throughout the country (Aga Khan Development Network, 2020). Another way to reduce carbon intensity is to create 'leaner' healthcare pathways. Lean healthcare has emerged as a strategy to reduce waste and activities that do not add value to the healthcare process. Poor patient flow and inadequate resource utilisation contribute to delays and overcrowding, affecting patient safety, patient and staff satisfaction, and the overall quality of care (Tlapa et al., 2020). An excellent example is India's 'Aravind Eye Clinic', which developed a highly carbon-efficient cataract surgery pathway through the use of domestic suppliers, a specialised workforce, and a standardised protocol-driven approach. This has drastically reduced the per-patient cataract carbon footprint to roughly 5% of the UK cataract footprint, whilst maintaining safety and quality (Thiel et al., 2017).

Other examples include reducing the number of consumables healthcare purchases and shifting away from single-use products where possible, minimising travel by offering phone appointments and home treatments for chronic conditions, and encouraging active travel and other low carbon transport choices. These interventions address the triple bottom line by saving money, reducing carbon, and, in turn, improving patient and staff experience. An example of the latter has been demonstrated by Waldhausen et al. (2010) when redesigning and implementing process changes to optimise ambulatory paediatric surgical outpatient clinics. This led to an increase in face-to-face staff-patient time, and median number of patients seen in a four-hour clinic, which improved overall staff teamwork and patient satisfaction, due to more time for joint decision making, and a deeper understanding of their care plan.

The COVID-19 response highlighted opportunities for the use of telecommunications rather than conventional face-to-face outpatient clinics, which reduces staff and patient travel and clinic waiting times (Kichloo et al., 2020). This has been particularly transformative in health service delivery in low- and middle-income countries which have fragile resource-limited health systems, high rate of infectious diseases, and a high mortality rate (Osei and Mashamba-Thompson, 2021). The advances in mobile technologies have led to a rise in the integration of mobile health (mHealth) into the existing electronic health services in low- and middle-income countries, by using voice calls, short message service (SMS), data transmission, and mobile phone applications, to support healthcare provision (Sondaal et al., 2016).

mHealth technologies and applications have been recognised as an avenue to support the screening of infectious diseases such as COVID-19, Ebola, and HIV. In Brazil, healthcare authorities have encouraged the use of mHealth for remote screening and detection of COVID-19 (Caetano et al., 2020). The Ebola and Zika virus epidemics in West Africa (Danquah et al., 2019) and Southern America (Ahmadi et al., 2018) have benefited from the use of mHealth applications in promoting early screening and testing. mHealth applications have also been used to support screening of non-infectious diseases like Hypertension, Diabetes, and Cancer (Zhang et al., 2020). There are several cases where mHealth has enhanced adherence with medication in low- and middle-income countries. For example, mHealth reminders have been shown to improve antiretroviral adherence in HIV-infected patients, in multiple countries including Vietnam and South Africa (Georgette et al., 2017; DeSilva et al., 2019). A similar study in Pakistan demonstrated that mHealth applications encouraged medication adherence in stroke patients (Kamal et al., 2015).

Whilst mHealth has the potential to reduce the overall healthcare carbon footprint by streamlining costly medical practices, such as disease screening and treatment support, there are barriers that hinder its implementation. These include geographical access and internet connectivity difficulties, policy/regulatory barriers, limited awareness of mHealth applications, limited healthcare workers' competence in mHealth, and lack of funding (Osei and Mashamba-Thompson, 2021).

Patient Empowerment

Traditionally, clinical medicine has been practiced in a paternalistic manner, whereby decision making is dependent on the expertise of the clinician (Gallagher, 1998). However, with internet access to medical information, many patients have become experts in their own conditions. Informing patients about their condition, supporting them to recognise deterioration, managing self-limiting episodes, and seeking help early improve outcomes and reduce the demand for healthcare.

Health systems can themselves facilitate patient empowerment and self-care practices. An example of this is giving patients access to their health records to increase knowledge of their own health conditions, and readily accessible details on diagnosis and treatment plans, effectively shifting control from the healthcare facility to the home. Patients can monitor their health and share relevant information with family members and providers such as pharmacists or community-based clinicians. Dijkstra et al. (2005) reported that diabetic patients in Denmark, who had access to their health records in the way of a Diabetes Passport, were found to have better long-term glucose control.

At the national level, patient empowerment includes assuring health literacy. In low- and middle-income countries, deploying community health workers with knowledge of local needs can foster self-care among underserved populations and complement large-scale health campaigns. For example, the Bangladesh Government's 'Expanded Programme on Immunisation' used community health workers and successfully reduced the mortality and morbidity from vaccine-preventable diseases such as Polio, Measles, and Diphtheria (Jamil et al., 1999). Similarly, ensuring school-based education on health, hygiene, and first aid enables young people to protect their health before healthcare becomes necessary.

For example, in Karachi, Pakistan, pictorial storybooks helped primary school children understand how to avoid road traffic incidents (Ahmad et al., 2018).

Prevention of Illness

The prevention of illness is a powerful way to reduce the frequency of hospital admissions and appointments and clinicians can be powerful advocates for this. The Lung Health Study conducted in North America randomised participants between a specialised 10-week smoking cessation programme versus usual care and demonstrated that the 14-year all-cause mortality for cardiovascular disease, including Coronary Heart Disease and Lung Cancer, was significantly lower in those who underwent the smoking cessation programme (Anthonisen et al., 2005). The US Centre for Disease Control and Prevention estimate that up to 40% of the five main causes of death (heart disease, stroke, cancers, lower respiratory disease, and unintentional injury) are preventable (Garcia et al., 2014). The figure in low- and middle-income countries is even higher, although difficult to quantify.

Prevention Beyond the Health System

Public health has a critical role to play beyond decarbonising the health system. Every carbon-reducing intervention has potential health co-benefits or co-harms (Rudolph et al., 2015). Public health must communicate the health implications of failure to act on climate change, assist all sectors of society adapt to the impacts of climate change, foster climate-resilient communities, and ensure that strategies to address climate change, also protect health, reduce health inequalities, and maximise health co-benefits.

An example of such an intervention is 'urban greening' or 'green infrastructure': strategies to increase tree cover and other green space (forests, parks, gardens, and farms) in cities and have both health and environmental benefits. Green spaces reduce urban heat islands by lowering surface and air temperatures, decreasing the risk of heat illness (Wong and Lau, 2013). Trees and plants remove pollutants such as ozone, nitrogen dioxide, and particulate matter from the air (Royal Society of Chemistry, 2020), reducing the incidence of asthma. They provide opportunities for physical activity, relaxation, social interaction, and improve quality of life, especially in low-income communities (Cohen et al., 2007). Access to green space lowers stress and even speeds up recovery times in hospitalised patients (Lottrup et al., 2013). Trees and greenery are associated with decreases in crime and increases in property value, although without attention to equity, these positive improvements lead to gentrification and displacement of lower-income residents (Kuo and Sullivan, 2001).

Urban greening and green infrastructure also have environmental benefits. Plants improve air circulation and shade, which in turn provide a cooling effect and assist to lower air temperatures. Sorensen et al. (1997) demonstrated that increasing tree cover in Chicago by 10% reduced the total energy for heating and cooling by 5–10%. In contrast, some carbon reduction strategies have negative effects on health or may exacerbate health inequalities. For example, a country may choose to build hundreds of nuclear power stations for fossil-fuel-free electricity and incentivise drivers to switch to electric vehicles. This would greatly reduce greenhouse gas emissions from vehicle travel, but it would do nothing to address the problem of illness, related to sedentarism.

Similarly, biofuel initiatives have produced diesel from plant matter. When burned, biofuels simply add to the atmosphere carbon, which was earlier absorbed by the plants, creating a net-zero emission equation. However, an enormous amount of land is required to produce biofuels, and this is either created by converting agricultural land to biofuel crops, resulting in lower food production, or by clear-felling forests for biofuel plantations, with a consequential decline in biodiversity, and the displacement of forest-dwelling communities (Jeswani et al., 2020). Unintended outcomes such as these can be avoided by using environmental impact assessments and health impact assessments to calculate the distribution of risks to vulnerable communities.

Conclusion

This chapter has explored the responsibility of the health sector to reduce the impacts of climate change by aligning its actions and development trajectory with the Paris Agreement. We have highlighted that increasing resilience to climate change will require adopting a culture of continual improvement in the value that health services provide, to maximise health outcomes, while reducing environmental, social, and financial costs ('triple bottom line' of sustainability). To achieve this in the context of rising demand and pressure on healthcare services, lean methodology, low carbon medical practice, and moving to a single-payer system may reduce administrative costs, governance-related waste, and help healthcare transition to net-zero emissions. Public health planners and policy makers at national, regional, and local levels need to consider health, a central dimension of climate change mitigation activities.

Research Points and Reflective Exercise

With reference to the discussions in this chapter, begin to reflect upon the following:

- In what ways is climate change a determinant of health?
- How are the climate and ecological crises related to the health sector?
- What are the components of a sustainable health system?
- What actions could be taken to ensure that the healthcare system in your country is sustainable?

Further Resources and Reading

NHS England and Improvement. (2020). *Delivering a 'Net Zero' National Health Service*. London: NHS England and NHS Improvement.

Githeko, A. K. and Woodward, A. (2003). "International Consensus on the Science of Climate and Health: The IPCC (Intergovernmental Panel on Climate Change) Third Assessment Report". In A. J. McMichael, D. H Campbell-Lendrum, C. F. Corvalan, K. L. Ebi, A., Githeko et al. (eds.) *Climate Change and Human Health: Risks and Responses*. Geneva: World Health Organization.

References

Aga Khan Development Network Publications (2020). "Inhalers and Anaesthetics Special Initiatives". Available at: https://www.akdn.org/our-agencies/aga-khan-health-services/climate-smart-health-care/specialenvironmentclimate (Accessed: 21 December 2021).

Ahmad, H., Naeem, R., Feroze, A., Zia, N., Shakoor, A. Khan U. R. et al. (2018) "Teaching Children Road Safety through Storybooks: An Approach to Child Health Literacy in Pakistan". *BMC Pediatrics*, 18 (1): 1–8. https://doi.org/10.1186/s12887-018-0982-5

Ahmadi, S., Bempong, N. E., De Santis, O., Sheath, D. and Flahault, A. (2018). "The Role of Digital Technologies in Tackling the Zika Outbreak: A Scoping Review". *Journal of Public Health and Emergency*, 2 (20): 1–15. https://doi.org/10.21037/jphe.2018.05.02

Anthonisen, N. R., Skeans, M. A., Wise, R. A., Manfreda, J., Kanner, R. E. et al. (2005). "For the Lung Health Study Research Group. The Effects of a Smoking Cessation Intervention on 14.5-Year Mortality". *Annals of Internal Medicine*, 142 (4): 233–239. https://doi.org/10.7326/0003-4819-142-4-200502150-00005

Caetano, R., Silva, A. B., Guedes, A. C. C. M., Paiva, C. C. N. D., Ribeiro, G. D. R. et al. (2020). "Challenges and Opportunities for Telehealth During the COVID-19 Pandemic: Ideas on Spaces and Initiatives in the Brazilian Context". *Cadernos de Saúde Pública*, 36. https://doi.org/10.1590/0102-311X00088920

Cohen D. A, McKenzie T. L, Sehgal, A., Williamson, S., Golinelli, D. et al. (2007). "Contribution of Public Parks to Physical Activity", *American Journal of Public Health*, 97 (3): 509–514. https://doi.org/10.2105/AJPH.2005.072447

COP26 Health Team. (2021). "COP26 Health Programme: Country Commitments to Build Climate Resilient and Sustainable Health Systems". Available at: https://cdn.who.int/media/docs/default-source/climate-change/cop26-health-programme.pdf?sfvrsn=cde1b578_5 (Accessed: 2 January 2022).

Danquah L, O., Hasham, N., MacFarlane, M., Conteh, F. E., Momoh, F. et al. (2019). "Use of a Mobile Application for Ebola Contact Tracing and Monitoring in Northern Sierra Leone: A Proof-Of-Concept Study". *BMC Infectious Diseases*, 19 (1): 1–12. https://doi.org/10.1186/s12879-019-4354-z

DeSilva, M., Vu, C. N., Bonawitz, R., Van Lam, N., Gifford, A. L. et al. (2019). "The Supporting Adolescent Adherence in Vietnam (SAAV) Study: Study Protocol for a Randomized Controlled Trial Assessing an mHealth Approach to Improving Adherence for Adolescents Living With HIV in Vietnam". *Trials*, 20 (1): 1–13. https://doi.org/10.1186/s13063-019-3239-1

Dijkstra R. F., Braspenning, J. C. C., Huijsmans, Z., Akkermans, R. P., Van Ballegooie, E. (2005). "Introduction of Diabetes Passports Involving Both Patients and

Professionals to Improve Hospital Outpatient Diabetes Care". *Diabetes Research and Clinical Practice*, 68 (2): 126–134. https://doi.org/10.1016/j.diabres.2004.09.020

Elkington, J. (1997). "The Triple Bottom Line". In *Environmental Management: Readings and Cases, 2*. Thousand Oaks, CA: Sage.

England NHS and Improvement. (2020). *Delivering a 'Net Zero' National Health Service*. London: NHS England and NHS Improvement.

Gallagher, S. M. (1998). "Paternalism in Healthcare Decision Making", *Ostomy/Wound Management*, 44 (4): 22–24.

Gandhi, V., Al-Hadithy, N., Göpfert, A., Knight, K., van Hove, M. et al. (2020) "Integrating Sustainability into Postgraduate Medical Education". *Future Healthcare Journal*, 7 (2): 102. https://doi.org/10.7861/fhj.2020-0042

Garcia, M. C., Macarena, C., Bastian, B., Rossen, L. M., Anderson, R. et al. (2014). "Potentially Preventable Deaths Among the Five Leading Causes of Death — United States, 2010 and 2014". *MMWR Morbidity and mortality weekly report*, 65: 1245–1255. https://doi.org/10.15585/mmwr.mm6545a1external icon.

Georgette, N., Siedner, M. J., Petty, C. R., Zanoni B. C., Carpenter, S. et al. (2017). "Impact of a Clinical Program Using Weekly Short Message Service (SMS) on Antiretroviral Therapy Adherence Support in South Africa: A Retrospective Cohort Study". *BMC Medical Informatics and Decision Making*, 17 (1): 1–9. https://doi.org/10.1186/s12911-017-0413-9

Health Care Without Harm (2019). "Healthcare Climate Footprint Report". Available at: https://noharm-global.org/documents/health-care-climate-footprint-report. (Accessed: 14 March 2021).

Jamil, K., Bhuiya, A., Streatfield, K. and Chakrabarty, N. (1999), "The Immunization Programme in Bangladesh: Impressive Gains in Coverage, but Gaps Remain", *Health Policy and Planning*, 14 (1): 49–58. https://doi.org/10.1093/heapol/14.1.49

Jeswani, H. K., Chilvers, A. and Azapagic, A. (2020). "Environmental Sustainability of Biofuels: A Review". *Proceedings of The Royal Society A, 476*: 20200351. http://doi.org/10.1098/rspa.2020.0351

Kamal, A. K., Shaikh, Q., Pasha, O., Azam, I., Islam, M. et al. (2015). "A Randomized Controlled Behavioral Intervention Trial to Improve Medication Adherence in Adult Stroke Patients with Prescription Tailored Short Messaging Service (SMS)-SMS4Stroke Study". *BMC Neurology*, 15 (1): 1–11. https://doi.org/10.1186/s12883-015-0471-5

Kichloo, A., Albosta, M., Dettloff, K., Wani, F., El-Amir, Z. et al. (2020). "Telemedicine, The Current COVID-19 Pandemic and the Future: A Narrative Review and Perspectives Moving Forward in the USA". *Family Medicine and Community Health*, 8 (3): e000530. https://doi.org/10.1136/fmch-2020-000530

Kuo, F. E. and Sullivan, W. C. (2001). "Environment and Crime in the Inner City: Does Vegetation Reduce Crime?". *Environment and Behaviour, 33* (3): 343–367. https://doi.org/10.1177/0013916501333002

La Placa, V., McVey, D. MacGregor, E., Smith, A. and Scott, M. (2013). "The Contribution of Qualitative Research to the Healthy Foundations Life-stage Segmentation". *Critical Public Health*, 24 (3): 266–282. https://doi.org/10.1080/09581596.2013.797068

Lottrup, L., Grahn, P. and Stigsdotter, U. K. (2013). "Workplace Greenery and Perceived Level of Stress: Benefits of Access to a Green Outdoor Environment at the Workplace". *Landscape and Urban Planning*, 110: 5–11. https://doi.org/10.1016/j.landurbplan.2012.09.002

Mortimer, F. (2010). "The Sustainable Physician". *Clinical Medicine*, 10 (2): 110. https://doi.org/10.7861/clinmedicine.10-2-110

Mortimer, F., Isherwood, J., Wilkinson, A. and Vaux, E. (2018). "Sustainability in Quality Improvement: Redefining Value". *Future Healthcare Journal*, 5 (2): 88. https://doi.org/10.7861/futurehosp.5-2-88

Osei, E. and Mashamba-Thompson, T. P. (2021). "Mobile Health Applications for Disease Screening and Treatment Support in Low- and Middle-Income Countries: A Narrative Review". *Heliyon*, 7 (3): p.e06639. https://doi.org/10.1016/j.heliyon.2021.e06639

Rasheed, F. N., Baddley, J., Prabhakaran, P., De Barros, E. F., Reddy, K. S. et al. (2021). "Decarbonising Healthcare in Low and Middle Income Countries: Potential Pathways to Net Zero Emissions". *BMJ*, 375: n1284. https://doi.org/10.1136/bmj.n1284

Royal Society of Chemistry. (2020). "How Do Trees Clean Our Air?" Available at: https://edu.rsc.org/feature/how-do-trees-clean-our-air/4010864.article (Accessed: 25 March 2020).

Rudolph, L., Gould. S. and Berko J. (2015). *Climate Change, Health, and Equity: Opportunities for Action*. Oakland, CA: Public Health Institute.

Sondaal, S. F. V., Browne, J. L., Amoakoh-Coleman, M., Borgstein, A., Miltenburg, A. S. et al. (2016). "Assessing the Effect of mHealth Interventions in Improving Maternal and Neonatal Care in Low-and Middle-Income Countries: A Systematic Review". *PloS One*, 11 (5): p.e0154664. https://doi.org/10.1371/journal.pone.0154664

Sorensen, M., Smit, J., Barzetti, V. and Williams J (1997). "Good Practices for Urban Greening", Inter-American Development Bank. Available at: http://www.iadb.org/sds/doc/ENV109KKeipiE.pdf (Accessed: 22 December 2021).

Thiel, C. L., Schehlein, E., Ravilla, T., Ravindran, R. D., Robin, A. L. (2017). "Cataract Surgery and Environmental Sustainability: Waste and Lifecycle Assessment of Phacoemulsification at a Private Healthcare Facility". *Journal of Cataract and Refractive Surgery*, 43 (11): 1391–1398. https://doi.org/10.1016/j.jcrs.2017.08.017

Tlapa, D., Zepeda-Lugo, C. A., Tortorella, G. L., Baez-Lopez, Y. A., Limon-Romero, J. et al. (2020). "Effects of Lean Healthcare on Patient Flow: A Systematic Review". *Value In Health*, 23 (2): 260–273. https://doi.org/10.1016/j.jval.2019.11.002

United Nations. (1987). "Report of the World Commission on Environment and Development: Our Common Future". Available at: https://sustainabledevelopment.un.org/content/documents/5987our-common-future.pdf (Accessed: 1 November 2021).

United Nations Development Programme. (2018). "Solar for Health". Available at: https://www.undp-capacitydevelopment-health.org/en/capacities/focus/solar-for-health/. (Accessed: 22 December 2021).

United Nations Framework Convention on Climate Change. (2015). "Report of the Structured Expert Dialogue on the 2013–2015 Review". Available at: https://unfccc.int/resource/docs/2015/sb/eng/inf01.pd). (Accessed: 26 December 2021)

Waldhausen, J. H., Avansino, J. R., Libby, A. and Sawin, R. S. (2010). Application of Lean Methods Improves Surgical Clinic Experience. *Journal of Paediatric Surgery*, 45 (7): 1420–1425. https://doi.org/10.1016/j.jpedsurg.2009.10.049

Wong, J. K. W and Lau, L. S. K. (2013). "From the 'Urban Heat Island' to the 'Green Island'? A Preliminary Investigation into the Potential of Retrofitting Green Roofs in Mongkok District of Hong Kong". *Habitat International*, 39: 25–35. https://doi.org/10.1016/j.habitatint.2012.10.005

World Health Organization News. (2021). "Countries Commit to Develop Climate-Smart Health Care at COP26 UN Climate Conference", 9 November. Available at:

https://www.who.int/news/item/09-11-2021-countries-commit-to-develop-climate-smart-health-care-at-cop26-un-climate-conference (Accessed: 26 December 2021).

Zhang, D., Advani, S., Waller, J., Cupertino, A. P., Hurtado-de-Mendoza, A. (2020). "Mobile Technologies and Cervical Cancer Screening in Low-and Middle-Income Countries: A Systematic Review". *JCO Global Oncology*, 6: 617–627. https://doi.org/10.1200/JGO.19.00201

12

VIOLENCE AND GLOBAL PUBLIC HEALTH

Julia Morgan and Clare Choak

Introduction

Violence is a major global public health problem (WHO, 2002) with some likening it to an epidemic being both contagious, as well as causing morbidity and mortality (Slutkin, 2013). Moreover, a public health approach to violence is highlighted as being important in relation to interventions. This chapter will explore violence and its impact on global public health before continuing to explore how an awareness of critical social theories such as structural and cultural violence contributes to a more in-depth understanding of violence. The impact of structural and cultural violence in relation to male violence towards women and girls, including femicide, will be focused upon, as well as a discussion of youth violence.

Violence and Public Health

The World Health Organization defines violence as 'the intentional use of physical force or power, threatened or actual, against oneself, another person, or against a group or community, that either results in, or has a high likelihood of resulting in injury, death, psychological harm, mal-development or deprivation' (WHO, 2002: 4). Violence is a leading cause of injury, disability, and death and causes fear within communities and homes. For example, 405,000 people died from homicide in 2017, which is more than double the number of people who died from terrorism, natural disasters, and armed conflicts; and in some countries, homicide is amongst the leading cause of death (Roth et al., 2018). In relation to suicides, there were a reported 793,823 deaths by suicide in 2017 (Roth et al., 2018). This is likely to be an underestimate, given the stigma attached to suicide in some countries. Comparing suicide rates from 1990 to 2017, it is

DOI: 10.4324/9781003128373-12

evident that many European countries have seen a decline in death by suicide across the period, but for some countries, for example, Zimbabwe and South Korea, there appears to be an increase (Our World in Data, 2021). Violence can also have many negative health impacts on those who experience it or witness it. For example, witnessing or experiencing violence increases the risk of mental health issues as well as increases in substance abuse (WHO, 2002). Violence has also been shown to increase the risk of chronic diseases, such as cardiovascular disease, as well as infectious diseases, for example, HIV, and sexually transmitted diseases (Houry and Mercy, 2016). Intimate partner violence (IPV) has been shown to increase the likelihood of infection with HIV in women and girls and has been associated with lower CD4 counts, higher viral loads, and lower adherence to HIV drugs (Li et al., 2014; Hatcher et al., 2015).

The World Health Organization (2002) identifies three categories of violence. These include self-directed violence such as self-harm or suicide; interpersonal violence including domestic violence or IPV, violence towards elders and child abuse, plus rape, gang violence, bullying, and institutional violence, for example, in care homes or prisons. Lastly, it identifies collective violence which is further subdivided into three types: social, political, and economic violence. This would include violence which has a social focus, including mob violence, and acts of terrorism; a political focus, including war and armed conflict, and an economic focus, including acts which disrupt economies. The World Health Organization (2002) also defines violence further according to the type of violence, which is used, into physical, sexual, psychological, and deprivation/neglect.

A public health approach to violence, as espoused by the World Health Organization (2017), is highlighted as being an appropriate approach in which to tackle violence. This approach focuses on violence being preventable and highlights the importance of the collection of data around violence, a focus on understanding the causes of violent acts, an exploration of what works in reducing violence, and, lastly, the implementation of effective violence prevention initiatives or interventions. This public health approach focusing on surveillance, tracking causes and interventions, is used generally in health protection and the tracking of epidemics, enabling a primary prevention response, which focuses on upstream (causal) factors, as well as policy interventions to prevent violence from occurring.

The social determinants of health are important in understanding violence, as they situate the violent acts within a potential causal framework, which can be used to explore upstream factors. The social determinants of health highlight that the conditions in which people live can influence their health outcomes and that to prevent negative outcomes and inequalities, we need to address their fundamental causes (Marmot and Wilkinson, 2006). For example, poverty and inequality as social determinants of health have been shown to be linked to numerous violent acts, including armed conflicts, as well as child maltreatment and street crime, which impact on health outcomes (Brainard and Chollet, 2007). Moreover, the social determinants of health are important in helping us understand how health inequalities per se can be perceived as a violent act.

For example, in relation to maternal mortality, the rate in Sierra Leone is 1,120 maternal deaths per 100,000 live births, compared to two maternal deaths per 100,000 live births in Norway (World Health Organization, 2021a). This inequality in global maternal mortality rates, which are both preventable and reflect social inequalities, is in themselves violent, as they cause both harm and death. In relation to policy, the Sustainable Development Goals (SDGs) highlight several targets that explicitly aim to reduce violence (United Nations, 2015). These are:

- SDG Target 5.2 Eliminate all forms of violence against women and girls;
- SDG Target 5.3 Eliminate all harmful practices, such as child, early and forced marriage, and female genital mutilation;
- SDG Target 16.1 Significantly reduce all forms of violence and related death rates everywhere;
- SDG Target 16.2 End abuse, exploitation, trafficking, and all forms of violence against children.

Moreover, other SDG goals also focus on reducing structural factors that relate to the social determinants of health, which are in turn implicated in direct acts of violence: this includes ending poverty in all its forms; zero hunger, improving health and wellbeing, reducing gender inequality, and inequalities in education.

Structural and Cultural Violence

Galtung's (1990) critical theory of violence identifies three categories of violence: direct or personal violence, structural violence, and cultural violence. Direct violence corresponds to the types of violence identified by the World Health Organization (2002) above in its definition. Structural violence, on the other hand, can be perceived as a form of oppression that prevents people from fulfilling their potential and negatively impacts their life-chances. In some ways this is like the social determinants of health; in that it highlights how structural factors such as poverty, for example, can result in higher deaths rates amongst poorer people because of a lack of access to health care, a lack of power, or other forms of neglect. However, the concept of structural violence goes further and highlights how those who are less powerful, or more vulnerable, can be reduced to the position of 'non-persons' (Scheper-Hughes, 2004) by social and government policies which become 'normalised' as part of the everyday taken for granted 'status quo'. Poverty, for example, can be perceived as just 'the way the world is', and this injustice results in the general acceptance, rather than outrage, of high death rates amongst women or children in many low-income countries because they are poor or from a particular ethnicity, social class, or religion. Structural violence, therefore, is structural because it is embedded in the political, legal, religious, cultural, and economic organisation of the social world; it is violent because it can cause injury, death, and a lack of opportunity for people. This inequality is then naturalised or justified, or unacknowledged or blamed on individuals, for their lifestyle choices without recognising how structural factors limit the options available to groups and constrain personal agency. It, thus, becomes an accepted part of 'normal ordinary life'.

Gilligan (1996) has highlighted how structural violence leads to high rates of disability and death amongst those in lower social classes, with the structural violence rendered invisible, and often attributed to other medical causes of death or disability. Others have highlighted how structural violence is the most 'lethal' form of violence (Butchart and Engström, 2002) and can lead to people dying from famines in a world of plenty (Sen, 1982); with Gandhi calling poverty 'the worst form of violence' (cited in Alger and Stohl, 1988). However, it is important to understand that both direct and structural violence are connected, and structural violence can impact directly on the likelihood of direct violence; and direct violence can, in turn, reinforce both structural and cultural violence (Gilligan, 1996).

Cultural violence, on the other hand, legitimatises and normalises both structural and direct violence through ideologies and discourses. Utilising a feminist critical theory lens, an example of this would be the mass media and film industry, which often depicts women as sexualised, emotive, 'other', vulnerable, invisible, and secondary. This type of cultural representation reinforces sexism and misogyny and forms the basis for the ideology of Patriarchy, to infiltrate social institutions and legitimise the domination of women by men. Cultural violence, therefore, refers to representations, thoughts, practices, and discourses and reinforces the structural position of women vis-à-vis men in society (structural violence) as well as direct violence against women (IPV, rape, and femicide). Because cultural violence normalises misogynistic discourses, it can be likened to Marx's idea of 'false consciousness' in that 'the most intolerable conditions of existence can so often be perceived as acceptable and even natural' (Bourdieu, 2001:1).

Bourdieu's theory of symbolic violence is relevant here and demonstrates how the symbolic, for example, knowledge, art, social life, science, religion, and language influence worldviews or societal views and reinforce domination. This domination or injustice is hidden as the 'natural way of things', what Bourdieu (2001) refers to as 'Doxa', and he highlights the importance of questioning the 'taken for grantedness' of the world (Bourdieu, 1977). Bourdieu (1977) states that rather than accepting the social order as the way things are, we need to critically understand that relations within society are the result of history, power, and contextual factors, and not the natural order of things. Critical Race Theory, with its emphasis on race and racial difference as social constructs, as opposed to biology, is also relevant. Race, like gender, can be perceived as a system of oppression, which is socially constructed, and is a product of social contexts, social relations, and social organisation, which privileges 'whiteness' (Delgado and Stefancic, 2001). Within such a system, structural, cultural, and direct violence can be used to maintain a social order of oppression vis-à-vis people of colour; this is evident in events in the USA in relation to endemic police violence against black people (Mesic et al., 2018).

Femicide and Male Violence against Women and Girls

Male violence against women and girls is a significant global issue and implicates both structural and cultural violence. For example, the World Health Organization (2021b) estimates that around 736 million women, or one in three, have been exposed to IPV or sexual violence from a non-partner. Another issue is femicide or feminicides, the misogynous killing of women and girls by men, which is often legitimised by patriarchal social, and cultural institutions. This can include both intimate-related and non-intimate-related murder: honour and dowry-related killings, homophobic, and transphobic murders; and gender-based pre-natal abortions, as well as infanticide of girls (Radford and Russell, 1992). Across the globe, femicide is increasing at the same time as the general murder rate is decreasing (United Nations, 2019) and in 2017, 87,000 women were murdered, with 58% killed by family members (24%) or intimate partners (34%) (UNODC, 2019).

Women are, therefore, more likely than men, to be killed by people they know, with much of this violence being perpetrated in the home. Looking at specific countries, we can detect high rates of femicides in Honduras (6.2 femicides per 100,000 women) (Economic Commission for Latin American and the Caribbean, 2021); whilst in the UK, during the period 2009 to 2018, at least 1,425 women were killed by men, meaning that a woman died every three days (Long et al., 2020). In relation to regions of the world and intimate partner femicide, the African region has the highest rate, with 3.1 deaths per 100,000 women (UNODC, 2019), whilst concern has also been raised about the racist femicide of Indigenous women; with Indigenous women in Canada being approximately six times more likely to be murdered than non-Indigenous women (Canadian Femicide Observatory for Justice and Accountability, 2021).

Structural and cultural violence are implicated in male direct violence towards women and girls. Feminist critical theory shows us that patriarchal societies can be perceived to represent women as 'other' to men (De Beauvoir, 1949), and the 'otherness' ascribed to women is often characterised by one of dehumanisation, as well as dominance, with women subordinated to male power, and the structures which support male power. The subordination of women to men constitutes structural violence, creating inequalities, a lack of access to resources, including land and money, gender pay gaps, the devaluing of women's contributions, limits on freedom in public spaces, a lack of representation in politics, as well as criminal justice systems, which are discriminatory. Cultural or symbolic violence is also implicated within representations of violence against women in the media and in film, as well as hegemonic ideological justifications, which devalue women, and support the position which is ascribed to them. Direct violence by men, towards women and girls, therefore, reflects both structural and symbolic/cultural violence and is an exertion of power over the subordinated or devalued (Bourdieu, 2001). It is also important to understand how intersectional identities, such as gender and ethnicity, can make it more likely that women and girls are subjected to violence by men. Racialised violence by white men towards Indigenous women often has at its core structural inequalities such as the women's poverty, as well as colonial narratives, that represent Indigenous women as 'other', perceiving them as more disposable (Razack, 2016). This dehumanisation, as well as their socio-economic position, i.e., structural, and cultural violence, is likely to explain, in part, the higher rates of direct violent femicide towards this group of women (Razack, 2016; García-Del Moral, 2018).

Youth Violence

Youth violence, defined as physical fighting, to more severe assaults and homicide, is a serious global public health problem (WHO, 2020). Around 200,000 homicides occur each year amongst young people (defined as ages between 10 and 29), which account for 42% of the global homicide rate (WHO, 2020). Almost all the perpetuators of youth violence are male who account for 84% of the victims, with most of these victims being in low- and middle-income countries (WHO, 2015; 2020). Globally, youth violence appears to be decreasing, but this decrease is greater in higher-income countries, as opposed to lower- and middle-income countries (WHO, 2020). Youth violence not only impacts on young people directly in relation to injury and death but also impacts on the health and wellbeing of young people and their communities, which can lead to increased feelings of fear and decreased community cohesion, including depleted levels of social capital (WHO, 2015).

Structural violence is a causal factor in youth violence and all studies highlight structural elements, such as poverty, lack of opportunity, access to resources and power, discrimination, and marginalisation, as key to understanding direct violence, such as youth violence (WHO, 2015; Hyman et al., 2016). The Children's Commissioner for England (2019), for example, reported how structural factors, such as family poverty, living in high crime areas, high unemployment, local illicit drug trades, and economic inequality, were associated with youth violence and gang membership. Furthermore, Nation et al. (2021) demonstrate how, for example, social and housing policies contribute to the marginalisation of people of colour in the USA, which increased rates of community youth violence. Moreover, they highlight how many violence prevention interventions focus on individual factors, rather than social and structural factors, perceiving violence as a personal or interpersonal failing, as opposed to a societal structural issue.

This discourse of individual failure or choice can be perceived as a form of cultural or symbolic violence which supports structural violence (Galteng, 1990; Bourdieu, 2001) by obscuring how structural forces such as poverty impact youth violence. This is apparent in Zoetti's (2020) research in the Brazilian city of Salvador and the north-eastern state of Bahia, which have prominent levels of youth homicide, and violence related to gangs and the drug trade. Violent young people in these areas are represented as 'other', which supports, in turn, the State's extremely violent response to young people, who are categorised in this way.

They 'deserve' the violence which is meted out to them by police because they 'chose' to be 'bandits'. Moreover, the Brazilian government and the criminal system accept 'the violence perpetrated and suffered by marginalised youths as an unalterable social fact, inherent to their, supposedly chosen, condition of sub-citizens' (Zoetti, 2020: 275). This normalisation of individual choice in relation to violence results in the structural social conditions in which young people live, including high crime environments, and elevated levels of marginalisation and poverty, being played down as causal factors in their violent behaviour. Instead, cultural or symbolic violence shifts the responsibility away from societal ine-quality onto the young people themselves, further marginalising, punishing, and demonising them (Bourdieu, 2001), whilst simultaneously upholding the status quo, and systems of oppression.

Conclusion

This chapter has highlighted how violence is a global public health issue, which has been likened to an epidemic, requiring a public health approach, in its pre-ventions and identification. Critical social theories of structural and cultural violence have been introduced, and we argue that an understanding of these theories is key to understanding direct violence, such as youth violence and male violence towards women and girls. We have also argued that structural violence is a violent act and can impact upon communities and individuals, directly re-stricting their capabilities and opportunities to live a fulfilled and healthy life. An understanding of structural and cultural violence is key to violence preven-tion per se and needs to underpin policies and interventions, aimed at reducing violence.

Research Points and Reflective Exercise

With reference to the discussions in this chapter, begin to reflect upon the following:

1   Reflect upon your own country and explore a) how structural and cultural violence impacts the health and wellbeing of individuals and communities and b) what violence prevention policies have been introduced and how far do they engage with the concepts of structural and cultural violence?
2   How far do you think public health approaches can reduce violence?

Further Resources and Reading

Farmer, P. (1999). *Infections and Inequalities: The Modern Plagues.* Berkeley: University of California Press.

Fregoso, R. and Bejarano, C. (2010). *Terrorizing Women: Feminicide in the Americas.* Dur-ham, NC; London: Duke University Press.

Hamed, S. Thapa-Bjorkert, S., Bradbury, H. and Maina Ahlberg, B. (2020). "Racism in European Health Care: Structural Violence and Beyond". *Qualitative Health Research*, 30, (11): 1662–1673. https://doi.org/10.1177/1049732320931430

References

Alger, C. and Stohl, M. (1988). *A Just Peace through Transformation: Cultural, Economic, and Political Foundations for Change*. London: Routledge.

Bourdieu, P. (1977). *Outline of a Theory of Practice*. Cambridge: Cambridge University Press.

Bourdieu, P. (2001). *Masculine Domination*. Stanford, CA: Stanford University Press.

Brainard, L. and Chollet, D. (2007). *Too Poor for Peace? Global Poverty, Conflict, and Security in the 21st Century*. Washington, DC: Brookings Institution Press.

Butchart, A. and Engström, K. (2002). "Sex- and Age-Specific Relations between Economic Development, Economic Inequality, and Homicide Rates in People Aged 0–24 Years: A Cross-Sectional Analysis". *Bulletin of the World Health Organization*, 80 (10): 797–805.

Canadian Femicide Observatory for Justice and Accountability. (2021). "Trends and Patterns in Femicide". Available at: https://www.femicideincanada.ca/about/trends (Accessed: 18 May 2021).

Children's Commissioner for England. (2019). *Keeping Kids Safe: Improving Safeguarding Responses to Gang Violence and Criminal Exploitation*. London: Office of the Children's Commissioner.

De Beauvoir, S. (1949). *The Second Sex*. London: Vintage.

Delgado, R. and Stefancic, J. (2001). *Critical Race Theory: An Introduction*. New York: NYU Press.

Galtung, J. (1990). "Cultural Violence". *Journal of Peace Research*, 27 (3): 291–305. https://doi.org/10.1177/0022343390027003005

García-Del Moral, P. (2018). "The Murders of Indigenous Women in Canada as Feminicides: Towards a Decolonial Intersectional Reconceptualization of Femicide". *Signs: Journal of Women in Culture and Society*, 43 (4): 929-954. https://doi.org/10.1086/696692

Economic Commission for Latin American and the Caribbean (2021). "Gender Equality Observatory for Latin America and the Caribbean, Femicide or Feminicide". Available at: https://oig.cepal.org/en/indicators/femicide-or-feminicide (Accessed: 16 May 2021).

Gilligan, J. (1996). *Violence: Our Deadly Epidemic and Its Causes*. New York, NY: Putnam.

Hatcher, A.M. et al. (2015). "Intimate Partner Violence and Engagement in HIV Care and Treatment among Women: A Systematic Review and Meta-Analysis". *AIDS*, 29 (16): 2183-2194. https://doi.org/10.1097/QAD.0000000000000842

Houry, D. E. and Mercy, J. A. (2016). "Preventing Multiple Forms of Violence: A Strategic Vision for Connecting the Dots". Available at: https://www.cdc.gov/violenceprevention/pdf/strategic_vision.pdf (Accessed: 15 May 2021).

Hyman, I., Vahabi, M., Bailey, A. et al. (2016). "Taking Action on Violence through Research, Policy, and Practice". *Global Health Research and Policy*, 1, 6: 1-9. https://doi.org/10.1186/s41256-016-0006-7

Li, Y. et al. (2014). "Intimate Partner Violence and HIV Infection among Women: A Systematic Review and Meta-Analysis". *Journal of the International AIDS Society*, 17 (1): 18845. https://doi.org/10.7448/IAS.17.1.18845

Long, J., Wertens, E., Harper, K., Brennan, D., Harvey, H. et al. (2020). "Ten Year Femicide Survey: UK Femicide 2009-2018". Available at: Femicide-Census-10-year-report.pdf (femicidecensus.org) (Accessed: 17 May 2021).

Marmot, M. and Wilkinson, R. (2006). *Social Determinants of Health*, 2nd edn. Oxford: Oxford University Press.

Mesic, A., Franklin, L., Cansever, A. et al. (2018). "The Relationship between Structural Racism and Black-White Disparities in Fatal Police Shootings at the State Level". *Journal of the National Medical Association*, 110 (2): 106-116. https://doi.org/10.1016/j.jnma.2017.12.002

Nation, M., Chapman, D. A., Edmonds, T., Cosey-Gay, F. N., Jackson et al. (2021). "Social and Structural Determinants of Health and Youth Violence: Shifting the Paradigm of Youth Violence Prevention". *American Journal of Public Health*, 111(Suppl 1): S28-S31. https://doi.org/10.2105/AJPH.2021.306234

Our World in Data. (2021). "Suicide Rate in 1990 vs. 2017". Available at: https://ourworldindata.org/grapher/suicide-rate-1990-2019 (Accessed: 15 May 2021).

Radford, J. and. Russell, D. E. H. (1992). *Femicide: The Politics of Woman Killing*. New York: Twayne.

Razack, S. (2016). "Gendering Disposability". *Canadian Journal of Women and the Law, 28* (2): 285–307. https://doi.org/10.3138/cjwl.28.2.285

Roth, G. A., Abate, D., Abate, K. H., Abay, S. M., Abbafati, C. et al. (2018). "Global, Regional, and National Age-Sex-Specific Mortality for 282 Causes of Death in 195 Countries and Territories, 1980–2017: A Systematic Analysis for the Global Burden of Disease Study 2017". *The Lancet*, 392 10159: 1736-1788. https://doi.org/10.1016/S0140-6736(18)32203-7

Scheper-Hughes, N. (2004). "Dangerous and Endangered Youth: Social structures and Determinants of Violence". *Annals of the New York Academy of Sciences, 1036*: 13-46. https://doi.org/10.1196/annals.1330.002

Sen, A. (1982). *Poverty and Famines: An Essay on Entitlement and Deprivation*. Oxford: Oxford University Press.

Slutkin, G. (2013). "Violence is a Contagious Disease". In D. M. Patel, M. A. Simon and R. M. Taylor (eds.) *Contagion of Violence: Workshop Summary*. Washington, DC: National Academies, 94-111.

United Nations. (2015). *"Transforming Our World: The 2030 Agenda for Sustainable Development*. Available at: https://sustainabledevelopment.un.org/post2015/transformingourworld/publication (Accessed: 14 May 2021).

United Nations. (2019). "Femicide Press Release Rising Rates", 26 September. Available at: https://www.un.org/press/en/2019/dsgsm1349.doc.htm (Accessed: 15 May 2021).

United Nations Office on Drugs and Crime. (2019). "Global Study on Homicide: Gender-Related Killing of Women and Girls". Available at: https://www.unodc.org/documents/data-and-analysis/GSH2018/GSH18_Gender-related_killing_of_women_and_girls.pdf (Accessed: 17 May 2021).

World Health Organization. (2002). *World Report on Violence and Health*. Geneva: World Health Organization.

World Health Organization. (2015). *Preventing Youth Violence: An Overview of Evidence*. Geneva: World Health Organization.

World Health Organization. (2017). "Violence Prevention Alliance: The Public Health Approach". Available at: http://www.who.int/violenceprevention/approach/public_health/en/ (Accessed: 14 May 2021).

World Health Organization. (2020). "Youth Violence", 8 June. Available at: https://www.who.int/news-room/fact-sheets/detail/youth-violence (Accessed: 14 May 2021).

World Health Organization. (2021a). "Maternal Mortality Ratio". Available at: https://www.who.int/data/gho/indicator-metadata-registry/imr-details/26 (Accessed: 17 May 2021).

World Health Organization. (2021b). *Violence against Women Prevalence Estimates 2018.* Geneva: World Health Organization.

Zoetti, P. A. (2020). "It's Wrong, But That's the Way It Is. Youth, Violence and Justice in North-Eastern Brazil". *Social and Legal Studies*, 30 2: 272-290. https://doi.org/10.1177/0964663920915967

13

EVERY CHILD AND ADOLESCENT, EVERYWHERE

Contemporary Issues in Child and Adolescent Health

Abidemi Okechukwu, Babasola O. Okusanya, and John Ehiri

Introduction

A child, as defined by the United Nations Convention on the Rights of the Child (1989), is 'a human being below the age of 18 years unless, under the law applicable to the child, majority is attained earlier' (OHCHR, 1989; UNICEF, 2021). Most countries consider the age of 18 years to be the legal threshold for childhood. Previously, children were regarded as 'little' adults, erroneously creating the impression that health and life outcomes largely depended on genetic factors (Kotch, 2013). However, over the last four decades, scientific evidence has shown that an individual's growth and development are mostly shaped by the environment in which the individual is born, grows, lives, plays, and attends school (Marmot et al., 2008). Adolescence is a phase of life between childhood and adulthood. The World Health Organization defines adolescence as a period between the ages of 10 and 19 years and youths as people between the ages of 10 and 24 years (WHO, n.d.). This chapter will explore theories and contemporary global health issues of children and adolescents and their intersections with social and structural determinants of health.

Theoretical Approaches to Child and Adolescent Health

To conceptualise theoretical underpinnings of child and adolescent health, we will explore the shared understandings of the Social Determinants of Health (SDOH) framework, the Rights-Based Approach, and the Life-Course Perspective to health, to describe the multisectoral factors that influence child and adolescent health and outcomes.

DOI: 10.4324/9781003128373-13

Social Determinants of Health Framework

Worldwide, challenges to child and adolescent health have root causes that are directly related to the SDOH framework. SDOH are non-medical conditions that drive health outcomes and equity. These are conditions in which people are born, grow, attend school, live, work, and age (Marmot et al., 2008). The World Health Organization Commission on SDOH categorises SDOH into three domains. The first domain consists of upstream factors that shape the political and socio-economic environment; these include governance and political stability, policies, cultural beliefs and practices, and societal norms and values. The second domain is the social position which describes stratifications within a societal context. These factors include educational status, income and employment, gender identity, ethnicity, and race. Social position is an important construct that aids our understanding of inequities in health (Braveman et al., 2011). According to Diderichsen et al.'s (2012) model of social stratification, these stratifications create differential exposures to risk and protective health factors, vulnerabilities to these factors, and differential consequences. The factors in the first and second domains of the SDOH Framework are termed 'structural' determinants of health. The effects of these structural determinants are observed within communities and families, and these include material and living circumstances, neighborhood, and built environment, social and community contexts, psychosocial factors, biological factors, and access to quality health care systems. These intermediary determinants of health comprise the third domain of the SDOH framework. The SDOH framework provides an overview of the interconnections of structural and intermediary-level factors that determine the health status and outcomes for individuals within a social group or context. Structural determinants are constructs within a context that generate social stratifications and which create inequalities in access to services, vulnerabilities, opportunities, and differential health outcomes, and status. The strongest structural determinants of children's and adolescents' health are national and family-level income, access to education and healthcare, social cohesion, and availability of safe and engaging schools (Viner et al., 2012).

The Life-Course Perspective on Child and Adolescent Health

The Life-Course Theory suggests that health and wellbeing are determined by lifelong experiences from life before birth into adulthood (Elder, 1998). The Life-Course Perspective examines and affirms the role of social context, agency, and intergenerational linkages of health across multiple life stages (Johnson et al., 2011). The Global Strategy for Women's, Child, and Adolescent Health (2016–2030) recognises that an integrated life-course approach that links health across the lifespan, linking multiple facets of life and development, will be key for improving health outcomes among children and adolescents. This is based on findings from extensive research in social epidemiology, which posit that risks and protective factors in early life, combine either cross-sectionally or cumulatively to influence current, future, and intergenerational health outcomes (Kotch, 2013). Furthermore, the Lancet Commission on Adolescent Health and Wellbeing underscores a 'triple dividend of benefits now, into the future adult life and, for the next generation of children' if global health policies and interventions focus on the health and development of adolescents (Patton et al., 2016: 74). These global reports highlight the imperative to continuously expand the understanding of emerging issues that affect the health of children and adolescents, particularly, within their environment and social context (Bhutta et al., 2020; Tomlinson et al., 2021).

Rights-Based Approach to Child and Adolescent Health

Challenges that impact children's and adolescents' health, such as globalisation, inequities in access to resources, violence, and the effects of climate change on communities, threaten the safety and survival of children and adolescents, particularly in low- and middle-income countries (LMICs). Ensuring the rights of children to protection and safety, and access to intermediary determinants of health, will promote health and wellbeing (Goldhagen et al., 2020). The United Nations Convention on the Rights of the Child (1989) recognises that a child needs special safeguards including 'appropriate legal protections' that provide a framework that will improve the living conditions of children across countries (OHCHR, 1989). A Rights-Based Approach to health is grounded on the principles of social justice and health equity, where structural determinants of health can be optimised at a public health scale, to improve health and outcomes for children and adolescents. Adolescents face unique health problems and bear a significant burden of disease from unplanned pregnancy, teenage childbirth, unsafe abortion, female genital mutilation, and sexually transmitted diseases (Chandra-Mouli et al., 2015). Risk and vulnerabilities mostly originate from biological differences and inequities that are driven by the SDOH. Adolescents' sexual and reproductive health rights provide a benchmark for minimum investments in adolescent health.

Contemporary Issues in Global Child and Adolescent Health

COVID-19 Pandemic, Children, and Adolescents

The unprecedented impact of the COVID-19 pandemic on health and wellbeing since March 2020 has called for a re-evaluation of issues that affect children and adolescents across countries around the world. The pandemic worsened social and environmental conditions that determine health particularly, socio-economic factors such as poverty and education. Although all children and adolescents across the world have been affected by the pandemic, the effects of the pandemic will vary across contexts for children, and for some, these effects may be permanent and lifelong.

The COVID-19 pandemic plunged global economies into recession. With many people losing their livelihoods, household-level poverty increased, putting about 800 million of the world's children and adolescents in households that live below the poverty line (UNICEF, 2021). Children living in poor households increasingly become deprived of necessities such as food, clothing, or housing. This increases the vulnerabilities of children and adolescents to malnutrition (Coker et al., 2020), abuse, violence, exploitation, and child marriage (UNICEF, 2021). The pandemic also worsened conditions for learning and the ability to access quality education (Racine et al., 2021). School closures, in response to the pandemic across countries, have created gaps in learning, limited access to remote learning, and widened the already significant inequities in education for children and adolescents (Parolin and Lee, 2021). This disruption to learning and routines created distress, anxiety, and exacerbated existing or latent medical conditions in children and adolescents, especially mental health disorders (Racine et al., 2021).

Although children appeared to have been spared from the severe medical complications of the SARS-COV-2 virus infection, they were indirectly affected by strains imposed on weak healthcare systems (Coker et al., 2020). These strains reduced access to immunisation for children, treatments for common infectious diseases, such as malaria, diarrhea, and pneumonia, and access to reproductive health services for adolescents, and affected access to life-saving treatments for HIV and Tuberculosis, for both children and adolescents (Coker et al., 2020).

The Double Burden of Malnutrition: Undernutrition and Obesity

Malnutrition infers deficits, excesses, or imbalances in the intake of nutrients and energy. The term broadly applies to two main conditions. Undernutrition implies deficiencies in height for age (stunting), weight for height (wasting), weight for age (underweight) and micronutrients, and overnutrition, which could be overweight and obesity (excess weight for height and age). These two conditions of malnutrition were previously thought to be mutually exclusive in populations differentiated by socio–economic conditions such as wealth and lifestyle. However, malnutrition is increasingly having double-burden effects within populations. This means that within populations, communities, families, or within the lifetime of an individual, under-, and over–nutrition could occur simultaneously (Wells et al., 2020).

The rising rates of the double burden of malnutrition are increasing the risks for developmental retardation, reduced cognitive achievement, and non-communicable diseases, such as diabetes and hypertension among children and adolescents (Popkin et al., 2020). Although the double burden of malnutrition in LMICs has been simplified by attributing it to increased access to processed meals and beverages and reduced access to physical activity and exercises, the etiology of this phenomenon is complex, interconnected with broader issues, and can only be fully understood when analyzed through the lens of broader social and structural determinants of health such as changing food environments, diet diversity, and food security (Popkin et al., 2020).

Mental Health and Wellbeing

Worldwide, about 20% of children and adolescents experience mental health disorders (Clark et al., 2020). It is estimated that about 15% of adolescents aged 10–19 years have been diagnosed at least once with a mental health disorder and over 450,000 adolescents die from suicide annually (UNCEF, 2021). Across LMICs, the prevalence of mental health issues in children and adolescents is largely unknown (Erskine et al., 2021) and is stigmatised. Even in affluent contexts and countries, investments in children's and adolescents' mental health and treatments are insufficient. A recent study on the prevalence of anxiety and depression symptoms among children and adolescents during the COVID-19 era, showed an approximate 25% prevalence among children and 21% among adolescents (Racine et al., 2021). Before the COVID-19 pandemic, prevalence rates were about 11% for children and adolescents (Glied and Cuellar, 2003).

Given that about 40% of the world's population are below the age of 24 years, and the majority live in LMICs, humanitarian investments in mental health are very limited (Lu et al., 2018). Governments of LMIC rarely make upstream investments in mental health, leading to gross neglect in diagnosing and treating mental health problems in low-income settings. Unfortunately, the pandemic has widened disparities in accessing treatments for mental health for children and adolescents. It is also important to note that globally, minority populations, and marginalised communities, are being disproportionately affected by events that precipitate mental health challenges in children and adolescents, such as the death of family members or poverty (Benton et al., 2021).

Common substances misused among children and adolescents include alcohol, tobacco, marijuana, and illicit drugs. Substance use disorders are considered forms of mental health disorders, contributing to the global burden of mental health diseases among adolescents (GBD, 2018). Although substance use often begins during adolescence, when the brain is undergoing rapid development, the patterns and types of substance use disorders vary by context and country (Degenhardt et al., 2016). The largest impact of substance use disorders is seen in other health outcomes such as HIV and sexually transmitted infections and accidental injuries that lead to death (GBD 2016 Alcohol and Drug Use Collaborator, 2018). However, global studies indicate that less than 12% of children and adolescents with substance use disorder have access to treatments (Nock et al., 2017).

Sexual and Reproductive Health

The determinants of risk and vulnerabilities in reproductive and sexual health of adolescents are influenced by complex interactions between rapidly evolving biological growth and the socio-cultural and economic environment. While sexual initiation and sexual activity may vary across contexts, adolescents generally are reaching sexual maturity, and engaging in sexual activities earlier, and having diversified experiences based on their gender identities, sexual orientation, and their immediate living circumstance.

Adolescents are at high risk of numerous reproductive health issues: sexually transmitted infections including HIV, unplanned or teenage pregnancy, pregnancy-related morbidity and mortality, and unsafe abortions (Patton et al., 2016). Worldwide, over 200 million women have unmet need for contraceptives and adolescents comprise a substantial portion of people with this need. The main outcome of this need is unplanned and unwanted pregnancies (Morris and Rushwan, 2015). Although variations exist globally, early pregnancy among adolescents is common in LMICs. Over 10% of childbirths worldwide are by girls aged 15–19 years (Morris and Rushwan, 2015). Unwanted pregnancies among very young mothers predispose them to seek unsafe abortions, or develop pregnancy and birth complications, that increase the risk of death or disabilities (Igras et al., 2014). In addition to direct pregnancy-related health risks, pregnancy and childbirth create disruptions in education and other personal attainments, particularly among girls (Morris and Rushwan, 2015). Social determinants such as education and employment moderate sexual and reproductive risks among adolescents (Viner et al., 2012). Adolescents with opportunities to be meaningfully engaged tend to avoid high-risk sexual behaviors (Hindin and Fatusi, 2009). Additionally, technology and social media have strong influences on children and adolescents' choices and decisions regarding their sexual health (Viner et al., 2012; Guthold et al., 2019).

Communicable Diseases of Poverty

While communicable diseases continue to threaten the health and wellbeing of every age group across the globe, children and adolescents are at increased risk of diseases that are strongly associated with poverty (Kyu et al., 2016). Diseases of poverty are communicable and non-communicable diseases that are influenced by the socio-economic conditions of families and communities (Patton et al., 2016). Although diseases of poverty become less prominent as countries experience demographic and epidemiological transitions, they still pose a risk to sub-populations such as children and adolescents.

Endemic or common infectious and vaccine-preventable diseases that are communicable diseases of poverty such as lower respiratory tract infections (pneumonia), diarrheal diseases, malaria, and HIV, still pose devastating health risks to children and younger adolescents (Kyu et al., 2016). Older adolescents have higher risks of sexually transmitted infections and HIV.

Recommendations

Social and structural determinants of health for children and adolescents are multi-sectorial, comprising factors that are beyond the health system. In tackling these determinants, upstream, country, or context-wide interventions are necessary to create systems that offer equitable resources and access to services that promote health and wellbeing. Health services are critical as points of care, but they are not the only solutions to health issues in children and adolescents. Effective strategies will need to focus on groups that are marginalised and, on the fringes, to improve equity and access. Attention should be paid to the social and economic needs of children and adolescents from minority and marginalised groups within countries and contexts (Clark et al., 2020).

Policies, Systems, and Opportunities

Global calls to action on child and adolescent health have raised awareness and created roadmaps for strengthening child and adolescent health. These mechanisms and other relevant partnerships with country policy and legislative organisations should be institutionalised to ensure long-lasting outcomes. This will enable improved evaluation of policies and the flexibility that enables policies to respond to their varying needs. Partnerships and investments in health should encompass proximal, intermediate, and structural determinants of health (Patton et al., 2016). Children and adolescents need to be prioritised within the goals of Sustainable Development Goals (SDGs) and other programs and policies that aim to improve living circumstances and health access and outcomes for children and adolescents (Requejo and Strong, 2021).

Enhanced Access to Treatments and Prevention Services

Healthcare should be centred on children and adolescents to ensure that there are provisions for funding quality healthcare and increasing access to universal healthcare. Healthcare should be responsive and proactive to the unique needs of adolescents. For instance, reproductive health care and counseling should be private and non-judgmental to increase demand for, and use of, essential reproductive health services. Increasingly, as noted earlier, technologies and social media are influencing the behaviors of families and adolescents. Therefore, online interventions and social marketing that promote positive and protective behaviors should be prioritised. Telemedicine and telehealth provide enhanced opportunities to expand access to care and alleviate the effects of health system challenges, encountered by families and adolescents in low-income contexts. It is necessary to expand systems of care by increasing funding for mental healthcare that can reach adolescents and families of children through online adaptations and telemedicine (Benton et al., 2021).

Conclusion

Children and adolescents have health challenges that are common to the adult population. In this chapter, we have discussed health challenges that children and adolescents uniquely encounter across global contexts through the lens of social and structural determinants of health. Multiple studies have shown that children or adolescents are not 'little' adults. Rather, they are individuals whose brains, minds, and physical development are dynamic and constantly interact with the enabling, protective, and risk factors within their contexts. To tackle these challenges more broadly, upstream approaches should be employed to create enabling environments, policies, and structures, that will improve health outcomes over the life course of children and adolescents.

Research Points and Reflective Exercise

With reference to the discussions in this chapter, begin to reflect upon the following:

1   What are the broader factors that influence the health of children and adolescents in your country?
2   How do these issues affect children and adolescents in marginalised communities?
3   What are the key structural and systems-level interventions that can improve the health of children and adolescents in your country?

Further Resources and Reading

Marmot, M., Friel, S. and Bell, R., Houweling, T. A. and Taylor, S (2008). "Closing the Gap in a Generation: Health Equity through Action on the Social Determinants of Health". *The Lancet*, 372 (9650): 1661–1669. https://doi.org/10.1016/S0140–6736(08)61690-6

References

Benton, T. D., Boyd, R. C., Njoroge, W. F. M. (2021). "Addressing the Global Crisis of Child and Adolescent Mental Health". *JAMA Pediatrics*, 175 (11): 1108–1110. https://doi.org/10.1001/jamapediatrics.2021.2479

Bhutta, Z. A., Yount, K. M., Bassat, Q. and Arikainen A. A. (2020). "Revisiting Child and Adolescent Health in the Context of the Sustainable Development Goals". *PLoS Medicine*, 17 (10). https://doi.org/10.1371/journal.pmed.1003449

Braveman, P. A., Egerter, S. A. and Mockenhaupt, R. E. (2011). "Broadening the Focus: The Need to Address the Social Determinants of Health". *American Journal of Preventive Medicine*, 40 (1 SUPPL. 1). https://doi.org/10.1016/j.amepre.2010.10.002

Chandra-Mouli, V., Svanemyr, J., Amin A., Fogstad, H., Say, L. et al. (2015). "Twenty Years After International Conference on Population and Development: Where Are We with Adolescent Sexual and Reproductive Health and Rights?" *Journal of Adolescent Health*, 56 (1 Suppl): S1–S6. https://doi.org/10.1016/j.jadohealth.2014.09.015

Clark, H., Coll-Seck, A. M., Banerjee, A., Peterson, S., Dalglish, S. L. et al. (2020). "A Future for the World's Children? A WHO–UNICEF–Lancet Commission". *The Lancet*, 395 (10224): 605–658. https://doi.org/10.1016/S0140-6736(19)32540-1

Coker, M., Folayan, M. O., Michelow, I. C., Oladokun, R. E., Torbunde, N. et al. (2020). "Things Must Not Fall Apart: The Ripple Effects of the COVID-19 Pandemic on Children in Sub-Saharan Africa". *Pediatric Research*, 89 (5): 1078–1086. https://doi.org/10.1038/s41390-020-01174-y

Degenhardt, L., Stockings, E., Patton, G., Hall, W. D. and Lynskey, M. (2016) "The Increasing Global Health Priority of Substance Use in Young People". *The Lancet Psychiatry*, 3 (3): 251–264. https://doi.org/10.1016/S2215–0366(15)00508-8

Diderichsen, F., Andersen, I., Manuel, C. et al. (2012). Health Inequality--Determinants and Policies. *Scandinavian Journal of Public Health*, 40 (8 Suppl): 12–105. https://doi.org/10.1177/1403494812457734

Elder, G. H. (1998). "The Life Course as Developmental Theory". *Child Development*, 69 (1): 1–12. https://doi.org/10.2307/1132065

Erskine, H. E., Baxter, A. J., Patton, G. et al. (2021). "The Global Coverage of Prevalence Data for Mental Disorders in Children and Adolescents". *Epidemiology and Psychiatric Sciences*, 26 (4): 395–402. https://doi.org/10.1017/S2045796015001158.

GBD 2016 Alcohol and Drug Use Collaborators. (2018). "Alcohol and Drug Use Collaborators. The Global Burden of Disease Attributable to Alcohol and Drug Use in 195 Countries and Territories, 1990–2016: A Systematic Analysis for the Global Burden of Disease Study 2016". *Lancet Psychiatry*, 5 (12): 987–1012. https://doi.org/10.1016/S2215-0366(18)30337-7

Glied, S. and Cuellar, A. E. (2003). "Trends and Issues in Child and Adolescent Mental Health". *Health Affairs*, 22 (5): 39–50.

Goldhagen, J. L., Shenoda, S., Oberg, C., Mercer, R., Kàdir, A. et al. (2020). "Rights, Justice, and Equity: A Global Agenda for Child Health and Wellbeing. *The Lancet Child and Adolescent Health*, 4 (1): 80–90. https://doi.org/10.1016/S2352-4642(19)30346-3.

Guthold, R., Moller., A. B. and Azzopardi, P. et al. (2019). "The Global Action for Measurement of Adolescent Health (GAMA) Initiative—Rethinking Adolescent Metrics". *The Journal of Adolescent Health*, 64 (6): 697. https://doi.org/10.1016/J.JADOHEALTH.2019.03.008

Hindin, M. J. and Fatusi, A. O. (2009). "Adolescent Sexual and Reproductive Health in Developing Countries: An Overview of Trends and Interventions". *International Perspectives on Sexual and Reproductive Health*, 35 (2): 58–62. https://doi.org/10.1363/IPSRH.35.058.09

Igras, S. M., Macieira, M., Murphy, E., and Lundgren, R. (2014). "Investing in Very Young Adolescents' Sexual and Reproductive Health". *Glob Public Health*, 9 (5): 555–569. https://doi.org/10.1080/17441692.2014.908230.

Johnson, M. K., Crosnoe, R. and Elder, G. H. (2011). Insights on Adolescence from a Life Course Perspective". *Journal of Research on Adolescence*, 21 (1): 273–280. https://doi.org/10.1111/J.1532-7795.2010.00728.X

Kotch, J. B. (2013). *Maternal Child Health Programs, Problems, and Policy in Public Health*. Burlington, MA: Jones and Bartlett Learning.

Kyu, H. H., Pinho, C., Wagner, J. A., Brown, J. C., Bertozz-Villa, A. et al. (2016). "Global and National Burden of Diseases and Injuries among Children and Adolescents between 1990 and 2013: Findings from the Global Burden of Disease 2013 Study". *JAMA Pediatrics*, 170 (3): 267–87. https://doi.org/10.1001/jamapediatrics.2015.4276.

Lu, C., Li, Z. and Patel, V. (2018). "Global Child, and Adolescent Mental Health: The Orphan of Development Assistance for Health". *PLoS (Public Library of Science) Medicine*, 15 (3): e1002524. https://doi.org/10.1371/journal.pmed.1002524.

Marmot, M., Friel, S. and Bell, R., Houweling, T. A. and Taylor, S (2008). "Closing the Gap in a Generation: Health Equity through Action on the Social Determinants of Health". *The Lancet*, 372 (9650): 1661–1669. https://doi.org/10.1016/S0140-6736(08)61690-6

Morris, J. L. and Rushwan, H. (2015). "Adolescent Sexual and Reproductive Health: The Global Challenges". *International Journal of Gynecology and Obstetrics*, 131: (S1): S40–S42. https://doi.org/10.1016/J.IJGO.2015.02.006

Nock, N. L., Minnes, S. and Alberts, J. L. (2017). "Neurobiology of Substance Use in Adolescents and Potential Therapeutic Effects of Exercise for Prevention and Treatment of Substance Use Disorders". *Birth Defects Research*, 109 (20): 1711–1729. https://doi.org/10.1002/bdr2.1182.

Office of the High Commissioner for Human Rights. (1989). "Convention on the Rights of the Child". Available at: https://www.ohchr.org/en/professionalinterest/pages/crc.aspx (Accessed: 21 December 2021).

Parolin, Z. and Lee, E. K. (2021). "Large Socio-Economic, Geographic, and Demographic Disparities Exist in Exposure to School Closures". *Nature Human Behaviour*, 5 (4): 522–528. https://doi.org/10.1038/s41562-021-01087-8

Patton, G. C., Sawyer, S. M, Santelli, J. S, Ross, D. A., Afifi, R. et al. (2016). "Our Future: A Lancet Commission on Adolescent Health and Wellbeing. *The Lancet*, 387 (10036): 2423–2478. https://doi.org/10.1016/S0140–6736(16)00579-1

Popkin, B. M., Corvalan, C. and Grummer-Strawn, L. M. (2020). "Dynamics of the Double Burden of Malnutrition and the Changing Nutrition Reality". *The Lancet*, 395 (10217): 65–74. https://doi.org/10.1016/S0140-6736(19)32497-3

Racine, N., McArthur, B. A., Cooke, J. E., Eirich, R., Zhu, J. et al. (2021). "Global Prevalence of Depressive and Anxiety Symptoms in Children and Adolescents during COVID-19: A Meta-Analysis". *JAMA Pediatrics*, 175 (11): 1142–1150. https://doi.org/10.1001/JAMAPEDIATRICS.2021.2482

Requejo, J. and Strong, K. (2021). "Redesigning Health Programmes for All Children and Adolescents". *BMJ*, 372. https://doi.org/10.1136/BMJ.N533

Tomlinson, M., Hunt, X., Daelmans, B., Rollins, N., Ross, D. et al. (2021). "Optimising Child and Adolescent Health and Development through an Integrated Ecological Life Course Approach". *BMJ*, 372. https://doi.org/10.1136/BMJ.M4784

Viner, R. M., Ozer, E. M., Denny, S., Marmot, M., Resnick, M. et al. (2012). Adolescence and the Social Determinants of Health. *The Lancet*, 379 (9826): 1641–1652. https://doi.org/10.1016/S0140-6736(12)60149-4

United Nations Children's Fund. (2021). "COVID-19 and Children UNICEF Data Hub". Available at: https://data.unicef.org/covid-19-and-children/ (Accessed: 20 December 2021).

Wells, J. C., Sawaya, A. L., Wibaek, R., Mwangome, M., Poullas, M. S. et al. (2020). "The Double Burden of Malnutrition: Aetiological Pathways and Consequences for Health". *The Lancet*, 395 (10217): 75–88. https://doi.org/10.1016/S0140-6736(19)32472-9.

World Health Organization (n.d.). "Adolescent Health in the South-East Asia Region". Available at: https://www.who.int/southeastasia/health-topics/adolescent-health#:~:text=Adolescent%20health%20in%20the%20South,15%2D24%20year%20age%20group. (Accessed: 1 September 2021).

14

ARMED CONFLICT AND THE MENTAL HEALTH OF CHILDREN

Julia Morgan and Constance Shumba

Introduction

Armed conflicts, defined as 'any organised dispute that involves the use of weapons, violence, or force, whether within national borders or beyond them, and whether involving state actors or nongovernment entities' (Kadir et al., 2018: 2), are said to impact one in ten children worldwide with estimates of around 230 million children living in areas affected by conflict (UNICEF, 2015). In this chapter, we will explore the impact of armed conflict on children's mental health briefly, outlining community-based and trauma-based psychosocial interventions. We conclude by offering a critique of Western-focused psychosocial interventions, highlighting the importance of culturally responsive interventions, which take on board, locally socially constructed ideas of healing and trauma.

Armed Conflict and Children's Mental Health

Armed conflicts impact on children directly, for example, through death, injury, illness, hunger, trauma, increased violence, including sexual trauma, separation from parents, and impacts on mental health but can also impact on children indirectly. Indirect effects can be a lack of access to medical and education services, poor living conditions, disrupted social orders, and unsafe environments. Moreover, armed conflicts can mean that many children will have to leave their home and seek sanctuary in another part of the country (internally displaced) or seek refuge in another country (refugees and asylum seekers). Armed conflicts also involve children because they can become involved in the fighting themselves, either as 'child soldiers' or as porters and cooks for armed groups. It is said that the

DOI: 10.4324/9781003128373-14

impact on children of armed conflicts can continue throughout the life-course and impact on life chances (Kadir et al., 2019).

Exposure to trauma from armed conflict is said to lead to several mental health issues in children including post-traumatic stress disorder (PTSD), depression, anxiety, and suicidal thoughts (Dimitry, 2012). The prevalence of PTSD in children, for example, was found to be 23%–70% in Palestine and 10%–30% in Iraq, whilst in Rwanda, it was estimated to be between 54% and 62% after the 1994 genocide (Dimitry, 2012). The literature highlights how armed conflict can lead to prolonged stress responses in children, resulting in toxic stress, with Feldman et al. (2013) identifying changes in cortisol and salivary amylase in children, because of war stress. This may be exacerbated for children who are in extremely difficult circumstances because of gender (girls), unaccompanied children (who have lost or been separated from their parents/carers), or children with disabilities (Ataullahjan et al., 2020).

Research demonstrates, for example, that in Syria, an estimated 30% of children experienced toxic stress due to the unstable environment (Raslan et al., 2021); this manifested itself in nervousness, nightmares, sadness, and aggression, as reported by their parents, increased bed-wetting at night, and during the day, and many became mute or developed speech issues such as stutters (McDonald et al., 2017). This prolonged exposure to toxic stress and cortisol activation is said to disrupt their developing neuro-endocrine-immune response and, in some instances, physiological development (Franke, 2014). Continual multiple causes of trauma and toxic stress, therefore, have been highlighted, as not only having an immediate impact but also life-long impact on children's socio-emotional and mental health development and increased risk of several chronic physical and mental health difficulties in later life (Franke, 2014; McDonald et al., 2017).

The number of children involved in armed conflict as 'child soldiers' is increasing (United Nations, 2018). Many of these children perpetrate violence themselves and, at the same time, are subjected to violent acts, including torture and rape (Betancourt et al., 2020). Research has indicated that both shorter-term and longer-term mental health issues, amongst this group of children and former 'child soldiers', are worryingly high. However, not all 'child soldiers' report long-term mental health issues, and this may be a result of the level of trauma that they were exposed to, as well as other factors, such as stigma and levels of community and family reintegration (Betancourt et al., 2020). Su et al. (2021) in their longitudinal study found that children who were 'soldiers' in Sierra Leone during the civil war were more likely to report mental health issues, including PTSD, as well as hyperarousal, and difficulties in controlling emotions, if they had experienced higher levels of war trauma, including the perpetration of violence, being a victim of violence, and the loss of loved ones. They highlight that this has important implications for interventions in low-resource countries and that 'child soldiers' who report elevated levels of war involvement should be prioritised in relation to interventions.

Mental Health and Psychosocial Support Interventions

Inter-Agency Standing Committee (IASC) (2016) guidelines for mental health and psychosocial support (MHPSS) in emergencies highlight the importance of creative expressive, psychoeducational, and cognitive behavioural strategies to support children's mental health in armed conflict situations. There is a growing body of evidence on MHPSS interventions and practice in conflict settings, particularly in sub-Saharan Africa, although these are not always adequately documented (Kamali et al., 2020). In relation to psychosocial and trauma-based interventions, the focus tends to be on supporting resilience, management of stress, and conflict resolution, as well as trauma-focused cognitive-behaviour therapy and psychotherapy. Mindfulness-informed interventions are also popular and focus on improving wellbeing and decreasing stress (Franke, 2014). Other therapies, which focus on decreasing heart and respiratory rates, as well as breathing techniques and guided imagery, have also shown to reduce toxic stress (Franke, 2014). Narrative Exposure Therapy and meditation-relaxation were also found to improve recovery rates for PTSD (Catani et al., 2009). In the Narrative Exposure Therapy, children gave a detailed account of their biography, with the traumatic experiences recorded into a coherent narrative by a therapist, enabling them to relive the emotions. With the meditation-relaxation intervention, children went through six sessions involving assessment, participation in psychoeducation, followed by breathing, meditation, and relaxation exercises, led by counsellors (Catani et al., 2009). Moreover, in the Democratic Republic of Congo, a 15-session, group-based, culturally adapted Trauma-Focused Cognitive-Behavioural Therapy (TF-CBT) intervention was found to be effective in reducing post-traumatic stress and psychosocial distress among 50 former 'child soldiers' and other war-affected boys in a randomised controlled trial (McMullen et al., 2013).

There are a limited number of community-based interventions that have been empirically evaluated, with most of the peer-reviewed literature mainly focused on school-based interventions (Betancourt et al., 2013). A greater focus on the evaluation of interventions that strengthen community and family support is, therefore, required (Jordans et al., 2016). Nonetheless, 'Child Friendly Spaces' (CFSs) are often highlighted by humanitarian organisations as being key to supporting children's psychosocial wellbeing in armed conflict settings. CFSs are 'safe' community-based spaces where children can engage in 'normal' fun activities such as play, arts and crafts, drama, and have opportunities to make friends. These activities are normally facilitated by trained practitioners often from the child's own community. Since 2011, 'Syria Relief' operates CFS through school platforms to address children's exposure to toxic stress (Raslan et al., 2021). They work with trained psychologists, counsellors, case managers, social workers, and caregivers to provide group and individual support using a four-tiered approach namely: (1) provision of clothing, food, hygiene packs, and financial vouchers for vulnerable children and families; (2) community engagement through psychosocial support (PSS) activities and awareness campaigns on the importance of MHPSS, identification, and referral of at-risk children; (3) non-specialised support activities, often implemented directly at the schools, including guided art, sport, play, peer interaction, and skills-building activities; and (4) specialised focused services and treatment (Raslan et al., 2021). Another example of the implementation of CFSs is by 'BRAC', in partnership with the LEGO Foundation, Sesame, and UNICEF, who have been implementing the Humanitarian Play Labs, an MHPSS model in Rohingya refugee camps in Bangladesh since 2018 (Frounfelker et al., 2019). The CFSs provide safe spaces for children aged 0–6 years to access free and structured play and learning activities with adult supervision. The model combines play and PSS to address the mental health needs of children, delivered by trained paraprofessional play leaders, and has been lauded for its novel approach in humanitarian settings (Frounfelker et al., 2019).

Other forms of community-based interventions include art-based services such as 'Save the Children's HEART' programme in Syria, which supports children to communicate their feelings, through activities such as drawing, music, role-play, and drama (McDonald et al., 2017). School-based activities are also used to support psychosocial wellbeing and mental health. One example of a school-based programme was implemented in the Gaza Strip for Palestinian children. This included teachers, parents, social workers, and counsellors working with children using cognitive-behavioural technique to discuss and work upon traumatic experiences. Other activities also included games, physical activities, and drama to increase self-esteem, wellbeing, relationships, and cooperation amongst children (El-Khodary and Samara, 2020). School-based programmes can also include mentoring, after-school clubs, and use of lay counsellors (Ataullahjan et al., 2020).

Culturally Responsive Interventions: Critique of Mental Health and Trauma Based Interventions

Universal ideas of mental health and trauma, based on Western socially constructed biomedical categories of health and wellbeing, have been critiqued by many social scientists (Torre et al., 2019). The main tenet of the critique highlights that 'mental health' is socially constructed and the 'way in which people express, embody, and give meaning to their afflictions are tied to specific social and cultural contexts' (Honwana, 2006: 150). It is argued that the contemporary western focus on the individual, or person-centred emotions, underpins the increased emphasis on psychosocial interventions, to support mental health in armed conflict and humanitarian non-Western settings. This is seen as problematic for several reasons. First, a focus on individual trauma or emotions may not be recognised by many non-Western societies, who may be more likely to focus on distress, in relation to what has happened to the moral and social order, as opposed to them individually (Kirmayer, 1989). Moreover, the description of communities or individuals as traumatised can in turn undermine agency and result in the community or individual viewing themselves in this way (Armstrong,

2008). Second, the focus on (emotional) vulnerability means that resilience can be ignored (Torre, 2019), which leads to an emphasis on therapeutic medicalised interventions, as opposed to reinforcing existing local support networks and empowering communities. Imposition of Western values of trauma and individual emotions on non-Western societies could be perceived as a form of modern global imperialism, where Western ways of thinking become dominant across cultures.

It is also argued that Western-focused mental health and trauma definitions, which are used by the international humanitarian and aid communities across the globe, lead to the 'psychologisation' of non-Western populations (Enomoto, 2011; Pupavac, 2005) and constitute modern-day 'international therapeutic governance' (Pupavac, 2001), a form of control whereby 'global social risk' is managed to support Western interests. Pupavac (2001) questions the relevance of Western-based psychosocial interventions for war trauma in non-Western countries and highlights the importance of culturally and locally relevant support systems and coping strategies. Moreover, the medicalisation of war trauma is said to lead to the pathologisation of communities and individuals as being 'unable to function', pathologising normal responses to distress. This results in externally programmed 'psychosocial interventions implicitly [denying] the capacity of populations for self-government' (Pupavac, 2001: 365) and undermining responses to conflict, grief, and pain, which may be appropriate to the situation.

Although therapeutic psychosocial interventions are a hegemonic discourse amongst international stakeholders and humanitarian aid workers, there is lack of evidence on which psychosocial interventions work (Torre et al., 2019). For example, the evidence for the success of CFSs is limited due to the poor evaluation design of the interventions (Ager et al., 2013). Whilst some evaluations of CFSs found some short terms benefits, they did not demonstrate any longer-term benefits to the children (Metzler et al., 2019). Furthermore, CFS models have been noted to have a weakness in terms of community engagement (UNICEF, 2018). Torre et al. (2019) claim further that, in many cases, Western psychosocial interventions can do more damage than good and can lead to people claiming symptoms that they do not feel, to fit in with the categories of trauma, which aid agencies support. This was found in Honwana's (2006) work with 'child soldiers' in Mozambique and Angola and describes how returning 'child soldiers' 'quickly understand that their status as victims is crucial to obtaining aid (from non-governmental agencies (NGOs)......and are likely to enhance their victim status in the presence of NGOs' (Honwana, 2006: 15). This resulted in them telling the stories that they believed the NGOs wanted to hear e.g., stories of trauma, helplessness, and need for support to access services such as education and health, as well as other poverty eradication interventions. Torre (2019: 14) argues that there is also very 'little evidence that war-affected individuals in non-Western countries have regarded their mental health as an issue or looked for specific treatment for it en masse' (Almedom and Summerfield, 2004). This is problematic due to increased focus from NGOs on offering these services to local populations. Many donors who fund NGOs are based in Western countries and may have visions of what needs to be the focus of humanitarian development initiatives; hence services provided in non-Western countries, for example, may be influenced more by international dictates than local need (Morgan, 2016). The relatively recent focus on armed conflicts as 'psychological emergencies' may be justification for the NGO's presence in armed conflict situations, as well as justification to funders that they are doing something about the issue (Torre, 2019).

Honwana (2006: 4) stresses that for interventions to be effective and sustainable, they need to be 'embedded in local world views and meaning systems'. If mental health definitions are socially constructed, so too is the treatment of distress. In the Africa context, for example, this tends to involve community responses, family support, the role of ancestral spirits, and traditional healing approaches, rather than an over-reliance on individual Western biomedical models (Boyden and Gibbs, 1997; Summerfield, 1999; Honwana, 2006). There is a need for improved cultural understanding and cultural sensitivity about the mental health of children in non-Western refugee contexts to improve the effectiveness and acceptability of tailored intervention programs (Im et al., 2017). As an example, the linguistic barrier between Rohingya terms and Western concepts of mental disorders is an impediment in ensuring delivery of culturally sensitive and contextually relevant MHPSS services (Tay et al., 2019). Culturally grounded interventions can be achieved by engaging with communities to understand perceptions, management, and impacts of mental health within their cultural contexts, taking into consideration, the cultural concept of distress, and integration of existing support systems, encompassing psychosocial, behavioural, biomedical, and traditional and religious approaches (Im et al., 2017). Tailored culturally relevant family-based support is also important, as in many cases, children's distress in conflict settings may be a direct result of the trauma they experience themselves, but also a result of the distress that their caregivers experience, with parental psychopathology being a strong predictor of children's mental health (Eruyar et al., 2018).

Conclusion

Although international humanitarian aid agencies acknowledge the need for culturally sensitive programmes to support children in armed conflicts, there is an over-reliance on Western-influenced trauma-based interventions. This is problematic, we argue, because it can ignore the lived experiences and the cultural context of children, meaning that Western ideas of mental health and trauma become hegemonic in non-Western contexts. Ideas about mental health, distress, and trauma are socially constructed within specific cultural contexts and hence, interventions which aim to support children, should reflect the relevant social context, including traditional and local understandings of distress and healing. Critical Public Health theory and Social Constructionism can also provide conducive theoretical frameworks to locate the issues within, particularly emphasis upon the socio-economic context of suffering, trauma, and grief.

Critical Public Health and Social Constructionist theory, for instance, would emphasise the need for practitioners, to reflect upon hegemonic socially constructed Western discourses, such as trauma and mental health, to critically explore, that what may be taken for granted in one context, may not be the case in another. Context and setting are key to supporting children in armed conflict situations, as contextual cultural factors interplay with mental health, and adaptive mechanisms in a unique manner within these settings. Key consideration should be given to cultural factors to enhance diagnosis and management of trauma in children and reduce the intergenerational transmission of trauma, leading to an improved quality of life, and lessen social suffering. Finally, it is also problematic to infer that everyone within a conflict zone will be traumatised as it can lead to the 'psychologising' of whole communities and obscure evidence of resilience and community agency.

Research Points and Reflective Exercise

Here are some questions for you to reflect upon after reading this chapter:

- How far do you think concepts of trauma are universal as opposed to being culturally specific?
- In what ways can psychosocial interventions better reflect the lived experiences and worldviews of children in armed conflict situations?
- What empirically supported strategies are effective for promoting resilience among children, families, and communities in conflict settings?

Further Resources and Reading

McDonald, A. (2017). *Invisible Wounds: The Impact of Six Years of War on the Mental Health of Syria's Children.* United Kingdom: Save The Children.

Torre, C. (2019). *Psychosocial Support (PSS) in War-Affected Countries: A Literature Review.* Politics of Return Working Paper No 3. Available at: http://eprints.lse.ac.uk/100199/1/Torre_PSSin_War_affectedCountries.pdf (Accessed: 5 October 2021).

References

Ager, A. Metzler, J. Vojta, M. and Savage, K. (2013). "Child Friendly Spaces: A Systematic Review of the Current Evidence-Base on Outcomes and Impact". *Intervention,* 11: 133–148.

Almedom, A. M. and Summerfield, D. (2004). "Mental Well-Being in Settings of 'Complex Emergency': An Overview". *Journal of Biosocial Science,* 36 (4): 381–388. https://doi.org/10.1017/s0021932004006832

Armstrong, K. (2008). "'Seeing the Suffering' in Northern Uganda: The Impact of a Human Rights Approach to Humanitarianism". *Canadian Journal of African Studies/Revue Canadienne des Études Africaines,* 42 (1): 1-32. https://doi.org/10.1080/00083968.2008.10751371

Ataullahjan, A., Samara, M. Betancourt, T. S. Bhutta, Z. A. (2020). "Mitigating Toxic Stress in Children Affected by Conflict and Displacement". *BMJ*, 3 (71): m2876. https://doi.org/10.1136/bmj.m2876

Betancourt, T. S., Meyers-Ohki, S. E., Charrow, A. P. and Tol, W. A. (2013). "Interventions for Children Affected By War: An Ecological Perspective on Psychosocial Support and Mental Health Care". *Harvard Review of Psychiatry*, 21 (2): 70-91. https://doi.org/10.1097/HRP.0b013e318283bf8f

Betancourt, T. S., Thomson, D. L., Brennan, R. T., Antonaccio, C. M., Gilman et al. (2020). "Stigma and Acceptance of Sierra Leone's Child Soldiers: A Prospective Longitudinal Study of Adult Mental Health and Social Functioning". *Journal of the American Academy of Child and Adolescent Psychiatry*, 59: 715–726. https://doi.org/10.1016/j.jaac.2019.05.026

Boyden, J. and Gibbs, S. (1997). *Children of War: Responses to Psycho-Social Distress in Cambodia*. Geneva: United Nations Research Institute for Social Development.

Catani, C., Kohiladevy, M., Ruf, M., Schauer, E., Elbert, T. et al. (2009). "Treating Children Traumatized by War and Tsunami: A Comparison between Exposure Therapy and Meditation-Relaxation in North-East Sri Lanka". *BMC Psychiatry*, 9, (22): 1-11. https://doi.org/10.1186/1471-244X-9-22

Dimitry L. (2012). "A Systematic Review on the Mental Health of Children and Adolescents in Areas of Armed Conflict in the Middle East". *Child Care Health Dev*, 3: 153–161. https://doi.org/10.1111/j.1365-2214.2011.01246.x

El-Khodary, B. and Samara, M. (2020). "Effectiveness of a School-Based Intervention on the Students' Mental Health after Exposure to War-Related Trauma". *Front Psychiatry*, 10 (1031): 1-10. https://doi.org/10.3389/fpsyt.2019.01031

Enomoto, T. (2011). "Revival of Tradition in the Era of Global Therapeutic Governance: The Case of ICC Intervention in the Situation in Northern Uganda". *African Study Monographs,* 32 (3): 111-134.

Eruyar, S., Maltby, J. and Vostanis, P. (2018). "Mental Health Problems of Syrian Refugee Children: The Role of Parental Factors". *European Child & Adolescent Psychiatry*, 27 (4): 401-409. https://doi.org/10.1007/s00787-017-1101-0.

Feldman, R., Vengrober, A., Eidelman-Rothman, M. and Zagoory-Sharon, O. (2013). "Stress Reactivity in War-Exposed Young Children with and Without Posttraumatic Stress Disorder: Relations to Maternal Stress Hormones, Parenting, and Child Emotionality and Regulation". *Development and Psychopathology*, 25, (4 Pt 1): 943–955. https://doi.org/10.1017/S0954579413000291

Franke, H. A. (2014). "Toxic Stress: Effects, Prevention and Treatment". *Children (Basel)*, 1 (3): 390-402. https://doi.org/10.3390/children1030390

Frounfelker, R. L., Islam, N., Falcone, J., Farrar, J., Ra, C. et al. (2019). "Living Through War: Mental Health of Children and Youth in Conflict-Affected Areas". *International Review of the Red Cross*, 101 (911): 481–506.

Honwana, A. (2006). *Child Soldiers in Africa*. Philadelphia: University of Pennsylvania Press.

Im, H., Ferguson, A. and Hunter, M. (2017). "Cultural Translation of Refugee Trauma: Cultural Idioms of Distress Among Somali Refugees in Displacement". *Transcultural Psychiatry*, 54 (5-6): 626-652. https://doi.org/10.1177/1363461517744989

Inter-Agency Standing Committee. (2016). *A Common Monitoring and Evaluation Framework for Field Test Version Mental Health and Psychosocial Support in Emergency Settings*. Geneva: IASC.

Jordans, M. J., Pigott, H. and Tol, W. A. (2016). "Interventions for Children Affected by Armed Conflict: A Systematic Review of Mental Health and Psychosocial Support in

Low- and Middle-Income Countries". *Current Psychiatry Reports*, 18 (1): 9. https://doi.org/10.1007/s11920-015-0648-z

Kadir, A., Shenoda, S., Goldhagen, J. and Pitterman, S. (2018). "The Effects of Armed Conflict on Children". *Pediatrics.* 20, 142(6):e20182586. https://doi.org/10.1542/peds.2018-2586

Kadir, A., Shenoda, S. and Goldhagen, J. (2019). "Effects of Armed Conflict on Child Health and Development: A Systematic Review". *PLoS ONE,* 14 (1): e0210071. https://doi.org/10.1371/journal.pone.0210071

Kamali, M., Munyuzangabo, M., Siddiqui, F. J., Gaffey, M. F., Meteke, S. et al. (2020). "Delivering Mental Health and Psychosocial Support Interventions to Women and Children in Conflict Settings: A Systematic Review". *BMJ global health*, 5 (3): e002014. https://doi.org/10.1136/bmjgh-2019-002014

Kirmayer, L. (1989). "Cultural Variations in the Response to Psychiatric Disorders and Emotional Distress". *Social Science and Medicine,* 29 (3): 327-339. https://doi.org/10.1016/0277-9536(89)90281-5

McDonald, A., Buswell, M., Khush, S. and Brophy, M. (2017). *Invisible Wounds, The Impact of Six Years of War on the Mental Health of Syria's Children.* Save the Children.

McMullen, J., O' Callaghan, P., Shannon, C., Black, A. and Eakin, J. (2013). "Group Trauma-Focused Cognitive-Behavioural Therapy With Former Child Soldiers and Other War-Affected Boys in the DR Congo: A Randomised Controlled Trial". *J Child Psychol Psychiatry*, 54 (11): 1231-1241. https://doi.org/10.1111/jcpp.12094

Metzler, J., Diaconu, K., Hermosilla, S., Kaijuka, R., Ebulu, G. et al. (2019). "Short- and Longer-Term Impacts of Child Friendly Space Interventions in Rwamwanja Refugee Settlement, Uganda". *Journal of Child Psychology and Psychiatry*, 60: 1152-1163. https://doi.org/10.1111/jcpp.13069

Morgan, J. (2016). "Participation, Empowerment and Capacity Building: Exploring Young People's Perspectives on the Services Provided to them by a Grassroots NGO in Sub-Saharan Africa". *Children and Youth Services Review*, 65: 175-182. https://doi.org/10.1016/j.childyouth.2016.04.012

Pupavac, V. (2001). "Therapeutic Governance: Psycho-Social Intervention and Trauma Risk Management". *Disasters,* 25 (4): 358-372. https://doi.org/10.1111/1467-7717.00184

Pupavac, V. (2005). "Human Security and the Rise of Global Therapeutic Governance: Analysis". *Conflict, Security and Development,* 5 (2): 161-181. https://doi.org/10.1080/14678800500170076

Raslan, N., Hamlet, A. and Kumari, V. (2021). "Mental Health and Psychosocial Support in Conflict: Children's Protection Concerns and Intervention Outcomes in Syria". *Conflict and Health*, 15: 19. https://doi.org/10.1186/s13031-021-00350-z

Su, S., Frounfelker, R. L., Desrosiers, A., Brennan, R. T., Farrar, J. et al. (2021), "Classifying Childhood War Trauma Exposure: Latent Profile Analyses of Sierra Leone's Former Child Soldiers". *Journal of Child Psychology and Psychiatry,* 62 (6): 51–761. https://doi.org/10.1111/jcpp.13312

Summerfield, D. (1999). "A Critique of Seven Assumptions Behind Psychological Trauma Programs in War-Affected Areas". *Social Science and Medicine*, 48: 1449-1462. https://doi.org/10.1016/s0277-9536(98)00450-x

Tay, A. K., Riley, A., Islam, R., Welton-Mitchell, C., Duchesne, B. et al. (2019). "The Culture, Mental Health and Psychosocial Wellbeing of Rohingya Refugees: A Systematic Review". *Epidemiology and Psychiatric Sciences*, 28 (5): 489-494. https://doi.org/10.1017/S2045796019000192

Torre, C. Mylan, S., Parker, M. and Allen, T. (2019). "Is Promoting War Trauma Such a Good Idea?" *Anthropology Today*, 35 (6): 3-6. https://doi.org/10.1111/1467-8322.12538

Torre, C. (2019). "Psychosocial Support (PSS) in War-Affected Countries: A Literature Review". Available at: at: http://eprints.lse.ac.uk/100199/1/Torre_PSSin_War_affected Countries.pdf (Accessed: 5 October 2021).

United Nations. (2018). "Children and Armed Conflict – Report of the Secretary-General (A/72/865-S/2018/465) (EN/AR), 16 May. Available at: https://reliefweb.int/report/world/children-and-armed-conflict-report-secretary-general-a72865-s2018465-enar (Accessed: 1 October 2021).

United Nations Children's Fund. (2015). *More than 1 in 10 Children Living in Countries and Areas Affected by Armed Conflict.* New York: United States Fund for UNICEF.

United Nations Children's Fund. (2018). *Operational Guidelines on Community Based Mental Health and Psychosocial Support in Humanitarian Settings: Three-Tiered Support for Children and Families (Field Test Version).* New York: UNICEF.

15

AGENTIC DYING

The Global Imperative to Acknowledge Socio-Anthropological Aspects in Palliative Care Services for All

Carlos J. Moreno-Leguizamon, Marcela Tovar-Restrepo, and Ana María Medina Chavez

Introduction

In Reimagining Global Health, Farmer et al. (2013) called for social theory to enrich the action orientation of the health sciences. They argue that theoretical work can inform health services research and training, including diverse populations' dying processes. Palliative care would benefit from incorporating the humanities and social sciences to complement the biological aspects of dying processes, dominated by medical science (Moreno-Leguizamon et al., 2015). This chapter proposes three socio–anthropological arguments to be inbuilt into palliative care. First, pain is a biological condition and a social intersubjective relation (Das, 1995; Kleinman et al., 1997; Djordjevic, 2021). Saunders (2006) reimagined and reconceptualised this complexity as 'total pain'.

Second, modern hospices and homes are not the only locations where people may die. They can be places where dying is treated more humanely and sympathetically (Sallnow et al., 2022). Third, the concept of agentic dying, based on Castoriadis' idea of autonomy (1987; 1991; 1992; 1997), opens the space for self-reflection about dying processes with the facilitation of health professionals and institutions, which help reduce suffering. In turn, this enables us to critically reflect upon how, where, and with whom, we wish to die. The United Kingdom (UK) and Colombia are used to illustrate these issues.

The Global Need for Palliative Care for All

Palliative care is formally defined by the World Health Organization (WHO) as:

> ...an approach that improves the quality of life of patients (adults and children) and their families who are facing problems associated with a

DOI: 10.4324/9781003128373-15

life-threatening illness. It prevents and relieves suffering through the early identification, correct assessment and treatment of pain and other problems, whether physical, psychosocial or spiritual.

(WHO, 2020)

Further, it is one of the latest-recognised medical specialisations globally. For example, it was recognised in 1987 in the UK, and 2008, in the United States of America (USA) (Moreno-Leguizamon et al., 2017). However, it lends itself to misinterpretation from health professionals and the public. It is commonly assumed to be the healthcare you receive when you are dying or the type of care provided in hospices, which are 'new' places where people die, at least in advanced economies.

In most advanced economies, palliative care, as a medical discipline, has progressed immensely in the last 50 years, to the extent that there is now a marked differentiation between 'palliative' and 'end-of-life' care in the UK. Palliative care is the care needed when facing a long-term chronic or severe disease, and end-of-life care occurs, when a person is facing the 'last year' of life (Moreno-Leguizamon et al., 2017). In contrast to advanced economies, in low- and middle-income countries, there is still a need to recognise palliative care, end-of-life care, hospices, or alternative places to die, besides hospitals. In Colombia, death is an event that occurs in hospitals (Colombian Palliative Care Observatory, 2020).

According to the World Health Organization (2020), the current global picture of palliative care shows insufficient access to this service. Of the people requiring this type of care globally, only 14% receive it. Similarly, of the estimated 40 million people who need it globally, 78% are in low- and middle-income countries. The overall need for palliative care for children in low- and middle-income countries could be up to 98% (WHO, 2020). Additionally, this need is greater in low-income countries, which are mainly situated in Africa. Nonetheless, independently of the needs of countries of different income levels, the ageing population is globally increasing demand for palliative care.

Furthermore, the World Health Organization (2020) states that the global barriers to overcoming the insufficiency of palliative care services mean addressing misconceptions and misunderstandings around it. For example, the lack of inclusion in health policies and systems; training for professionals; access to opioid pain relief; awareness among policy makers, professionals, and the public; and education and self-reflection about death and dying from a cultural and social perspective, are missing from current debates around palliative care. The social sciences and humanities can contribute to the socio-anthropological aspects related to pain and dying, that palliative care, as a new medical discipline, does not currently include.

Social scientists have agreed extensively that pain and dying are events that, far from being merely biological and individual, are emotional, psychological, and cultural processes, which involve various intersectional identity markers, such as gender, ethnicity, class, sexual orientation, disability, age, location, and religion

(Moreno-Leguizamon et al., 2017). For example, ethnic minorities in the UK and USA have less access to palliative care services, due to lack of information, resources, and limited linguistic skills (Moreno-Leguizamon et al., 2017). Also, among certain ethnic groups in the UK, British Punjabi women indicated a preference for dying in hospital, while men's preference was for dying at home, implicitly revealing the type of care expected. Women expected better care in hospitals, while men expected care at home, by their carer/wife/partner (Smith et al., 2015).

Using Castoriadis' philosophical concepts (1987; 1991; 1992; 1997), pain, death, and dying can be defined as social imaginary significations, which provide meaning, and sense to the individual's lives. Social imaginary significations constitute the web of meanings that permeate, orient, and direct social life, providing internal cohesion, and routinised means of behaviour and culture. They produce what we call 'reality' or 'rationality' in our social and psychical life. Therefore, social imaginary significations are socio-historical meanings that give society norms, values, procedures, and methods to understand and construct lived experience (Castoriadis, 1987). It is through these, that processes of pain and death, are represented and managed.

Consequently, the social imaginary significations give meaning and identity to social institutions, which are defined as sanctioned symbolic networks, which function among human collectives. The social construction of social institutions is continuously in a state of contingency by individuals and collective discourses and directed by human agency and intentions. Therefore, social institutions never exhaust the creations of their social and functional roles (Castoriadis, 1997). As social constructions, both the social imaginary significations, and its produced social institutions, are not fixed. They are historically and contextually informed and are constantly changing, through significations and resignifications. Gawande (2014), in his account of recent history of healthcare and hospitals as social institutions, to cope with death and dying processes, illustrates this fact. For him, recent dying practices developed in hospitals do not produce the most effective outcomes.

The socio-historical meanings of pain and death can be questioned and altered by individuals and collective institutions, which are capable of self-reflection, to redefine, and manage 'quality of life' and 'quality of dying'. A current illustrative example in the UK is the grassroots movement, 'My Death, My Decision', which seeks compassionate legislation for greater choice in assisting dying adults with sound minds, who are terminally ill, or suffering from pain to an intolerable point (My Death, My Decision, 2022). Saunders (2006), the founder of the modern hospice movement, in her reimagining of a more sympathetic signification around treatments for cancer patients in the 1970s, revolutionised biomedicine with (1) the reconceptualisation of pain as total pain; (2) the creation of the hospice as an alternative institutional space to die; and (3) the opening of debates about more compassionate and sympathetic choices for dying (Moreno-Leguizamon et al., 2017). This is elaborated below.

Total Pain and Dying as Social Imaginary Significations

Moreno-Leguizamon et al. (2017) argue that Saunders's construction of the concept of total pain witnessed the emergence of the social, cultural, psychological, and spiritual dimensions that were rarely conceptualised by conventional biomedicine. The fact that she initially studied philosophy, later nursing and social work, and finally medicine, probably assisted her in designating the comprehensive and intersectional conceptualisation of total pain (Moreno-Leguizamon et al., 2017). This critical philosophical concept animates the modern hospice movement. However, this resignification of pain has had a limited impact on other areas of biomedicine, in which the conceptualisation of pain is still constructed, as a biological event, for example, pain clinics.

Total pain can be seen as an intersubjective relationship, where different intersectional identity markers are at stake, in addition to its biological condition (Das, 1995; 1996; Kleinman et al., 1997; Djordjevic, 2021). As ethnographic research in different contexts has shown, pain talk (Djordjevic, 2021) is related, not only to knowledge (as a medical object), but it is also associated with recognition and acknowledgement, or the lack of it (as an intersubjective relation) of the others' experience of pain. No one can communicate or transmit the experience of pain but through pain talk (Djordjevic, 2021). Since one cannot experience another's sensations, one must comprehend and apprehend pain through a narration of it. For this reason, empathy and compassion become central to the way pain is experienced, expressed, and acknowledged by others (i.e., medical doctors, nurses, carers, and institutions). Thus, understanding and acknowledging pain, when dying, is an intersubjective experience, informed by cultural content, and intersectional positionality.

Djordjevic (2021) has recently argued for a further conceptualisation that reimagines and recognises pain for its productivity, rather than a malfunction, to be eradicated from the body. For example, certain ethnic groups have rites of passage in which pain is inflicted to prove one can be regarded as an adult by others in the community; this illustrates that pain can be traded for belonging and coming of age (Djordjevic, 2021). Furthermore, he perceives in pain, political and transformative possibilities, such as in the recollection by Rev. Dr Martin Luther King Jr, of African Americans walking deliberately into fire hoses and vicious dogs during the 1950s–1960s, when the Civil Rights movement redefined politics in the USA. Hence, it is possible to observe how pain works as a symbol, which enables new and different expressions of identity, subjective content, and a sense of community.

Thus, concepts of pain and suffering, either as total pain or as productive pain, within palliative care for all, are strengthened, when partnered with the social sciences and humanities. Such acknowledgement will enable the development of the intersubjective, political, and productive dimensions of pain within the living-dying process, the place where we wish to die, and, finally, the concept that is proposed in this chapter: 'agentic dying'.

Hospices and Homes as Alternative Dying Institutions

Kakar (2014) has pointed out the intrinsic difficulty of admitting the complexity of dying as a multidimensional, inescapable human condition. As he points out, 'Death is not mysterious… yet the mystery of death lies everywhere' (Kakar, 2014: 17). Commonly, people only embrace death when it becomes imminent. This is due not only to the inherent emotional and psychical difficulties in accepting our finitude but also to the lack of social institutions, in most cultures, to prepare us to accept death. However, as this article attempts to demonstrate, the modern hospice, as reimagined by Saunders (2006), is a social institution, where people die, not only in an almost 'de-medicalised' way but also in a more compassionate and empathetic way (du Boulay, 2007).

'Home' was the oldest and most traditional location of death until its relocation, to mainly hospitals. However, when people use the word 'home', they seem to mean a familiar site (dwelling) rather than people's houses in the physical sense. Home as a familiar site has a long socio-cultural and historical history, in contrast to the hospital. As Gawande (2014) demonstrates, the hospital is a recent invention, or social imaginary signification, and one that is unlikely to be effective in terms of dying. Nonetheless, despite the similarities, the two locations operate differently. While hospices provide some minimum medical technology and facilities for daily care, such as symptom management and adapted facilities (beds, baths, and showers), homes can appear precarious or lack adequate infrastructure (Hoare et al., 2019). What seems clear is that these two institutions are serious alternatives to the traditional hospital, and its deficiencies, because of their new and radical approaches. Heubber and Sellschopp (2014: 215) note that Saunders stated: 'Hospice is not a place to go to die, but rather a concept of care based on the promise that when medical science can no longer add days to life, more life will be added to each day'.

In Colombia, for example, death at home may imply radically different meanings and symbols for various intersectional groups. For instance, for the poorest, it means a lack of essential public services, home adaptations for end-of-life care, and the presence of a caregiver, who is usually a woman. The general health system does not pay for direct and indirect costs to caregivers. Although Colombia is unique among non-industrialised economies with legislation regulating palliative care services, with the Law 1733 of 2014 (Congress of Colombia, 2014), the hospice has not become a recognised institution. Access to this type of care is limited and concentrated in urban centres (Hernández-Rico and Ballén-Vanegas, 2021).

A six-year research project attempted to understand the palliative and end-of-life care of black, Asian, and ethnic minorities in the Southeast of England through a Learning Alliance – LAPCEL (2019). Various groups of local stakeholders familiarised themselves with the hospice as an institution (Smith et al., 2015) through collaboration, training, public engagement, and dissemination of research findings through pictograms (LAPCEL, 2019). Overall, it was observed that the hospice, as a provider of care at the end of life, was friendly and sympathetic. As Djordjevic (2021: 11) clarifies, 'etymologically the root of 'empathy' 'is to feel with', to enter into another's pain and inhabit it with [them]'. Thus, the need for both the public and health professionals to familiarise themselves with the hospice, as an alternative institution for dying is urgent, as is the 'reimagining' of the hospice, or its equivalent in middle- and low-income countries.

In the UK, hospices have lately developed the infrastructure to support people dying at home, and this could also be a positive development for middle- and low-income countries where resources are scarce. Posing the question about 'dying institutions' and provision of care, nonetheless, raises the urgent need to challenge the unpaid or underpaid care work that the dying process implies. Globally, this work is mainly done by women, ethnic minorities, and migrants. This is another socio-anthropological aspect which needs to be explored as studies of dying and palliative care develop. The social sciences and humanities can assist here to affect all the socio-cultural, social, and even economic aspects of these two alternative institutions. In the UK, comparative studies of the costs for people dying in a hospital, hospice, or home are emerging, and they illustrate their financial viability, from the perspectives of governments, and health authorities. The case of the My Death, My Decision movement in the UK, sheds light on the perspective of 'public choice'. It includes advocacy for a place to die, and for agentic dying, which refers to the right to make decisions about one's dying process.

Agentic Dying as a Self-Reflection on How to Die

Societies have traditionally remained closed to discussing the processes of death and dying as social imaginary significations. They seek to defend themselves from a fear or the abyss of uncertainty of dying (Tovar-Restrepo, 2012). However, contesting the prolongation of life for the sake of it, as in the case of some biomedical practices, is an issue which contemporary discussions are challenging, as in the case with euthanasia, too. Only a few countries have legislated for euthanasia, including, among high-income countries: Belgium, Luxembourg, Canada, New Zealand, Spain, the Netherlands, and some states in the USA. Among middle- and low-income countries, Colombia is the only one to do so (Moreno-Leguizamon et al., 2017).

The concept of death revolves around a circle of heteronomy (e.g., subjection to religion or science) and the idea that death and dying institutions are self-instituted by society is emerging in social sciences (Castoriadis, 1987; Tovar-Restrepo, 2012). Castoriadis (1997) asserts, that even though heteronomy is socially present, there will always be an openness, which is a creative power, called the instituting imaginary, which opposes heteronomy. Autonomy, according to him, is the appropriation of creative capacity, or the power of self-institution, to provide meaning and sense, to central social imaginary significations and institutions, such as in the cases of death and dying. This is the reflective capacity of self-regulation and the deliberate actions and creation of our own laws, agency, and social significations, about death and dying practices. The concept of agentic dying proposed here is based on Castoriadis' notion of autonomy.

In practice, agentic dying requires the acknowledgment that the meanings, practices, understandings, institutional procedures, and regulatory frameworks of death and dying be collectively defined, to enable utmost autonomy for individuals, as opposed to prescriptive cultural or religious frameworks, such as 'intervention from God' (Tovar-Restrepo, 2012). The right to autonomously decide when to die, and how to die, lays at the centre of this discussion, as My Death, My Decision in the UK, illustrates. It also includes promoting and creating institutions that provide palliative care health services to plan (as much as possible) our individual deaths in ways that respect carers' and family members' rights. For example, this may include (1) death with dignity and autonomy, (2) identification of wishes and preferences of the dying individual (part of patient-centred care), and (3) decisions on the preferred site of death (Moreno-Leguizamon et al., 2017).

Recent debates on euthanasia have emerged globally, showing how important it is to collectively discuss it, especially within multicultural societies. The debate about legislation on euthanasia is also crucial to agentic dying as is death literacy (Sallnow et al., 2022). Agentic dying compels us to autonomously approach the psychical anxiety created by our human finitude, a human sentiment that we are more familiar with, than we might like to acknowledge. As unbearable as they might be, death and finitude are more frequent than one would like to accept, be conscious of, or be responsible for. Health professionals are only facilitators of the processes that are our responsibility and autonomy.

Conclusion

To conclude, following Farmer et al. (2013), this article has presented three critical socio-anthropological issues which underpin the recently founded science of palliative care. This paper discussed the need to complement the approach reimagined by Saunders with perspectives from the social sciences and humanities, which will enable the creation of social imaginary significations, and institutions around pain, death, and dying, and that will provide autonomy and responsibility, as suggested by Castoriadis (1987; 1991; 1992; 1997). This is called agentic dying. This chapter illustrated cases in the UK and Colombia where additional aspects related to palliative care are being discussed. It showed that pain, death, and dying can be resignified. Saunders reimagined these aspects: (1) the re-conceptualisation of pain as total pain; (2) the creation of hospices as alternative institutional spaces for dying; and (3) the opening of debates about more compassionate and sympathetic choices regarding the processes of dying (Moreno-Leguizamon et al., 2017). With the risk of more pandemic threats like COVID-19, climate and environmental disasters, structural violence, and health inequalities, we are being challenged to reflect on our dying processes and, by default, about quality of life and dying.

As this article was being submitted for publication on the 31st of January 2022, the Lancet Commission launched a report that validates the socio-anthropological arguments raised in this article. To quote from the report, this calls for:

> ...radically reimagining a better system for death and dying, the Lancet Commission on the Value of Death has set out the five principles of a real-istic utopia: a new vision of how death and dying could be. The five prin-ciples are: the social determinants of death, dying, and grieving are tackled; dying is understood to be a relational and spiritual process rather than simply a physiological event; networks of care lead support for people dy-ing, caring, and grieving; conversations and stories about everyday death, dying, and grief become common; and death is recognised as having value'.
>
> *Sallnow et al., 2022:1*

Research Points and Reflective Exercise

With reference to the discussions in this chapter, begin to reflect upon the following:

- How far do concepts of total pain and dying need to be researched further by social and health scientists?
- Is the concept of 'agentic dying' useful in thinking about dying processes?
- How far are debates around euthanasia relevant in middle- and low-income countries?

Further Resources and Reading

Sallnow, L. Smith, R., Ahmedzai, S. H., Bhadelia, A., Chamberlain, C. et al. (2022). "Report of the Lancet Commission on the Value of Death: Bringing Death Back into Life". *The Lancet*, 31 January 2022. (London, England), S0140–6736(21)02314-X. Advance online publication. https://doi.org/10.1016/S0140-6736(21)02314-X

References

Castoriadis, C. (1987). *The Imaginary Institution of Society*. Cambridge: The MIT Press.
Castoriadis, C. (1991). *Philosophy, Politics, Autonomy: Essays in Political Philosophy*. Oxford: Oxford University Press.
Castoriadis, C. (1992). "Logic, Imagination, Reflection". *American Imago*, 49 (1): 3–33.
Castoriadis, C. (1997). "Radical Imagination and the Social Instituting Imaginary". In. D. Curtis (ed). *The Castoriadis Reader*. Oxford: Blackwell Publishers, 319–338.
Colombian Palliative Care Observatory. (2020). "Educación". Available at: https://occp. com.co/dominios/educacion/ (Accessed: 23 February 2022).
Congress of the Republic of Colombia, Law 1733 of 2014". (2014). Available at: http:// www.secretariasenado.gov.co/senado/basedoc/ley_1733_2014.html (Accessed: 4 Jan-uary 2022)

Das, V. (1995). *Critical Events: An Anthropological Perspective on Contemporary India*. Delhi: Oxford University Press.

Das, V. (1996). "Language and the Body: Transactions in the Construction of Pain". *Daedalus*, 125 (1): 67–91.

du Boulay, S. (2007). *Cicely Saunders: The Founder of the Modern Hospice Movement*. London: Society for Promoting Christian Knowledge.

Djordjevic, C. (2021). 'The Politics In/Of Pain". *Philosophy and Social Criticism*, 47 (3): 362–388. https://doi.org/10.1177/0191453720912291

Farmer, P., Kim, J. Y., Kleinman, A. and Basilico, M. (2013). *Reimagining Global Health: An Introduction (Vol. 26)*. Berkeley: University of California Press.

Gawande, A. (2014). *Being Mortal: Mortal: Medicine and What Matters in the End*. New York: Picador, Metropolitan Books, Henry Holt and Company.

Hoare, S., Kelly, M. P. and Barclay, S. (2019). "Home Care and End-of-Life Hospital Admissions: A Retrospective Interview Study in English Primary and Secondary Care". *British Journal of General Practice*, 69 (685): 561–569. https://doi.org/10.3399/bjgp19X704561

Hernández-Rico, A. N. and Ballén-Vanegas, M. A. (2021). "Palliative Care in Colombia: Home Care Services, Access Barriers and Progress in the Implementation of these Programs during the COVID-19 Pandemic". *Revista de la Facultad de Medicina*, 70 (4). https://doi.org/10.15446/revfacmed.v70n4.95147

Heubber, P. and Sellschopp, A. (2014). "Adding Life to the Dying: Palliative Care and Psycho-Oncology" In. S. Kakar (ed.) *Death and Dying*. New Delhi: Penguin India, 213–222.

Kakar, S. (2014). *Death and Dying*. New Delhi: Penguin India.

Kleinman, A., Das, V., Lock, M. and Lock, M.M. (1997). *Social Suffering*. Berkeley: University of California Press.

Learning Alliance for Palliative and End of Life Care (LAPCEL). (2019). "Palliative Care and End of Life Practises". Available at: https://www.diversityhouse.org.uk/portfolio-items/palliative-care-end-of-life-practises-among-black-minority-ethnic-bme-groups/ (Accessed: 5 February 2022).

Moreno-Leguizamon, C. J., Patterson, J. J. and Gómez Rivadeneira, A. (2015). "Incorporation of Social Sciences and Humanities in the Training of Health Professionals and Practitioners in Other Ways of Knowing". *Research and Humanities in Medical Education*, 2: 18–23. https://doaj.org/article/711d3e763d4a4592911958a27f54de75

Moreno-Leguizamon C., Smith. D. and Spigner. C. (2017). "Positive Aging, Positive Dying: Intersectional and Daily Communicational Issues Surrounding Palliative and End of Life Care Services in Minority Groups". In. R. Docking and J. Stock J (eds.) *International Handbook of Positive Aging*. London: Routledge, 21–37.

My Death, My Decision. (2022). "What We Stand For". Available at: https://www.mydeath-mydecision.org.uk/ (Accessed: 5 February 2022).

Sallnow, L. Smith, R., Ahmedzai, S. H., Bhadelia, A., Chamberlain, C. et al. (2022). "Report of the Lancet Commission on the Value of Death: Bringing Death Back into Life". *The Lancet*, 31 January 2022. (London, England), S0140–6736(21)02314-X. Advance online publication. https://doi.org/10.1016/S0140-6736(21)02314-X

Saunders, D. C. M. (2006). *Cicely Saunders: Selected Writings 1958–2004*. Oxford: Oxford University Press.

Smith, D., Moreno-Leguizamon, C., Grohmann, S. (2015). "End of Life Practices and Palliative Care among Black and Minority Ethnic Groups (BME). Health Education Kent Surrey and Sussex Vision". Available at: http://www.diversityhouse.org.uk/

wp-content/uploads/2017/07/REPORT-End-of-Life-BME-Groups-101115-submitted.pdf (Accessed: 21 February 2022).

Tovar-Restrepo, M. (2012). *Castoriadis, Foucault and Autonomy: New Approaches to Subjectivity, Society and Social Change.* London: Continuum Press.

World Health Organisation (WHO). (2020). "WHO Definition of Palliative Care". Available at: http://www.who.int/cancer/palliative/definition/en/ (Accessed: 11 May. 2020).

16

NOMADIC PEOPLES AND ACCESS TO HEALTHCARE

Julia Morgan and Tumendelger Sengedorj

Introduction

Nomadic peoples are diverse and heterogenous groups who have high levels of mobility and move from place to place, often with their livestock, in search of resources, work, and food. Examples of nomadic or mobile peoples are African pastoralist groups such as the Turkana, as well as the Bedouin, and Mongolian Herders. It is difficult to estimate the number of nomadic peoples globally, due to their high level of mobility, and because they often inhabit remote and isolated places (Wild et al., 2019). In relation to nomadic pastoralists, some estimates put the number at 20 million pastoral households (de Haan et al., 1997: cited in FAO, 2016) or 200 million pastoralist individuals (Rota and Sperandini, 2009). These latter numbers, however, do not include other nomadic peoples, such as San hunter gatherers or groups such as Gypsies, Roma, and Travellers who have cultural traditions of nomadism. Access to healthcare is often highlighted as being problematic for nomadic peoples and is said to contribute to poor health outcomes. This chapter will explore access to healthcare for nomadic peoples, and link this to critical theory in relation to marginalisation, invisibilisation, and social justice.

Marginalisation, Invisibilisation, Health Inequalities, and Nomadic Peoples

Nomadic peoples are often described as marginalised (Moazzam et al., 2019; Shibli et al., 2021). Marginalisation is defined as 'a process...in which certain groups of people are pushed to the margins of society, and thus excluded from the mainstream' (Thompson, 2011: 92). Marginalisation can occur because of many factors such as socio-economic status, poverty, discrimination, ethnicity,

DOI: 10.4324/9781003128373-16

religion, geography or physical location, sexuality, culture, language, way of life, gender, illness, and disability (Thompson, 2011). Another term, often used for marginalisation, is 'social exclusion' (Duffy, 1995). Marginalisation is said to be problematic, because it can lead to inequalities between groups and individuals, which can impact upon quality of life and wellbeing. Social justice, which is often said to relate to the Rawlsian concept of 'fairness' (Rawls, 1972), is an issue in relation to marginalisation (please see Chapter 6 for a discussion of social justice). Marginalisation of groups and individuals can mean that they do not have 'fair' access to services that others have access to. Nomadic peoples, for example, often have difficulty accessing healthcare services, which impacts on health outcomes and increases health inequalities. This is true for Gypsies, Roma, and Travellers in Europe, also reported to have worse health outcomes, compared with the majority population, and poorer access to healthcare (McFadden et al., 2018). From a social justice and health rights perspective this is challenging, as health is perceived as 'one of the fundamental rights of every human being without distinction of race, political belief, economic or social condition' (WHO, 1946). It is also important to note how intersectionality can increase the effects of marginalisation and discrimination; Bedouin women, for example, can be marginalised not only because of being Bedouin but also because of their gender (Queder, 2007; Shibli et al., 2021). Crenshaw's (2019) theory of intersectionality is relevant, particularly the emphasis on group-oriented and structuralist approaches towards social change and how discrimination and disadvantage may be contingent upon other applicable intersecting categories. The intersectionality of ethnic group and gender can in turn further reduce access to healthcare services and increase health inequalities (for a discussion of intersectionality, please see Chapter 5).

The concept of 'invisibilisation' is also relevant to marginalisation. Invisibility can result from belonging to a marginalised social group, which reduces the group's social influence in society, and can impact upon the ability, as agents, to precipitate change. This simultaneously results in the group's needs, voices, and representation, not being mainstream priorities. Biehl (2005:259) defines this process as 'technologies of invisibility' and using the work of Foucault (1991) demonstrates how 'bureaucratic procedures, informational difficulties, sheer medical neglect, and moral contempt... all mediate the process by which (marginalised) people are turned into 'absent things''. Through 'technologies of invisibility', marginalised groups become ignored; they become invisible to mainstream society, and as a result, their needs are not recognised, increasing their marginalisation. Technologies of invisibility can, therefore, be perceived as forms of structural and symbolic violence, which renders injustices and people invisible (Bourdieu, 1977; Galtung, 1990). Please see Chapter 12 for a discussion of structural and symbolic violence.

Nomadic Peoples and Barriers in Accessing Healthcare

The World Health Organisation (2007) identified six building blocks which are essential to strengthening health systems. These include efficient, effective, and accessible health services, availability of well-trained staff, and the availability of medicines, vaccines, and medical technologies to all. Access to healthcare is a social justice issue and is important in improving health inequalities, reducing marginalisation, and supporting universal health coverage for essential health services. The United Nations' Sustainable Development Goal 3.8 target aims to 'achieve universal health coverage, including financial risk protection, access to quality essential healthcare services, and access to safe, effective, quality, and affordable' essential medicines and vaccines for all' (United Nations, 2015: 18). Access to comprehensive primary healthcare (PHC) is seen as one way in which this target can be achieved, especially for those who are socially or geographically marginalised (Sacks et al., 2020). However, there are issues in achieving this target, with more than half of people lacking access to universal essential health services worldwide (WHO, 2017) and primary care facilities still too far away for many isolated groups (Sacks et al., 2020). This is problematic as access to healthcare has been on the global health radar since at least the Declaration of Alma Ata (WHO, 1978: 1), which asserts that access to appropriate healthcare was essential to achieve 'health for all' by 2000. This focus on health for all, and the importance of access to healthcare, was reiterated in the Declaration of Astana in 2018 (WHO, 2018).

Nomadic peoples mostly have lower access and uptake of healthcare services than the general population (Sheik-Mohamed and Velema, 1999; Moazzam et al., 2019). For example, nomadic peoples in Eastern Africa were found to have lower access to maternal health provision, which contributed to higher rates of maternal mortality (van der Kwaak et al., 2012), whilst Roma in Europe were found to be three times more likely to have unmet health needs (Cook et al., 2013). There are many barriers to accessing health services, for nomadic peoples, including geographical location, lifestyles factors, affordability, language, and cultural norms, poor quality services, as well as marginalised status, which leads to their needs not being prioritised by governments and policy makers (Moazzam et al., 2019). The World Health Organization's (2007) six building blocks for health systems also identify the importance of health information systems, which capture reliable data, to inform service provision and delivery; however, there is a lack of data and academic literature on nomadic peoples and healthcare, which supports their invisibility and marginalisation in relation to service planning and provision (Randall, 2015). For example, Wild et al. (2020) found in their systematic review of the literature on nomadic health, that most academic studies were conducted in East Africa (64%), mainly in Ethiopia (30%), with the focus primarily on maternal health and TB. Sternberg et al. (2021) also note that nomadic peoples tended not to be included in COVID-19 assessments. Given that nomadic peoples are diverse groups, and live in most areas of the world, this lack of representation, or 'technology of invisibility', to quote Biehl (2005), is problematic, contributing further to their invisibilisation, marginalisation, and poorer health outcomes.

As was mentioned, one of the main barriers to accessing healthcare services for nomadic peoples is that of geography and mobility. Many nomadic peoples live in remote or isolated places, with very little healthcare provision available to them, as most healthcare provision is focused on urban areas and static populations (Moazzam et al., 2019). As a result, nomadic peoples may have to travel long distances to access healthcare; this is compounded by transportation issues (poor roads and lack of transport), having no one to look after their animals, whilst attending provision, and the cost of transportation to health centres, which means that accessing healthcare is often impossible (Caulfield et al., 2016; Jackson et al., 2017; Government of Mongolia, 2021). Moreover, geographical and mobility issues can result in services being too expensive to be provided directly to nomadic peoples in their own location (Schelling et al., 2008). Local provision of services is also challenging because many nomadic peoples live in areas with high levels of armed conflict, and this too can further impact the direct provision of services (Moazzam et al., 2019). Nomadic peoples are often missed by health and immunisation campaigns (Wild et al., 2020) with some research showing, for example, that among the Nigerian Fulani group, 99% of children were not immunised (Gidado et al., 2014). Movement throughout the year, because of their nomadic lifestyles, can also mean that they are absent during routine outreach community health interventions, especially if their needs and mobile lifestyles are not accounted for by service providers (Wild et al., 2020).

The quality of services can also be poor, which impacts on the take-up of services by these groups. Health services not only need to be accessible, but to ensure take-up, those provided need to be of effective quality, responsive, and acceptable to the local community. Shibli et al. (2021) highlight the importance of cultural competency for practitioners in their work with Bedouin women in Israel and detail how one woman, for example, was told to improve her diet by changing her traditional foods to blended drinks of bananas and cherries. Unfortunately, this was problematic advice for this group of Bedouin women, who did not have access to electricity for the proposed blender, or access to these fruits in their vicinity. Moreover, this advice devalued their traditional foods. The language of the Bedouin women was also not effectively accommodated for in healthcare settings and many of the women, especially the older women, did not speak Hebrew or Arabic, which impacted upon experiences of the services provided (Shibli et al., 2021). Affordability of healthcare is also an issue given that many nomadic groups do not have the financial means to take up healthcare services if they must pay 'out of pocket' expenses (Moazzam et al., 2019).

Marginalisation impacts on nomadic groups' access to healthcare services because their needs are often not prioritised by government or other agencies (Moazzam et al., 2019). Furthermore, the resulting discrimination against nomadic groups, who are often ethnic minorities within their country, can mean that services, when available, are poorly resourced and poor quality. This discrimination, in turn, can make it more likely that they did not take up services. For example, Caulfield et al. (2016) reported that pastoralist women in Kenya felt they would be shamed, or verbally or physically abused, if they went to hospital during childbirth. Whilst Wilunda et al. (2014) found comparable results with pastoralist peoples in Uganda, who reported negative attitudes towards them from hospital staff, and lack of respect. For the Bedouin of southern Israel, it was reported that there was 'bi-directional distrust between them and health institutions' (Hermesh et al., 2020: 1) and institutional healthcare discrimination was found to be widespread and a significant issue for Bedouin peoples in Lebanon (Chatty et al., 2013).

Improving Provision of Healthcare to Nomadic Peoples

Healthcare for nomadic peoples needs to be accessible, affordable, acceptable, of good quality, and culturally appropriate. It has been stated, in relation to educational provision for nomadic peoples, that this needs to be 'complementary to, rather than in competition with' pastoralist livelihoods (Dyer, 2014: 180). Similarly, healthcare should be understanding of nomadic lifestyles and livelihoods and be conducive to the continuation of nomadic lifestyles. Training of healthcare providers and policy makers around nomadic healthcare issues, cultural sensitivity, and lifestyles is, therefore, a priority. Moreover, the strengthening of rural healthcare facilities that cater to nomadic peoples is also a key consideration to ensure sustainability and coverage. This includes ensuring that awareness of healthcare services is increased amongst nomadic people, as there is often low awareness of provision, amongst some groups (Moazzam et al., 2019). The participation of nomadic peoples in the planning and implementation of healthcare provision is important to ensure that services are culturally appropriate and accessible.

Mobile healthcare or outreach services have been highlighted as one way in which to support the uptake of healthcare services for nomadic peoples (Moazzam et al., 2019; Wild et al., 2020). The Government of Mongolia introduced the 'Expanding use of mobile health technology in PHC towards universal health coverage in Mongolia' or M-Health' initiative, where PHC services were offered in remote areas to Mongolian Herders, through home visits, mobile health services, as well as a fixed health centre service (WHO, 2021). The use of telemedicine was also utilised, and Mongolian Herders used their phones to access information about healthcare services and preventative services. Other examples of mobile services include the Ng'adakarin Bamocha intervention for the Turkana nomadic groups of Kenya, whereby container health clinics were moved to the traditional migratory routes of the group, so that health services were within walking distance (Jillo et al., 2015). The use of Health Extension Workers including 'traditional birth attendants', who are local people from the same communities, is also recommended. These workers are trained to offer local healthcare services, which are safe and of good quality to nomadic groups (Kikuku Kawai, 2012; Umer, 2012). Mongolia has also introduced 'maternity waiting homes' for herder women in remote areas, who are at high risk of a problematic pregnancy, to stay in before they give birth, so that they can be monitored and transferred, more easily, to a health facility if needed (Maternal Health Task Force, 2018).

However, to achieve improved health outcomes, and health access to services for nomadic peoples, it is important that governments and policy makers ensure that the needs of these groups become visible and address their marginalisation. Their invisibility in relation to data collection and government priorities is an issue and contributes further to their marginalisation. For example, Gypsies, Roma, and Travellers in the UK are not included in the NHS data dictionary as an ethnic group, resulting in their needs not being recognised or well understood. Malagi (2012) reports of a community-based health management information system, used in Tanzania for nomadic peoples, that could be of use. This consisted of local people being trained to record information about key events in their lives, including deaths and births, as well as reproductive health, which was then shared with the Ministry of Health and community workers. Community-based initiatives, such as this, not only build local capacity but are also important to ensure data is available for remote, marginalised, and invisible groups, so services can respond to their healthcare needs. However, these types of initiatives do not absolve governments and policy makers (both international and national) from their responsibility to ensure that social justice measures such as universal health coverage, including data collection, are a priority for all including nomadic peoples.

Conclusion

Globally, there are many barriers for nomadic peoples in accessing healthcare services, and this may impact on health outcomes and increase health inequalities. We have argued, in this chapter, that it is important to understand how processes, such as marginalisation and invisibilisation, impact on the exclusion of nomadic peoples from healthcare provision. Nomadic peoples tend to be invisible to governments and practitioners, as well as invisible in relation to healthcare policy and data collection. This invisibility can impact on the healthcare provision that is available to them and, as a result, impact on their health and wellbeing. Sustainable, culturally appropriate initiatives, and interventions to support nomadic peoples, are required, as well as a commitment from governments and policy makers, to ensure the needs of nomadic peoples become visible, and are perceived as important. Access to healthcare is a social justice issue and is key to ensuring universal health coverage to reduce health inequalities and inequalities in access to healthcare provision.

Research Points and Reflective Exercise

With reference to the discussions in this chapter, begin to reflect upon the following:

• Reflect upon some of the barriers to healthcare for nomadic or semi-nomadic groups in your own country.

- How could these barriers be overcome?
- How is invisibilisation a factor in healthcare access for these groups and other marginalised non-nomadic groups?

Further Resources and Reading

Ajala, A. and Onyima, B. N. (2020). "Public Health Care Access: Burdens and Adaptation in Ibarapa Nomadic Community of Southwestern Nigeria". *Journal of Asian and African Studies*, 56 (7): 1590-1606. https://doi.org/10.1177/0021909620975806

McFadden, A., Siebelt, L. Jackson, C. Jones, H. Innes, N. et al. (2018). *Enhancing Gypsy, Roma, and Traveller Peoples' Trust: Using Maternity and Early Years' Health Services and Dental Health Services As Exemplars of Mainstream Service Provision.* University of Dundee. https://doi.org/10.20933/100001117

van der Kwaak, A. and Maro, G. (2012). *Understanding Nomadic Realities: Case Studies on Sexual and Reproductive Health and Rights in Eastern Africa.* Amsterdam: Royal Tropical Institute Press KIT.

References

Biehl, J. (2005). *Technologies of Invisibility: Politics of Life and Social Inequality, Anthropologies of Modernity: Foucault, Governmentality and Life Politics.* Oxford: Blackwell.

Bourdieu, P. (1977). *Outline of A Theory of Practice.* Cambridge: Cambridge University Press

Caulfield, T., Onyo, P., Byrne, A., Nduba, J., Nyagero, J. et al. (2016). "Factors Influencing Place of Delivery for Pastoralist Women in Kenya: A Qualitative Study". *BMC Women's Health,* 16: 52. https://doi.org/10.1186/s12905-016-0333-3

Chatty, D. Mansour, N. and Yassin, N. (2013). "Bedouin in Lebanon: Social Discrimination, Political Exclusion, and Compromised Health Care", *Social Science and Medicine,* 82: 43-50. https://doi.org/10.1016/j.socscimed.2013.01.003

Cook, B., Wayne, G. F., Valentine, A., Lessios A. and Yeh, E. (2013). "Revisiting the Evidence on Health and Health Care Disparities among the Roma: A Systematic Review 2003-2012". *International Journal of Public Health,* 58 (6): 885-911. https://doi.org/10.1007/s00038-013-0518-6

Crenshaw, K. (2019). *On Intersectionality: The Essential Writings of Kimberlé Crenshaw.* New York: The New Press.

Duffy, K. (1995). *Social Exclusion and Human Dignity in Europe.* Strasbourg: Council of Europe.

Dyer, C. (2014). *Learning and Livelihoods: Education for All and the Marginalisation of Mobile Pastoralists.* London: Routledge.

Food and Agricultural Organization of the United Nations. (FAO). (2016). *Guidelines for the Enumeration of Nomadic and Semi-Nomadic (Transhumant) Livestock.* Rome: FAO.

Foucault, M. (1991). "Governmentality". In G. Burchell, C. Gordon, P. and Miller, P. (eds.). *Governmentality, The Foucault Effect: Studies in Governmentality.* Chicago: University of Chicago Press, 87-104.

Galtung, J. (1990). "Cultural Violence". *Journal of Peace Research,* 27 (3): 291–305.

Gidado, S. O., Ohuabunwo, C., Nguku, P. M., Ogbuanu, U. I., Waziri, E. N. et al. (2014). "Outreach to Underserved Communities in Northern Nigeria, 2012-2013". *The Journal of Infectious,* 210 (1): 118-124. https://doi.org/10.1093/infdis/jiu197

Government of Mongolia. (2021). *Gender Analysis of Young Male and Female Herders Livelihoods*. Ulaanbaatar: Government of Mongolia.

Hermesh, B., Rosenthal, A. and Davidovitch, N. (2020). "The Cycle of Distrust in Health Policy and Behaviour: Lessons Learned from the Negev Bedouin". *PLoS One*, 15 (8): e0237734. https://doi.org/10.1371/journal.pone.0237734

Jackson, R., Tesfay, F. H., Gebrehiwot, T. G. and Godefay, H. (2017). "Factors that Hinder or Enable Maternal Health Strategies to Reduce Delays In Rural and Pastoralist Areas In Ethiopia". *Tropical Medicine & International Health*, 22 (2): 148–160. https://doi.org/10.1111/tmi.12818

Jillo, J. A., Ofware, P. O., Njuguna, S. and Mwaura-Tenambergen, W. (2015). "Effectiveness of Ng'adakarin Bamocha Model in Improving Access to Ante-Natal and Delivery Services Among Nomadic Pastoralist Communities of Turkana West and Turkana North Sub-Counties of Kenya". *The Pan African Medical Journal*, 20: 403. https://doi.org/10.11604/pamj.2015.20.403.4896

Kikuku Kawai, D. (2012). "The Role of Traditional Birth Attendants in Perinatal Care among the Nomads: A Case Study of the Maasai of Magadi, Kenya". In A. van der Kwaak A. and G. Maro (eds.) *Understanding Nomadic Realities: Case Studies on Sexual and Reproductive Health and Rights in Eastern Africa*. Amsterdam: Royal Tropical Institute Press KIT, 73-78.

Malagi, H. E. (2012). "Community-Based Health Information: A Key to Harmonizing Tradition and Formal Health Systems". In A. van der Kwaak A. and G. Maro (eds.) *Understanding Nomadic Realities: Case Studies on Sexual and Reproductive Health and Rights in Eastern Africa*. Amsterdam: Royal Tropical Institute Press KIT, 81-84.

Maternal Health Taskforce. (2018). "How Mongolia Revolutionized Reproductive Health for Nomadic Women". Available at: https://www.mhtf.org/2018/02/13/how-mongolia-revolutionized-reproductive-health-for-nomadic-women/ (Accessed: 26 May 2021).

McFadden, A. Siebelt, L. Gavine, A. Atkin, K. Bell, K. et al. (2018). "Gypsy, Roma, and Traveller Access to and Engagement with Health Services: A Systematic Review". *European Journal of Public Health*, 28: 74–81, https://doi.org/10.1093/eurpub/ckx226

Moazzam, A., Cordero, J. P., Khan, F. and Folz, R. (2019). "'Leaving No One Behind': A Scoping Review on the Provision of Sexual and Reproductive Health Care to Nomadic Populations". *BMC Women's Health*, 19 (161): 1–14. https://doi.org/10.1186/s12905-019-0849-4

Queder, S. A. R. (2007). "Permission to Rebel: Arab Bedouin Women's Changing Negotiation of Social Roles". *Feminist Studies*, 33: 161–187. https://doi.org/10.2307/20459128

Rawls, J. (1972). *A Theory of Justice*. Oxford: Oxford University Press.

Randall, S. (2015). "Where Have All the Nomads Gone? Fifty Years of Statistical and Demographic Invisibilities of African Mobile Pastoralists". *Pastoralism*, 5: 22. https://doi.org/10.1186/s13570-015-0042-9

Rota, A. and Sperandini, S. (2009). *Livestock and Pastoralists*. Rome: International Fund for Agricultural Development.

Sacks, E., Schleiff, M., Were, M., Chowdhury, A. M. and Perry, H. B. (2020). "Communities, Universal Health Coverage and Primary Health Care". *Bulletin of the World Health Organization*, 98 (11): 773–780.

Schelling, E., Weibel, D. and Bonfoh, B. (2008). *Learning from the Delivery of Social Services to Pastoralists: Elements of Good Practice*. Nairobi: International Union for Conservation of Nature.

Sheik-Mohamed, A. and Velema, J. P. (1999). "Where Health Care Has No Access: The Nomadic Populations of sub-Saharan Africa". *Tropical Medicine & International Health*, 4 (10): 695–707. https://doi.org/10.1046/j.1365-3156.1999.00473.x

Shibli, H., Aharonson-Daniel, L. and Feder-Bubis, P. (2021). "Perceptions about the Accessibility of Healthcare Services Among Ethnic Minority Women: A Qualitative Study Among Arab Bedouins in Israel". *International Journal for Equity in Health*, 20: 117 https://doi.org/10.1186/s12939-021-01464-9

Sternberg, T., Batbuyan, B., Battsengel, B. E. and Sainbayar, E. (2021). "Research Report: Covid 19 Resilience in Mongolian Pastoralist Communities". *Nomadic Peoples*, 25 (1): 141–147. https://doi.org/10.3197/np.2021.250117

Thompson, N. (2011). *Promoting Equality: Working with Diversity and Difference*, 3rd edn. London: Palgrave Macmillan.

Umer, J. Y. (2012). "The Contribution of Health Extension Workers in the Formal Maternal health Care Service in Afar, Ethiopia". In A. van der Kwaak A. and G. Maro (eds.) *Understanding Nomadic Realities: Case Studies on Sexual and Reproductive Health and Rights in Eastern Africa*. Amsterdam: Royal Tropical Institute Press KIT, 67–71.

United Nations. (2015). "Transforming Our World: The 2030 Agenda for Sustainable Development". Available at: https://sustainabledevelopment.un.org/post2015/transformingourworld/publication (Accessed: 14 May 2021).

van der Kwaak, A., Baltissen, G., Nduba, J., van Beek, W., Ferris, K. et al. (2012). "Sexual and Reproductive Health of Nomadic Peoples in East Africa: An Overview". In A. van der Kwaak A. and G. Maro (eds.) *Understanding Nomadic Realities: Case Studies on Sexual and Reproductive Health and Rights in Eastern Africa*. Amsterdam: Royal Tropical Institute Press KIT, 11–19.

Wild, H., Glowacki, L., Maples, S., Mejía-Guevara, I., Krystosik, A. et al. (2019). "Making Pastoralists Count: Geospatial Methods for the Health Surveillance of Nomadic Populations". *The American Journal of Tropical Medicine and Hygiene*, 101 (3): 661–669. https://doi.org/10.4269/ajtmh.18-1009

Wild, H., Mendonsa, E., Trautwein, M., Edwards, J and Jowell, A. et al. (2020). "Health Interventions among Mobile Pastoralists: A Systematic Review to Guide Health Service Design". *Tropical Medicine & International Health*, 25 (11): 1332–1352. https://doi.org/10.1111/tmi.13481

Wilunda, C., Quaglio, G., Putoto, G., Lochoro, P., Dall'Oglio, G. et al. (2014). "A Qualitative Study on Barriers to Utilisation of Institutional Delivery Services in Moroto and Napak Districts, Uganda: Implications for Programming". *BMC Pregnancy and Childbirth*, 14: 259. https://doi.org/10.1186/1471-2393-14-259

World Health Organization. (1946). '*Constitution*', *International Health Conference*. New York: WHO.

World Health Organization. (1978). *Declaration of Alma-Ata. International Conference on Primary Health Care*. Alma-Ata, USSR: WHO.

World Health Organization. (2007). "Everybody's Business: Strengthening Health Systems to Improve the Health Outcomes", WHO's Framework for Action, Geneva. Available at: https://www.who.int/healthsystems/strategy/everybodys_business.pdf (Accessed: 24 May 2021).

World Health Organization. (2018). *Declaration of Astana*. Geneva: WHO.

World Health Organization. (2021). "Mongolia's Mobile Health Clinics Bring Primary Health Care to Vulnerable Communities". Available at: https://www.who.int/news-room/feature-stories/detail/mongolia-s-mobile-health-clinics-bring-primary-health-care-to-vulnerable-communities (Accessed: 23 May 2021).

World Health Organization and the World Bank. (2017). "Tracking Universal Health Coverage: 2017 Global Monitoring Report". Available at: https://apps.who.int/iris/bitstream/handle/10665/259817/9789241513555-eng.pdf (Accessed: 24 May 2021).

17

LIVING IN A FOREIGN LAND

Refugee and Migrant Health and Related Health Inequalities

Floor Christie-de Jong

Introduction

Migration is not new and has been a global phenomenon throughout history. However, the number of people migrating has increased in the last five decades. There is no universally agreed definition of the term 'migrants', who are a heterogeneous group, and include refugees, persons seeking asylum, as well as documented and undocumented economic migrants. They range from individuals, who have recently settled in their country of residence, to those who have been resident for many years. Key definitions are presented in Table 17.1. The terms 'refugees' and 'migrants', preferred by the United Nations, are used here (UNHCR, 2021a; 2021b). Refugees and migrants face unique challenges through the process of migration and experience health inequalities as a result. Multiple barriers to accessing healthcare exist for them, including structural, economic, legal, cultural, and social factors. This chapter offers an overview of refugee and migrant health and health inequalities and uses a Socio-Ecological perspective to discuss barriers to accessing healthcare.

Migration

The International Organization for Migration (IOM) estimates that in 2020 there were 281 million international migrants (McAuliffe and Triandafyllidou, 2021). This is equivalent to 3.6% of the world's population or one in 30 people who do not reside in the country in which they were born. The number of international migrants has steadily risen; the IOM reported 128 million international migrants in 1990, 173 million in 2000, and 221 million in 2010. The proportion of international female migrants in 2020 was 48% and males 52%. The proportion of international migrants who are children is estimated at 14.6%.

DOI: 10.4324/9781003128373-17

TABLE 17.1 UNHCR Definitions (adapted from UNHCR, 2021b).

International migrants	Individuals born outside their country of residence including asylum seekers, refugees as well as documented and undocumented economic migrants.
Refugees	• Persons outside their countries of origin who are in need of international protection because of fear persecution, or a serious threat to their life, physical integrity or freedom in their country of origin as a result of persecution, armed conflict, violence, or serious public disorder.
Economic migrants	• Persons who leave their countries purely for economic reasons, unrelated to the refugee definition, or in order to seek material improvements in their livelihood.
Person seeking asylum	• Someone whose request for sanctuary has yet to be processed.
Internally Displaced Person (IDP)	• A person who has been forced or obliged to flee from their home or place of habitual residence, in particular as a resolute of or in order to avoid the effects of armed conflicts, situations of generalised violence, violations of human rights, or natural or human-made disasters, and who has not crossed an internationally recognised State border.

Of the 281 million international migrants reported in 2020, 89.4 million people were living in displacement, which includes 26.4 million refugees, and almost two thirds, 169 million, were recorded as economic migrants (McAuliffe and Triandafyllidou, 2021).

The USA is the top destination for migration over the last five decades, with Germany and Saudi Arabia in second and third places (McAuliffe and Triandafyllidou, 2021). Turkey hosts the largest number of refugees with 3.7 million people, followed by Colombia (1.7), Uganda (1.5), Pakistan (1.4), and Germany (1.2) (UNHCR, 2021a). India has the largest emigrant population with nearly 18 million people living abroad. The Syrian Arab Republic has over eight million people living abroad, mainly as refugees (6.8 million). A large proportion of refugees come from just five countries: the Syrian Arab Republic (6.8 million), Venezuela (4.1), Afghanistan (2.6), South Sudan (2.2), and Myanmar (1.1) (UNHCR, 2021a).

People migrate for a multitude of reasons, including economic, political, environmental, and social factors (Bhugra and Becker, 2005). These factors can be multifaceted and interrelated; migration is an immensely complex issue. Migration can be forced and can result from a range of extreme circumstances, such as war, natural disaster, or famine. Forced migration refers to movement that migrants such as refugees or IDPs make. Migration could also be perceived to be a voluntary process, for example, labour migration, for those in pursuit of better economic opportunities. The 2030 Agenda for Sustainable Development recognises that migration is a key component of sustainable development.

For example, migration can strengthen the global workforce and facilitates the transfer of skills and financial resources (McAuliffe and Triandafyllidou, 2021). International remittances are financial or in-kind transfers made by migrants directly to families or communities in their countries of origin and can be an important source of a country's economy (McAuliffe and Triandafyllidou, 2021). In 2020, India, China, Mexico, the Philippines, and Egypt were respectively the top five remittance recipient countries, with China receiving $83 billion remittances (McAuliffe and Triandafyllidou, 2021).

Labour migration does need to be viewed in context. For example, it could be disputed whether a low-skilled worker, living in poverty, with a lack of opportunity in their own country, who migrates and leaves their family behind for a low-paid job, truly has a choice. Individuals may not have choices. Rather, they have chances in life. Refugees and migrants may not experience having a choice as a realistic possibility in their everyday life, as their choices are shaped by life chances, which are embedded in structural and social contexts (Watson and Platt, 2002). Structural mechanisms such as social class, ethnicity, occupation, income, education, and gender lead to unequal distributions of power and health and relevant cultural resources in society. These structural mechanisms are the social determinants of health inequalities. Migration has become a social determinant of health and refugees and migrants face barriers in accessing appropriate levels of healthcare, which are detrimental to health and result in health inequalities.

Refugee and Migrant Health Inequalities

Not only do refugees and migrants often come from countries affected by poverty or conflict, but the process of migration also impacts significantly on health and wellbeing (WHO, 2018). The mental health of refugees and migrants is a major health concern and can be severely impacted by stressful events before, during, or after migration (WHO, 2021a). Refugees may have been exposed to armed conflict, violence, extreme poverty, and/or persecution pre-migration. The process of migration travel and transit could expose both to immense stress and even life-threatening conditions. For example, consider the tragedy in November 2021 when 27 refugees died when crossing the Channel between France and the UK (Refugee Council, 2021). Post migration refugees and migrants can also experience significant stress, for example, due to difficulties with social and cultural integration, or feelings of loneliness and missing loved ones (Bhugra and Becker, 2005; WHO, 2021a). Refugees and people who seek asylum have been found to have increased levels of post-traumatic stress, depression, anxiety, and suicidal thoughts (Shawyer et al., 2017; Blackmore et al., 2020).

Refugees and migrants also face other health inequalities. For example, both are exposed to an increased risk of infectious diseases, such as respiratory diseases, HIV/AIDS, Tuberculosis, and Hepatitis B, through the process of migration and overcrowded, poor living conditions, and inadequate hygiene services (WHO,

2021a). COVID-19 has posed additional challenges to refugees and migrants and the pandemic has had a disproportionate impact on these populations. A World Health Organization survey of 30,000 refugees and migrants suggested they were at increased risk of COVID-19 due to lack of social distancing measures through their living and working conditions (WHO, 2020). Increased feelings of anxiety and depression were reported. Lack of financial means, fear of deportation, lack of availability of healthcare providers, or uncertainty about entitlement to healthcare were reasons for not seeking medical care in case of (suspected) COVID-19 infection (WHO, 2020).

Refugees and migrants from low-income countries are also at increased risk of childhood preventable diseases, particularly, Measles, Rubella, Tetanus, and Diphtheria, due to insufficient immunisation and often lack immunisation records (WHO, 2021a). Furthermore, they are at risk of inadequate nutrition and lack of sufficient physical activity, potentially associated with an increased risk of non-communicable diseases (WHO, 2021a). Similarly, refugees and migrants have been reported to experience inequalities in disease prevention. For example, refugees and migrants engage less with cancer screening services than citizens in their host country, putting them at risk of higher cancer morbidity and mortality (Campbell et al., 2020; Fang and Ragin, 2020). There are indications that refugees and migrants experience poorer oral health outcomes compared to people in their host countries (WHO, 2021a). Additionally, both face inequalities in sexual and reproductive health. Refugee women face increased risks of unintended pregnancies, poor birth spacing, adverse pregnancy outcomes, higher rates of maternal death and morbidity, higher rates of postnatal depression, and increases in congenital abnormalities (WHO, 2021a).

A Socio-Ecological Perspective

Applying a Socio-Ecological conceptual framework to refugee and migrant health helps us understand the context and multitude of factors involved that impact the health of refugees and migrants. The Socio-Ecological conceptual framework for public health is a multi-level and interactive framework. The framework proposes that a single factor is not sufficient in explaining health behaviour and is founded on the idea that in population health, individual outcomes, or health problems, are complex and cannot be investigated, explained, or improved without examining multiple layers of influence on health outcomes, including the larger social context in which these individual outcomes were created (Rimer and Glanz, 2018). Although Socio-Ecological models differ somewhat in their presentation, they are consistently underpinned by the assumption of a structure-agency approach and an interplay between multiple factors as levels of influence on determinants of health and health behaviour, all embedded in a broader structural context. The Socio-Ecological model has been described as 'Russian dolls', in which each layer is nested within a broader level of influence (Reifsnider, Gallagher and Forgione, 2005). As a result, it is often subsumed under Critical Public Health frameworks but illustrates ways of viewing the structure and agency dualism, discussed in previous chapters.

The Socio-Ecological model uses four levels of influence on health: (1) individual factors, (2) social and cultural factors, (3) institutional factors, and (4) structural factors. Individual factors at the micro level, sometimes referred to as intrapersonal factors, are individual and demographic characteristics, such as age, ethnicity, or health beliefs, which may impact uptake on refugee and migrant health. Social and cultural factors include interpersonal factors, such as cultural health practices, or social support networks, that influence health and health behaviour. At the next level of the framework are institutional factors, which include access to healthcare, as well as interaction with the health workforce. The outer layer presents the macro level and broader context in which all other factors are embedded. Structural context could include larger economic factors, such as living and working conditions, which may directly or indirectly influence health, as well as larger societal, legal, and political factors, such as policies and regulations, regarding healthcare for refugees and migrants.

Barriers to Accessing Healthcare for Refugees and Migrants

Countries differ in their migration policies and the type of healthcare they allow refugees and temporary migrants to access. Policy settings and national legal frameworks can exclude certain migrant populations from accessing mainstream health services in their host countries (WHO, 2021a). Migration issues, such as achieving universal health coverage (UHC) and the promotion of a safe and secure working environment for all workers, including refugees and migrants, have been included in the UN 2030 Agenda for Sustainable Development (UN Sustainable Development Goals 3 and 8) (Ang et al., 2017). Whether refugees and migrants are included in UHC or whether UHC systems pertain to universal coverage for citizens of countries only is an important issue, and non-inclusion of refugees and migrants in UHC can be an important barrier to accessing healthcare (Guinto et al., 2015). UHC is a fundamental component of the World Health Organization's 'Health for All' (2012) objective, which is defined as 'the attainment of all people of the highest possible level of health and that as a minimum all people in all countries should have at least such a level of health that they are capable of working productively and of participating actively in the social life of the community in which they live' (WHO, 2012: 15). Host countries have a duty to refugees and migrants to ensure equitable access to healthcare, and human rights may be affected if the 'rights for all' are not adhered to.

Even if access to healthcare is granted by the host country, other barriers to accessing healthcare exist. Key barriers include language and cultural differences, lack of culturally appropriate services, low levels of health literacy, and inadequate use of interpreting services (WHO, 2021a). In accordance with the Socio-Ecological model, barriers do not stand by themselves but interact with barriers at other levels. For example, the post migration social conditions of refugees and migrants often place them at the lower end of the social gradient (Hynie, 2018) and refugees and migrants have been described as marginalised and stigmatised by their ethnic identity, as well as their temporary status (individual and structural factors). Health literacy, defined as 'the ability to find, understand and use information to promote and maintain good health' (UNICEF, 2021), is low for refugees and migrants and has been related to poor health outcomes (WHO, 2021a). Part of low health literacy is the lack of understanding of the host country's healthcare system, leading to refugees and migrants experiencing difficulties in navigating healthcare systems. Difficulties in making appointments, not knowing where to go, or ability to pay for transport have been reported as barriers (Cheng et al., 2015; van der Boor and White, 2020), (individual, institutional and structural factors).

Health literacy cannot be perceived separately from language, and by nature, refugees, and migrants experience language barriers. If health information is accessible (institutional factor) to them, this increases confidence, autonomy, and agency. In the absence of such information, refugees and migrants rely on their social networks or interpreters, although these can lead to feelings of disempowerment (Au et al., 2019). For example, refugees or migrants relying on children to translate information to healthcare providers can be stressful to both parties and can lead to children feeling overburdened or preventing refugees or migrants from disclosing sensitive health issues (BMA, 2022). Availability of interpreting services is limited in some countries, linked to structural factors, such as government policies, and lack of subsidies (WHO, 2021a). Additionally, refugees have been concerned about interpreters not telling their stories adequately and have reported confidentiality concerns about using interpreters (Cheng et al., 2015; Au et al., 2019). Fear of unknown consequences has also been reported as a barrier to accessing healthcare, such as fear of deportation (van der Boor and White, 2020).

Furthermore, refugees and migrants may possess other health beliefs and practices (individual, social and cultural factors) than their host country, and a disjuncture may exist with the host country's health system (institutional factors), which may lead to more stress and an increase in their perception of marginalisation, impacting health. Culturally appropriate healthcare and caring communication are important aspects of healthcare for them (WHO, 2021a). Interactions with the health workforce (institutional factors) can be an important influence on refugees and migrants, impacting on trust and confidence in the healthcare system and health workforce, and in turn, influencing future health behaviour. Experiences of discrimination due to ethnicity, accent, or language barriers have been reported for refugees and migrants (Cheng et al., 2015).

Case Study: Overseas Filipino Workers

In 2020, it was estimated that 2.2 million Overseas Filipino Workers (OFWs) were working abroad (Philippine Statistics Authority, 2020). It is estimated that OFWs typically support five individuals back home in the Philippines. Saudi Arabia was recorded as the country with the highest proportion of OFWs (22.4%), followed by the United Arab Emirates (13.2%), Hong Kong (7.5%), and Taiwan (6.7%). More than half (58.7%) of female OFWs were recorded to perform low-skilled jobs, such as domestic work (Philippine Statistics Authority, 2020). Domestic workers are vulnerable to abuse as they are often based in employers' private home and access to healthcare may be limited (Hall et al., 2019). There is limited research into the health of OFWs, but existing research suggests that OFWs may experience health inequalities.

A mixed-method study conducted regarding cervical cancer screening with 480 female OWFs based in 28 countries found low rates of uptake of cervical screening. Barriers to uptake of screening were complex and were found at all levels of the Socio-Ecological model. These included lack of in-depth knowledge of screening, limited access to healthcare, not knowing where to go, cost, fear, and lack of time. Poverty was found an underpinning and structural barrier to screening. Women reported that they had left their families and children behind to financially provide for them by sending money home. Most women had not seen their children for several years. Women expressed how this separation impacted on their mental health, describing feelings of sadness and loneliness. Women feared finding out the outcome of a cervical screening test, and worried about the financial implications of potential health issues, limiting their ability to send money home.

Women also described difficult living and working conditions, limited time off, and opportunity to attend cervical screening, or being scared to ask their employer, underpinned by fear of deportation (Christie-de Jong and Reilly, 2020). This study illustrates the complexity of migrant health, the many Socio-Ecological factors involved, and the interaction between these factors, ultimately underpinned by the structural factor poverty. The study also shows it is vital to view health behaviour in the context of the wider circumstances in which we are born, grow, live, work, and age in, the social determinants of health.

Action

Almost 12 years after the first World Health Organization consultation on the health of refugees and migrants in 2008, a WHO Global Action Plan: Promoting the health of refugees and migrants (the Global Action Plan) was agreed upon by the 72nd World Health Assembly in 2019 (WHO, 2019). The plan is a clear attempt to prioritise refugees and migrant health, prevent health inequalities, strengthen international collaboration to protect refugees' and migrants' health and wellbeing, and contribute to the 2030 Agenda for Sustainable Development. The plan has been critiqued for lacking a clear direction for accountability (Onarheim and Rached, 2020). In 2021, the World Health Organization released their Global Competency Standards for Refugee and Migrant Health Services, acknowledging the pressing need to develop cultural competency in the global health workforce, invest in community-centred approaches to support refugees and migrants appropriately, and manage health systems' responsiveness to refugee and migrant health needs (WHO, 2021b). Health inequalities need to be tackled at all levels of the Socio-Ecological model, including tackling structural mechanisms at the root causes of health inequalities related to migration, for example, by adopting a 'Health in All Policies' approach, as essential steps in protecting refugees' and migrants' health.

Conclusion

With vast numbers of refugees and migrants worldwide, migrant health and equity to healthcare are more important than ever. Refugees and migrants face challenges throughout the migration process, that may affect their health, and access to healthcare may become compromised, resulting in health inequalities. Migration is complex and a Socio-Ecological approach ensures health inequalities are tackled at all levels. Refugees and migrants have the fundamental right to the enjoyment of the highest attainable standard of health. Healthcare systems need to be sensitive and appropriate to the needs of refugees both and developing health workforces' cultural competency is an essential part of protecting their health. The process of migration is a social determinant of health and preventing health inequalities for refugees and migrants must be achieved through a community centred and 'Health for All' approach, essential in assuming a Critical Public Health approach.

Research Points and Reflective Exercise

With reference to the discussions in this chapter, begin to reflect upon the following:

1 What are some of the factors that contribute to increased health inequities for refugees and migrants?

2 Who do you think is responsible for the health of refugees and migrants?
3 Which approach is most likely to achieve health equity for refugees and migrants?

For full definitions please refer to the United Nation High Commissioner for Refugees (UNHCR) Glossary (see reference list)

Resources and Further Reading

Hynie, M. (2018). 'The Social Determinants of Refugee Mental Health in the Post-Migration Context: A Critical Review". *The Canadian Journal of Psychiatry*, 63 (5): 297–303. https://doi.org/10.1177/0706743717746666
World Health Organization. (2021). "Common Health Needs of Refugees and Migrants: Literature Review". Available at: https://www.who.int/publications/i/-item/9789240033108 (Accessed: 4 January 2022).

References

Ang, J. W., Chia, C., Koh, C. J., Chua, B. W. B., Narayanaswamy, S. et al. (2017). "Healthcare-Seeking Behaviour, Barriers and Mental Health of Non-Domestic Migrant Workers in Singapore". *BMJ Global Health*, 2 (2): e000213. https://doi.org/-10.1136/bmjgh-2016-000213.
Au, M., Anandakumar, A. D., Preston, R., Ray, R. A. and Davis, M. et al. (2019). "A model Explaining Refugee Experiences of the Australian Healthcare System: A Systematic Review of Refugee Perceptions". *BMC International Health and Human Rights*, 19: 22. https://doi.org/10.1186/S12914-019-0206-6/TABLES/4.
Bhugra, D. and Becker, M. A. (2005). "Migration, Cultural Bereavement and Cultural Identity". *World Psychiatry: Official Journal of the World Psychiatric Association (WPA)*, 4 (1): 18–24.
Blackmore, R., Boyle, J. A., Fazel, M., Ranasinha S., Gray, K. M. et al. (2020). "The Prevalence of Mental Illness in Refugees and Asylum Seekers: A Systematic Review and Meta-Analysis. *PLoS (Public Library of Science) Med*, 21 (17): 9:e1003337. https://-doi.org/10.1371/journal.pmed.1003337. PMID:
British Medical Association. (2022). "Managing Language Barriers for Refugees and Asylum Seekers - Refugee and Asylum Seeker Patient Health Toolkit". Available at: https://www.bma.org.uk/advice-and-support/ethics/refugees-overseas-visitors-and-vulnerable-migrants/refugee-and-asylum-seeker-patient-health-toolkit/managing-language-barriers-for-refugees-and-asylum-seekers' (Accessed: 7 January 2022).
Campbell, C., Douglas, A., Williams, L., Cezard, G., Brewster, D. H. et al. (2020). "Are There Ethnic and Religious Variations in Uptake of Bowel Cancer Screening? A Retrospective Cohort Study Among 1.7 million People in Scotland". *BMJ Open*, 7 (10): 10 e037011. https://doi.org/10.1136/bmjopen-2020-037011.
Cheng, I. H., Drillich, A. and Schattner, P. (2015) "Refugee Experiences of General Practice In Countries of Resettlement: A Literature Review". *British Journal of General Practice*, 65 (632): 171–176. https://doi.org/10.3399/bjgp15X683977.
Christie-de Jong, F. and Reilly, S. (2020) "Barriers and Facilitators to Pap-Testing Among Female Overseas Filipino Workers: A Qualitative Exploration". *International Journal of Human Rights in Healthcare*, 17 (1): 16–34. https://doi.org/10.1108/ijhrh-01-2020-0006.

Fang, C. Y. and Ragin, C. C. (2020). "Addressing Disparities in Cancer Screening among U.S. Immigrants: Progress and Opportunities". *Cancer Prevention Research,* 13 (3): 253–260. https://doi.org/10.1158/1940-6207.CAPR-19-0249.

Guinto, R. L., Curran, U. Z., Suphanchaimat, R. and Pocock, N. S. (2015). "Universal Health Coverage in 'One ASEAN': Are Migrants Included?" *Global Health Action,* 8: 25749. https://doi.org/10.3402/gha.v8.25749

Hall, B. J., Pangan, C. A. C., Chan, E. W. W. and Huang, R. L. (2019). 'The Effect of Discrimination on Depression and Anxiety Symptoms and the Buffering Role of Social Capital Among Female Domestic Workers in Macao, China". *Psychiatry Research,* 271: 200–207. https://doi.org/10.1016/j.psychres.2018.11.050.

Hynie, M. (2018). "The Social Determinants of Refugee Mental Health in the Post-Migration Context: A Critical Review". *Canadian journal of psychiatry,* 63 (5): 297–303. https://doi.org/10.1177/0706743717746666.

McAuliffe, M. and Triandafyllidou, A. (2021). *World Migration Report 2022.* Geneva: IOM.

Onarheim, K. H. and Rached, D. H. (2020). "Searching For Accountability: Can the WHO Global Action Plan for Refugees and Migrants Deliver?" *BMJ Global Health,* 5 (6): e002095. https://doi.org/10.1136/BMJGH-2019-002095.

Philippine Statistics Authority. (2020). "2019 Overseas Filipino Workers (OFWs) Survey". Available at: https://psa.gov.ph/statistics/survey/labor-and-employment/survey-overseas-filipinos/title/Total' Number of OFWs Estimated at 2.2 Million (Accessed: 4 January 2022).

Refugee Council. (2021). "Refugee Council Pays Tribute to 27 People who Died Last Night". Refugee Council, 25 November. Available at: https://www.refugeecouncil.org.uk/latest/news/refugee-council-pays-tribute-to-27-people-who-died-last' night/?__cf_chl_f_tk=VXSYK509KL2J6DpGrgOeThsLnRC4tEF43of8t90F5ZM-1642264814-0-gaNycGzNCL0 (Accessed: 15 January 2022).

Reifsnider, E., Gallagher, M. and Forgione, B. (2005) "Using Ecological Models in Research on Health Disparities". *Journal of Professional Nursing,* 21 (4): 216–222. https://doi.org/10.1016/j.profnurs.2005.05.006.

Rimer, B. K. and Glanz, K. (2018). *Theory at a Glance: A Guide for Health Promotion,* 2nd edn. Bethesda, MD: US Department of Health and Human Services, National Cancer Institute (NCI).

Shawyer, F., Enticott, J. C., Block, A. A. Cheng, I. H and Meadows, G. N. (2017). "The Mental Health Status of Refugees and Asylum Seekers Attending A Refugee Health Clinic Including Comparisons With A Matched Sample of Australian-Born Residents". *BMC Psychiatry,* 17: 76. https://doi.org/10.1186/s12888-017-1239-9

United Nations Children's Fund. (2021). "Improving Health Literacy Among Refugee and Migrant Children". Available at: https://www.unicef.org/eca/stories-region/improving-health-literacy-among-refugee-and-migrant-children (Accessed: 15 January 2022).

United Nations High Commissioner for Refugees. (2021a). "UNHCR - Refugee Statistics". Available at: https://www.unhcr.org/refugee-statistics/ (Accessed: 5 January 2022).

United Nations High Commissioner for Refugees. (2021b). *UNHCR* "Master Glossary of Terms". Available at: https://www.unhcr.org/glossary/ (Accessed: 7 January 2022).

van der Boor, C. F. and White, R. (2020). "Barriers to Accessing and Negotiating Mental Health Services in Asylum Seeking and Refugee Populations: The Application of the Candidacy Framework". *Journal of Immigrant and Minority Health,* 22 (1): 156–174. https://doi.org/10.1007/s10903-019-00929-y.

Watson, J. and Platt, S. (2002). *Researching Health Promotion.* London: Routledge.

World Health Organization. (2012). "Global Strategy For Health For All By The Year 2000". Available at: https://www.who.int/publications/i/item/9241800038 (Accessed: 16 January 2022).

World Health Organization. (2018). "Health Promotion For Improved Refugee and Migrant Health". Available at: https://www.euro.who.int/__data/assets/pdf_file/0004/388363/ tc-health-promotion-eng.pdf (Accessed: 5 January 2022).

World Health Organization. (2019). "Promoting the Health of Refugees and Migrants: Draft Global Action Plan, 2019–2023". Available at: https://www.who.int/publications/ i/item/promoting-the-health-of-refugees-and-migrants-draft-global-action-plan-2019-2023 (Accessed: 9 January 2022).

World Health Organization. (2020). "Apart Together Survey-Preliminary Overview of Refugees and Migrants Self-Reported Impact of COVID-19". Available at: https://www. who.int/publications/i/item/9789240017924 (Accessed: 4 January 2022).

World Health Organization. (2021a). *Common Health Needs of Refugees and Migrants: Literature Review.* Geneva. Available at: https://www.who.int/publications/i/item/ 9789240033108 (Accessed: 4 January 2022).

World Health Organization. (2021b). *Mapping Health Systems' Responsiveness to Refugee and Migrant Health Needs.* Available at: https://www.who.int/publications/i/item/ 9789240030640 (Accessed: 9 January 2022).

18

UNRAVELLING DIETARY ACCULTURATION IN THE 21ST CENTURY

Amanda Rodrigues Amorim Adegboye, Amanda P. Moore, Claudia Stewart, and Gulshanara Begum

Introduction

Dietary acculturation is a dynamic and complex process and poorly understood (Blanchet et al., 2018). Studies demonstrate that these changes can have short- and long-term health consequences for migrants globally. This chapter describes dietary changes related to migration and the subsequent health consequences associated with them. This chapter also covers aspects of dietary changes related to globalisation, including the increased consumption of processed foods, which have a high content of calories, saturated fat, sugar, and salt. Global consumption of processed foods has been associated with poor diet and obesity, which have a significant impact on global public health (Pingali, 2007).

Terminology: Migrant Versus Immigrant

The words migrant and immigrant are often used interchangeably, and clarification is useful, as it impinges upon patterns of dietary change. The word migrant is commonly used to characterise people who voluntarily and temporarily moved from one region to another within the borders of their own country of origin (internal migration) or to another country (international migration) (Scagliusi et al., 2018). This movement of people, in the short-term, may occur due to the need for medical treatment, temporary, or fixed-term employment, education, or travel for business.

The word immigrant characterises individuals who have voluntarily left their countries of origin and legally moved to another country to live permanently or for long-term. The main reasons for migration are usually related to economic prosperity, career opportunities, a better education and quality of life, or a family reunion. Immigrant communities may encompass both first-generation (born overseas) and second-generation (parents born overseas) (Anderson and Blinder, 2019).

DOI: 10.4324/9781003128373-18

Patterns of Dietary Change and Dietary Patterns before Migration

Dietary acculturation is described as the shift in dietary patterns, as populations encounter a new culture and are exposed to new foods and food acquisition practices (Berry and Sam, 1997). However, the term acculturation was originally defined as a bi-directional term, meaning either the host population or migrating group can experience changes due to the influence of each other's culture (Redfield et al., 1936). Technically, the term assimilation more accurately describes the process of dietary change amongst immigrants and migrants, from traditional dietary patterns, towards food habits of the majority culture (Berry and Sam, 1997). Food practices are learned mainly through transmission from parents to children; this learning journey has both explicit (i.e., verbal communication about what to eat) and implicit (i.e., daily routines structured for children) aspects (Savage et al., 2007). Food flavours and seasoning play a part in food acceptance and preferences among children.

Traditional dietary patterns in non-Western countries are often considered healthier than modern dietary patterns (Bhopal, 2014). The West African diet before migration has been reported to be high in vegetables, fruits, root tubers, vegetable oils, and low in sugar. Similarly, in South Asian communities, the traditional diet includes starchy staples, such as rice and traditional bread like roti and paratha, eaten with vegetables, beans, and pulses (Leung and Stanner, 2011), a diet relatively high in fibre, and low in fat (Wyke and Landman, 1997). The protective effects of this type of whole-grain diet, on reducing deaths due to inflammation, oxidative stress, and infections, have been reported consistently (Jacobs and Gallaher, 2004; Jacobs et al., 2007; Aune et al., 2016).

Nutrition Transition and Increasing Urbanisation

Despite some benefits of traditional dietary patterns of many immigrant groups, nutritional transition is a common phenomenon in many low- and middle-income countries (Popkin, et al., 2012). This model is used to describe the shifts in diet, physical activity, and causes of disease, that follow changes in economic development (Popkin, 1993). Globally, the new trend of fast-food chains and mass food production is replicated such, that a person does not need to live in a high-income country to adopt Western food assimilation. This creates negative health consequences in many countries as populations become more urbanised; the RODAM study tracked dietary change and associated health consequences in urban and rural Ghanaian communities and noted an increase in obesity, hypertension, and type-2 diabetes, associated with nutrition transition in the urban setting (Agyemang et al., 2016). A study by Pingali (2007) also identified patterns of the westernisation of Asian diets among the urban middle-class moving away from staples (e.g., rice), towards livestock and dairy products, vegetables, fruits, fats, and oils.

A subsequent review of changes in Asian food systems, driven by transnational food and beverage corporations in the retail, manufacturing, and food-service sectors, found that ultra-processed food sales increased rapidly in most middle-income countries. Carbonated/fizzy drinks were leading products, in which Coca-Cola and PepsiCo had a regional oligopoly (Baker and Friel, 2016). Ultra-processed foods are designed for consumption anywhere and anytime. The idea of eating on the move can be attractive when time is at a premium, and the accessibility and availability of fresh food are scarce in the local environment (Yoon et al., 2018). This pressure towards increased westernisation of the diet is not always the case, however. In some low-income countries, fast-food chains are expensive and unaffordable for most. When available and accessible, fast food may also be culturally and socially controlled and regarded as a 'weekend treat' rather than an everyday indulgence (Martínez, 2013).

Post-Migration Dietary Patterns

Post-migration dietary changes commonly include increased consumption of fat, sugar, and salt. This consumption pattern of energy-dense foods combined with reduced physical activity increases the risk of chronic diseases, associated with immigrant populations (Renzaho and Burns, 2006; Gilbert and Khokhar, 2008; Shetty, 2013; Babatunde-Sowole et al., 2018). With increasing immigration generational status, there is a common trend towards less healthy food habits, due to acculturation and adoption of a 'modern' lifestyle (Figure 18.1). This phenomenon has been observed in mainland Europe, the UK, the USA, Canada, and Australia (Gilbert and Khokhar, 2008). Age and generational status are the major factors accounting for changes in dietary habits (Stirbu et al., 2006; Koya and Egede, 2007). This is prominent in younger generations within migrant communities, as they have experienced rapid social and cultural changes, with exposure to global influences, and fast-food chains (Gilbert and Khokhar, 2008). The Social Determinants of Health Framework can be useful in providing a theoretical framework to underpin this, with its emphasis upon inter-related upstream factors and social stratifications, as discussed in Chapter 13. Stratifications generate differential exposures to risk and protective health factors. Vulnerabilities to these produce differential consequences among social groups, and which assist to understand health inequalities, and critically frame solutions.

In the UK, younger generations within the southeast Asian community change their eating habits by including foods that are available and popular in this context (such as crisps, sandwiches, pastries, baked potatoes, and pizzas), as they are perceived to be convenient and associated with the host country (Jamal, 1998; Gilbert and Khokhar, 2008). A review of South Asian dietary habits after migration to Europe showed similar trends in terms of a substantial increase in energy and fat intake (Holmboe-Ottesen and Wandel, 2012). Studies amongst African Heritage communities in high-income countries highlight particularly the difficulties to maintain or adopt a healthy dietary habit faced, especially by

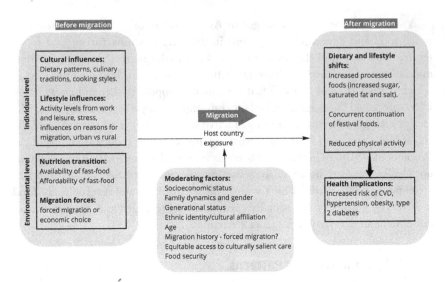

FIGURE 18.1 Factors influencing dietary acculturation.

young people because of the urban food environment, providing enticing and affordable fast-food (Ngongalah et al., 2018).

The pull towards cultural food traditions is strong, however, especially for first-generation immigrants who show stronger ethnic identity. Older women in particular act as gatekeepers of cultural food habits (Gerchow et al., 2014). Migrating individuals in unfamiliar environments can feel isolated and alone (Carballo and Nerukar, 2001). Cultural foods can provide a tangible link to home (Gunew, 2000), help maintain cultural identity (Wright et al., 2021), and provide a sense of comfort (Ore, 2018). Quandt et al. (2001) highlighted how food plays a wider social role; cooking and sharing of food can strengthen social relations and cultural norms. This can create challenges when healthy dietary advice conflicts with cultural traditions (Osokpo et al., 2021). The adoption of non-traditional dietary habits may not solely explain new dietary patterns among immigrants. Inclusion of specific ethnic traditions, alongside the incorporation of new food habits, for example, processed food, can compound each other, to contribute to health implications. For example, high consumption of ethnic festival foods (high in carbohydrates, animal protein, sugar, and fat) is noted to increase the risk of non-communicable diseases (Azar et al., 2013).

The experiences of forced migration due to persecution, war, or natural disaster may introduce additional complexities. Dietary changes experienced by forced migrants, living in emergency accommodation, can significantly impact traditional meals and meal patterns (Harris, 2009). Food experiences of asylum seekers in the UK suggest that single males often have limited or no cooking skills on arrival and were more likely to rely on fast-food outlets. Social isolation among those living in hostels, including single males and females, as well as married couples, resulted in a lack of autonomy over food pathways, coupled with depression, leading to increased weight gain, and obesity (Harris, 2009).

A range of other socio-cultural factors can shape food choices. Amongst the Latina immigrant population living in the US, the complex psychology behind healthy food choices was influenced by socio-economic status and family dynamics (Gerchow et al., 2014). Similarly, food insecurity and perceptions of healthy nutrition advice perceived to be culturally irrelevant were noted to influence dietary choices in UK African and Caribbean communities (Ochieng, 2011; Osei-Kwasi et al., 2019). These findings point towards the complexity of underlying factors, impacting post-migration changes, including country of origin, urban/rural residence, socio-economic, and cultural factors (Holmboe-Ottesen and Wandel, 2012).

Health Implications of Dietary Acculturation

The importance of diet and lifestyle in the aetiology of many chronic diseases is well recognised. A correlation is evident between the increasing consumption of processed food and the manifestation of major health problems, such as higher rates of obesity, cardiovascular disease (CVD), diabetes, and hypertension (Gilbert and Khokhar, 2008). A review investigating the obesity risk in migrant groups, particularly in countries with a lower prevalence of obesity, to a higher prevalence, confirmed the hypothesis that migrants arrive in new countries with a health advantage, including healthier body weight (Murphy et al., 2017). Gilbert and Khokhar (2008) observed that dietary components, such as grains and legumes, may be associated with a reduced risk of chronic diseases in the home country. However, this health advantage declines progressively over time and the health status of migrant communities becomes worse than the host population (Barozzino, 2010). This unhealthy weight gain can lead to similar or enhanced obesity risk in migrant populations, compared with native populations, and such differences in health outcomes may be a result of interactions between diet, other health behaviours, genetic predisposition, and developmental programming (Leung and Stanner, 2011). Similarly, whilst West African immigrants in the UK exhibit a lower risk of CVD than the majority population (Health Survey for England, 2006), there is evidence that this protective effect is lost amongst subsequent generations (Donin et al., 2010). These risks are likely to be exacerbated by poverty and discrimination.

Supporting the Health of Immigrants and Minority Communities

Cultural Competency in Healthcare

Providing dietary and lifestyle advice, which is culturally salient for minority communities living in high-income countries, is a key healthcare priority (WHO, 2018). Yet dietary practices are deeply entrenched in the culture of communities, providing a symbol of cultural identity, that goes beyond simply providing sustenance, and that prove resistant to change (Goody and Drago, 2009). Thus, delivering culturally competent care requires practitioners to understand dietary norms, traditions, and practices, within which to base their advice. Dietary traditions that are beneficial or neutral in their effect on health should be encouraged, and behaviours that require modification should be considered within the historical and cultural framework, within which they have developed (Airhihenbuwa, 1995); suggesting that traditional dishes cooked with high fat should be avoided, when an individual considers the food aligned to their cultural identity is unlikely to be effective. In Europe and the USA, healthcare practitioners identify barriers to supporting immigrants, include basic knowledge about cultural dietary practices, as well as language and communication barriers, and lack of time and resources (Zeh et al., 2018; Goff et al., 2020).

Culturally Sensitive Dietary Intervention

Culturally tailored dietary interventions are shown to improve engagement and health outcomes in immigrant populations (Liu et al., 2012). Culturally sensitive dietary interventions involve not only providing detailed dietary information relevant to cultural habits but also providing it in a culturally salient way, addressing wider socio-cultural factors specific to a particular cultural group. This includes understanding socio-economic influences, migration history, family structures and roles, and other cultural constructs (Kreuter et al., 2003). For instance, African culture is collectivist, which is a social pattern where individuals view themselves as an integral part of a group (Osokpo and Riegel, 2021). Collectivist behaviour in families' meal social interactions, a key cultural construct for many ethnic minorities, can make dietary change difficult, for example, as assuring family harmony is prioritised over individual dietary requirements (Osokpo and Riegel, 2021). Behaviour change involves consideration of capability, motivation, and environmental influences (Michie et al., 2014). For immigrant populations, this means healthcare advice needs to provide individuals with dietary knowledge that incorporates cultural food preferences; addresses motivational issues, such as compatibility of advice with cultural identity, and belief in the health benefits of dietary change; and accommodates environmental factors – such as social influences, the local food environment, and financial constraints (Moore et al., 2019).

Conclusion

This chapter explored the components of acculturation and captured pre- and post-migration dietary patterns. The importance of improving health inequalities amongst minority/immigrant communities was highlighted, with emphasis on cultural competency and sensitivity when designing health setting interventions. Although many studies have been conducted in this area, dietary acculturation is a dynamic and complex process that is still poorly understood (Blanchet et al., 2018). More research is required to establish a global association of increased prevalence of non-communicable diseases and food acculturation, and disentangle the role of dietary habits, socio-economic status, access to healthcare, health literacy, and genetics.

Research Points and Reflective Exercise

Here are some questions for you to reflect upon after reading this chapter:

- Why is it important to clarify terminology when working with migrant communities?
- What are common dietary patterns and health consequences reported from research among migrant communities?
- What are some of the key components to think about when working towards designing effective health support programmes for migrants?

Further Resources and Reading

Bhopal, R. S. (2014). *Migration, Ethnicity, Race and Health in Multicultural Societies*, 2nd edn. Oxford: Oxford University Press.

Leung, G. and Stanner, S. (2011). "Diets of Minority Ethnic Groups in the UK: Influence on Chronic Disease Risk and Implications for Prevention". *Nutrition Bulletin*, 36 (2): 161-198. https://doi.org/10.1111/j.1467-3010.2011.01889.x

References

Agyemang, C., Meeks, K., Beune, E., Owusu-Dabo, E., Mockenhaupt, F. P. et al. (2016). "Obesity and Type 2 Diabetes in Sub-Saharan Africans–Is the Burden in Today's Africa Similar to African Migrants in Europe? The RODAM Study". *BMC Medicine*, 14 (1): 1-12. https://doi.org/10.1186/s12916-016-0709-0

Airhihenbuwa, C. O. (1995). *Health and Culture: Beyond the Western Paradigm*. London: Sage.

Anderson, B. and Blinder, S. (2019). *Who Counts As A Migrant? Definitions and Their Consequences. Migration Observatory Briefing, COMPAS*. Oxford: University of Oxford.

Aune, D., Keum, N., Giovannucci, E., Fadnes, L. T., Boffetta, P. et al. (2016). "Whole Grain Consumption and Risk of Cardiovascular Disease, Cancer, and all Cause and Cause Specific Mortality: Systematic Review and Dose-Response Meta-Analysis of Prospective Studies". *BMJ*, 353: i2716. https://doi.org/10.1136/bmj.i2716

Azar, K. M. J., Chen, E., Holland, A. T. and Palaniappan, L. P. (2013). "Festival Foods in the Immigrant Diet". *Journal of Immigrant and Minority Health*, 15 (5): 953-960. https://doi.org/10.1007/s10903-012-9705-4

Babatunde-Sowole, O. O., Power, T., Davidson, P., Ballard, C. and Jackson, D. (2018). "Exploring the Diet and Lifestyle Changes Contributing to Weight Gain Among Australian West African Women Following Migration: A Qualitative Study". *Contemporary Nurse*, 54 (2): 150-159. https://doi.org/10.1080/10376178.2018.1459760

Baker, P. and Friel, S. (2016). "Food Systems Transformations, Ultra-Processed Food Markets and the Nutrition Transition in Asia". *Globalization and Health*, 12 (1): 1-15. https://doi.org/10.1186/s12992-016-0223-3

Barozzino, T. (2010). "Immigrant Health and the Children and Youth of Canada: Are We Doing Enough?" *Healthcare Quarterly (Toronto, Ont.)*, 14 (1): 52-59. https://doi.org/10.12927/hcq.2010.21983

Berry, J. and Sam, D. (1997). *Handbook of Cross-Cultural Psychology: Social Behavior and Applications*. Boston: Allyn and Bacon.

Bhopal, R. (2014). *Migration, Ethnicity, Race and Health in Multicultural Societies*. Oxford: Oxford University Press.

Blanchet, R., Nana, C. P., Sanou, D., Batal, M. and Giroux, I. (2018). "Dietary Acculturation Among Black Immigrant Families Living in Ottawa—A Qualitative Study". *Ecology of Food and Nutrition*, 57 (3): 223-245. https://doi.org/10.1080/03670244.2018.1455674

Carballo, M. and Nerukar, A. (2001). "Migration, Refugees, and Health Risks". *Emerging Infectious Diseases*, 7 (3): 556–560. https://doi.org/10.3201/eid0707.017733

Donin, A. S., Nightingale, C. M., Owen, C. G., Rudnicka, A. R., McNamara, M. C., et al. (2010). "Nutritional Composition of the Diets of South Asian, Black African-Caribbean and White European Children in the United Kingdom: The Child Heart and Health Study in England (CHASE)." *British Journal of Nutrition*, 104 (2): 276-285. https://doi.org/10.1017/s000711451000070x

Gerchow, L., Tagliaferro, B., Squires, A., Nicholson, J., Savarimuthu, S. M. et al. (2014). "Latina Food Patterns in the United States: A Qualitative Metasynthesis". *Nursing Research*, 63 (3): 182-193. https://doi.org/10.1097/NNR.0000000000000030

Gilbert, P. A. and Khokhar, S. (2008). "Changing Dietary Habits of Ethnic Groups in Europe and Implications for Health". *Nutrition Reviews*, 66 (4): 203-215. https://doi.org/10.1111/j.1753-4887.2008.00025.x

Goff, L. M., Moore, A., Harding, S. and Rivas, C. (2020). "Providing Culturally Sensitive Diabetes Self-Management Education and Support for Black African and Caribbean Communities: A Qualitative Exploration of the Challenges Experienced by Healthcare Practitioners in Inner London". *BMJ Open Diabetes Res Care*, 8 (2): e001818. https://doi.org/10.1136/bmjdrc-2020-001818

Goody, C. M. and Drago, L. (2009). "Using Cultural Competence Constructs to Understand Food Practices and Provide Diabetes Care and Education". *Diabetes Spectrum*, 22 (1): 43-47. https://doi.org/10.2337/diaspect.22.1.43

Gunew, S. (2000). "Introduction: Multicultural Translations of Food, Bodies, Language". *Journal of Intercultural Studies*, 21 (3): 227-237. https://doi.org/10.1080/713678979

Harris, A. (2009). Seminar: Food Experiences of Forced Migrants in the UK, Food and Migration Workshop, Centre for Migration and Diaspora Studies, SOAS, London, delivered 2-3 February 2009.

Health Survey for England. (2006). *The Health of Minority Ethnic Groups, Volume 1*. London: National Centre for Social Research.

Holmboe-Ottesen, G. and Wandel, M. (2012). "Changes in Dietary Habits After Migration and Consequences for Health: A Focus on South Asians in Europe". *Food & Nutrition Research*, 56 (1): 18891. https://doi.org/10.3402/fnr.v56i0.18891

Jacobs, D. R., Andersen, L. F. and Blomhoff, R. (2007). "Whole-Grain Consumption Is Associated With A Reduced Risk of Noncardiovascular, Noncancer Death Attributed to Inflammatory Diseases in the Iowa Women's Health Study". *The American Journal of Clinical Nutrition*, 85 (6): 1606-1614. https://doi.org/10.1093/ajcn/85.6.1606

Jacobs, D. R., Jr. and Gallaher, D. D. (2004). "Whole Grain Intake and Cardiovascular Disease: A Review". *Curr Atheroscler Rep*, 6 (6): 415-423. https://doi.org/10.1007/s11883-004-0081-y

Jamal, A. (1998). "Food Consumption Among Ethnic Minorities: The Case of British-Pakistanis in Bradford, UK". *British Food Journal*, 100 (5): 221-227. https://doi.org/10.1108/00070709810221436

Koya, D. L. and Egede, L. E. (2007). "Association Between Length of Residence and Cardiovascular Disease Risk Factors Among An Ethnically Diverse Group of United

States Immigrants". *Journal of General Internal Medicine,* 22 (6): 841-846. https://doi.org/10.1007/s11606-007-0163-y

Kreuter, M. W., Lukwago, S. N., Bucholtz, R. D., Clark, E. M. and Sanders-Thompson, V. (2003). "Achieving Cultural Appropriateness in Health Promotion Programs: Targeted and Tailored Approaches". *Health Education & Behavior,* 30 (2): 133–146. https://doi.org/10.1177/1090198102251021

Leung, G. and Stanner, S. (2011). "Diets of Minority Ethnic Groups In the UK: Influence on Chronic Disease Risk and Implications for Prevention". *Nutrition Bulletin,* 36 (2): 161-198. https://doi.org/10.1111/j.1467-3010.2011.01889.x

Liu, J., Davidson, E., Bhopal, R., White, M., Johnson, M. et al. (2012). "Adapting Health Promotion Interventions to Meet the Needs of Ethnic Minority Groups: Mixed-Methods Evidence Synthesis". *Health Technol Assess,* 16 (44): 1-469. https://doi.org/10.3310/hta16440

Martínez, A. D. (2013). "Reconsidering Acculturation in Dietary Change Research Among Latino Immigrants: Challenging thePpreconditions of US Migration". *Ethnicity and Health,* 18 (2): 115-135. https://doi.org/10.1080/13557858.2012.698254

Michie, S., Atkinson, L. and West, R. (2014). *The Behaviour Change Wheel: A Guide To Designing Interventions.* London: Silverback Publishing.

Moore, A. P., Rivas, C. A., Stanton-Fay, S., Harding, S. and Goff, L. M. (2019). "Designing the Healthy Eating and Active Lifestyles for Diabetes (HEAL-D) Self-Management and Support Programme for UK African and Caribbean Communities: A Culturally Tailored, Complex Intervention Under-pinned By Behaviour Change Theory". *BMC Public Health,* 19 (1): 1-14. https://doi.org/10.1186/s12889-019-7411-z

Murphy, M., Robertson, W. and Oyebode, O. (2017). "Obesity in International Migrant Populations". *Current Obesity Reports,* 6 (3): 314-323. https://doi.org/10.1007/s13679-017-0274-7

Ngongalah, L., Rankin, J., Rapley, T., Odeniyi, A., Akhter, Z. et al. (2018). "Dietary and Physical Activity Behaviours In African Migrant Women Living in High Income Countries: A Systematic Review and Framework Synthesis". *Nutrients,* 10 (8): 1017. https://doi.org/10.3390/nu10081017

Ochieng, B. M. N. (2011). "Factors Influencing the Diet Patterns and Uptake of Physical Activity Among Black Families." *International Journal of Health Promotion and Education,* 49 (4): 140-145. https://doi.org/10.1080/14635240.2011.10708221

Ore, H. (2018). "Ambivalent Nostalgia: Jewish-Israeli Migrant Women 'Cooking' Ways to Return Home." *Food, Culture and Society,* 21 (4): 568-584. https://doi.org/10.1080/15528014.2018.1481332

Osei-Kwasi, H. A., Nicolaou, M., Powell, K. and Holdsworth, M. (2019). "'I Cannot Sit Here and Eat Alone When I Know A Fellow Ghanaian Is Suffering'": Perceptions of Food Insecurity Among Ghanaian Migrants". *Appetite,* 140: 190-196. https://doi.org/10.1016/j.appet.2019.05.018

Osokpo, O., James, R. and Riegel, B. (2021). "Maintaining Cultural Identity: A Systematic Mixed Studies Review of Cultural Influences on the Self-Care of African Immigrants Living With Non-Communicable Disease". *Journal of Advanced Nursing,* 77 (9): 3600-3617. https://doi.org/10.1111/jan.14804

Osokpo, O. and Riegel, B. (2021). "Cultural Factors Influencing Self-Care By Persons With Cardiovascular Disease: An Integrative Review". *International Journal of Nursing Studies* 116: 103383. 10.1016/j.ijnurstu.2019.06.014

Pingali, P. (2007). "Westernization of Asian Diets and the Transformation of Food Systems: Implications for Research and Policy". *Food Policy,* 32 (3): 281-298. https://doi.org/10.1016/j.foodpol.2006.08.001

Popkin, B. M. (1993). "Nutritional Patterns and Transitions". *Population and Development Review,* 19 (1): 138-157. https://doi.org/10.2307/2938388

Popkin, B. M., Adair, L.S., and Ng, S. W. (2012). "Global nutrition transition and the pandemic of obesity in developing countries". Nutrition Reviews, 70(1):3-21. https://doi.org/10.1111/j.1753-4887.2011.00456.x

Quandt, S. A., Arcury, T. A., Bell, R. A., McDonald, J. and Vitolins, M. Z. (2001). "The Social and Nutritional Meaning of Food Sharing Among Older Rural Adults". *Journal of Aging Studies,* 15 (2): 145-162. https://doi.org/10.1016/S0890-4065(00)00023-2

Redfield, R., Linton, R. and Herskovits, M. J. (1936). "Memorandum for the Study of Acculturation". *American Anthropologist,* 38 (1): 149-152. https://doi.org/10.1525/aa.1936.38.1.02a00330

Renzaho, A. M. N. and Burns, C. (2006). "Post-Migration Food Habits of Sub-Saharan African Migrants in Victoria: A Cross-Sectional Study". *Nutrition and Dietetics,* 63 (2): 91-102. doi10.1111/j.1747-0080.2006.00055.x

Savage, J. S., Fisher, J. O. and Birch, L. L. (2007). "Parental Influence on Eating Behavior: Conception to Adolescence". *Journal of Law, Medicine, and Ethics,* 35 (1): 22-34. https://doi.org/10.1111/j.1748-720X.2007.00111.x

Scagliusi, F. B., Porreca, F. I., Ulian, M. D., de Morais Sato, P. and Unsain, R. F. (2018). "Representations of Syrian Food by Syrian Refugees in the City of Sao Paulo, Brazil: An Ethnographic Study". *Appetite,* 129: 236-244. https://doi.org/10.1016/j.appet.2018.07.014

Shetty, P. (2013). "Nutrition Transition and Its Health Outcomes". *The Indian Journal of Pediatrics,* 80 Suppl 1 (1): S21-S27. https://doi.org/10.1007/s12098-013-0971-5

Stirbu, I., Kunst, A. E., Vlems, F. A., Visser, O., Bos, V. et al. (2006). "Cancer Mortality Rates Among First and Second Generation Migrants in the Netherlands: Convergence Toward the Rates of the Native Dutch Population". *International Journal of Cancer,* 119 (11): 2665-2672. https://doi.org/10.1002/ijc.22200

World Health Organization. (2018). *Report of the Health of Refugees and Migrants in the WHO European Region: No Public Health Without Refugee and Migrant Health.* WHO: Regional Office for Europe.

Wright, K. E., Lucero, J. E., Ferguson, J. K., Granner, M. L., Devereux, P. G. et al. (2021). "The Influence of Cultural Food Security On Cultural Identity and Wellbeing: A Qualitative Comparison Between Second-Generation American and International Students in the United States". *Ecology of Food and Nutrition* 60, (6): 636-662. https://doi.org/10.1080/03670244.2021.1875455

Wyke, S. and Landman, J. (1997). "Healthy Eating? Diet and Cuisine Amongst Scottish South Asian People". *British Food Journal,* 99 (1): 27-34. https://doi.org/10.1108/00070709710158852

Yoon, N.-H., Yoo, S. and Kwon, S. (2018). "Influence of Highly Accessible Urban Food Evironment on Weight Management: A Qualitative Study in Seoul". *International Journal of Environmental Research and Public Health,* 15 (4): 755. https://doi.org/10.3390/ijerph15040755

Zeh, P., Cannaby, A. M., Sandhu, H. K., Warwick, J. and Sturt, J. A. (2018). "A Cross-Sectional Survey of General Practice Health Workers' Perceptions of Their Provision of Culturally Competent Services to Ethnic Minority People With Diabetes". *Primary Care Diabetes,* 12 (6): 501-509. https://doi.org/10.1016/j.pcd.2018.07.016

19

TRANSGENDER, GENDERQUEER, AND NON-BINARY IDENTITIES

Social and Structural Inequalities in Public Health

Danielle J. Roe, Jason Schaub, Jessica Lynn, and Panagiotis Pentaris

Introduction

Whilst there have been advances in policy and practice, transgender and genderqueer (TGD) populations continue to experience health inequalities, often deriving from a misunderstanding or generalisation of TGD needs. TGD people, for example, those who are not cisgender, are often grouped with gay, lesbian, and bisexual individuals. This intersection of gender and sexual orientation is problematic as the emphasis often focuses on sexual orientation, leaving challenges faced by TGD people to be poorly understood (Matsuno and Budge, 2017). The dearth of empirical evidence about TGD healthcare (Institute of Medicine, 2011) facilitates such generalisations, meaning the impact for the individual needs a more detailed analysis (Reisner et al., 2016). These knowledge gaps further perpetuate stigma and discrimination. This stigma is central to health outcomes and is a key driver of HIV disparities within TGD populations (Hughto et al., 2015; Poteat et al., 2016a; 2016b), highlighting the need for better knowledge about lived experience to improve services. This chapter recognises that transgender individuals are more likely to have multiple chronic conditions than their cisgender peers (Downing and Przedworski, 2018) and discusses the inequalities that link interventions and outcomes for TGD individuals.

Language and Definitions

It is important to think about the forms and use of language when examining TGD people's lives. Language is central to how societal gendered expectations are formed, reformed, and performed, to uphold structural inequalities in public health (Pearce et al., 2020). Giddens' (1984) theory of 'Structuration' is useful in this context. As was mentioned in Chapter 2, social structures are both the

DOI: 10.4324/9781003128373-19

medium and outcome of the practices they organise and perform. For instance, to communicate, one mobilises discourses around TGD people through language (structure) to articulate meaning. As a result, employing the rules that govern articulations of discourses through language reproduces it as an outcome/structure of communication which reinforces other social structures such as discrimination and health inequalities more broadly. Through language, we consistently construct broader structures which then feed into the revision and construction of language by individuals, through the use of agency and consciousness, a duality of structure and agency.

In this chapter, we use TGD as an umbrella term, inclusive of gender identities which do not align with the assignment made at birth, or shortly thereafter, any identity outside of, or between, binary categorisations of man/woman, such as non-binary and/or genderqueer (Matsuno and Budge, 2017), and which is independent of any gatekeeping through required diagnosis of dysphoria or medical transition. Although popular in contemporary discourse, Trans-Exclusionary Radical Feminists or TERFs (Smythe, 2018) will be referred to as 'gender critical' as some consider TERF to be a slur (Pearce et al., 2020) despite strong opposition to this claim. We also recognise that terminology and definitions are changing on a regular basis (Matsuno and Budge, 2017). We invite readers to consider this text in line with what language is used at a given time, and drawing on the descriptor above, as well as how language can reflect and reproduce social structures, and provide alternatives for further changes in meaning and discourses.

Whilst there is no one agreed definition of transphobia, as it is not a singular phenomenon with one uniform account (Bettcher, 2014), transphobia can be contextualised as the broad social context in which TGD people, or those perceived to be TGD, are systematically disadvantaged (Hopkins, 1996). The synergistic relationship of transphobia and homophobia dictate nonheterosexual and noncisgender individuals as 'deviant' (Tewksbury, 2015), creating a rationality of 'acceptable prejudice' that supports systemic disadvantages (Schilt and Westbrook, 2009). Health-related stigma is complex and multiple micro, meso, and macro inequalities should be viewed through a lens of intersectionality (Crenshaw, 2017) rather than as independent, separate entities (Rai et al., 2020).

Gender Critical and Trans Affirming: Socio-Political Context

Despite the heterogeneous nature of TGD identities in society (Bettcher, 2014), TGD literature is overbalanced throughout particular areas and topics. The blending of socially constructed Westernised ideals, notions, and understandings of gender, sex, and sexuality suggest a permeation of colonialised legacies, nationhood, and globalisation in gender and health studies, situating 'the West' as a perceived cultural 'centre' to the Majority World's supposed 'periphery' (Bhanji, 2013; Pearce et al., 2020). This over-emphasis complicates any attempt to authoritatively describe the challenges TGD people face globally. However, Giddens and Sutton (2021) highlight how a global outlook of experiences is emerging from 'cosmopolitanism'. The flow of information via the internet encourages the co-existence of differently positioned knowledge claims (Pearce et al., 2020) providing an understanding of TGD experience in a more globalised context.

Knowledge availability and access through cosmopolitanism, and the resulting cosmopolitan overload (Giddens and Sutton, 2021), are perceived through contemporary proliferations of distrust and misinformation within TGD public discourses (Pearce et al., 2020). This phenomenon enables conceptualisations of differences of opinion regarding TGD to be operationalised in public health contexts. On both occasions, the concept of intersected identities is essential. The 'cosmopolitisation' of sex and gender is by virtue shaped by an intersectional framework (Crenshaw, 2017), which highlights the complex and multiple dimensions of identity and the way it is experienced by individuals. Pearce et al. (2020) identify two core pillars of this debate: the operationalisation of sex and gender and identity self-determination.

As an example, in the United Kingdom (UK), anti-trans sentiment has increased over the last five years (Pearce et al., 2020). Those holding gender critical views often cite Raymond's (1994) position of trans women as male appropriation of the female body to infiltrate women's spaces with the intent to cause harm. Increasing social acceptance of TGD therefore challenges gender critical beliefs about biologically immutable conceptualisations of 'womanhood' and 'femaleness', providing the justification for gender critical actions to reassert essentialist values, reacting in part to cosmopolitan overload (Pearce et al., 2020).

In contrast to gender critical views, trans affirmative views and trans allyship suggest that sex and gender are culturally constituted and performative rather than biologically essentialist (Butler, 1990). From an affirmative view, gender critical approaches are therefore dissonant with how TGD people theorise, identify, and describe their experiences. Pearce et al. (2020) note that the majority of TGD public health (written about' rather than 'by, with or for' TGD people, further compounding health inequality) is characterised by the absence of robust data on TGD populations (Government Equalities Office, 2018). Despite the rapid growth of the TGD health research field (Thorne et al., 2018), gaps remain, such as non-binary identity needs (Clark et al., 2018) and a lack of research on TGD experiences in low- and middle-income countries (Reisner et al., 2016) especially transmasculine experiences (Scheim et al., 2020). This can lead to ineffective care experiences for TGD people, when individuals/organisations tasked with policy-making decisions, have insufficient scientific and/or personal knowledge of TGD needs (Clark et al., 2018). The use of a public inquiry case study will help further explore the differences between trans affirmative and gender critical views and how they relate to TGD public health.

Tavistock Inquiry

England's only gender-identity development service, the Tavistock Centre, was the focus of a public inquiry in 2020 after BBC Newsnight shared preliminary findings of an investigation into treatment at the Centre (BBC News, 2020; Carmichael et al., 2020), discussing that 98% of patients taking hormone blockers progress on to cross-sex hormones (Carmichael et al., 2020). This case rose to prominence in a suit, filed on behalf of Keira Bell, for the provision of misleading advice about hormone therapy, and the provision of puberty blockers (Bell v. Tavistock, 2020). The suit claimed true informed consent could not be given as the patient, Keira Bell, was 16 years of age at the time (Bell v. Tavistock, 2020). The High Court eventually ruled in favour of Bell, stating those under 16 are unlikely to be able to give informed consent, based upon Gillick competence (Gillick v West Norfolk and Wisbech AHA, 1986), with the Tavistock immediately suspending referrals for under-16s (BBC News, 2020).

Following the ruling, there was swift opposition from trans affirmative care specialists, trans activists, and trans-inclusive Feminists. They stated that TGD youth usually wait to seek help until at a crisis point (McDermott and Roen, 2012), despite evidence of TGD youth being at particular risk for discrimination, violence, rejection, depression, suicidal ideation, and suicide (Taylor et al., 2020). Psychological and social intervention evidence indicates health professionals should not impose binary categories of gender or sex (Clark et al., 2018) and affirmative models of care provide opportunities for resilience and positive mental health for TGD youth (Costa et al., 2015). This stance directly opposes that of gender critical views, which refutes the high risk of suicide among TGD youth, as trans activist 'scare tactics' (Hendley, 2019). The outcome of the original case was overturned by the Court of Appeal in September 2021, suggesting that the High Court should have dismissed the case when it ruled the Tavistock guidance was lawful and that it is the role of clinicians to exercise judgment in relation to puberty-blocking treatment (Thornton, 2021). In March 2021, a separate case involving the Centre also supported trans affirmative care, ruling that parents can consent to their child taking puberty-delaying drugs without a judge's approval, save where the parents and the child are in opposition (AB and CD v. Tavistock, 2021; Greenhalgh, 2021).

Health Inequalities for Transgender, Genderqueer, and Non-Binary Individuals

Like lesbian, gay, and bisexual people, trans people often meet with discrimination and prejudice in their everyday lives. Many, regardless of social position or class, experience isolation and face limited understanding of their lives (Fish 2007). The Stonewall Trans Report in the UK (Bachmann and Gooch, 2018) outlined ongoing discrimination and oppressive behaviours experienced by TGD individuals – 12% of participants were physically attacked in the last year; 25% have experienced homelessness; 41% felt that healthcare professionals lacked understanding; 50% hide their gender identity at work, fearing discrimination; and 7% have been refused healthcare because of their gender identity. Such evidence raises further concerns about the appropriateness of professionals' skills, primarily on the level of values and ethics, that appear to interfere with their duty of care. These experiences increase the risk for trans people of alcohol abuse, depression, suicide, self-harm, violence, substance abuse, and HIV (Kenagy, 2005).

Further, considerable extant literature prior to the COVID-19 pandemic consistently demonstrates TGD experience multiple health inequalities (Fish and Karban, 2015) leading to an increased prevalence of poor mental and physical health (Wagaman, 2014). The recent pandemic predominantly heightened the need for action (Pentaris, 2021) rather than caused the issues to hand. As a way of conceptualising the healthcare experiences of TGD individuals, some knowledge reviews show a clear link between stigma and healthcare issues. Winter et al. (2016) showed how this stigma complicates the healthcare experiences of TGD patients, calling it the 'stigma to sickness slope' (Winter et al., 2016: 394).

Mental Health Challenges

TGD individuals have higher rates of mental health issues than the general population. Many of these issues are understood to be in response to the widespread discrimination and abuse experienced from both wider society and those closest to them (Reisner et al., 2016). However, there is surprisingly little research looking at the impact of trauma on transgender people's mental health, but those studies that exist suggest widespread and sustained emotional distress, following discrimination both at home, and in social settings (Fish, 2007). For example, a study in Haiti (Joshi et al., 2021) linked an increase in mental health issues for transfeminine individuals to experiences of extreme sexual and non-sexual violence, which was perpetuated against them in hostile environments. Persistent discrimination, and the resulting stress, have been linked to a range of mental health issues including depression, suicidality, anxiety, as well as increased substance misuse as a coping mechanism (Reisner et al., 2014).

These higher rates of mental health issues have specific presentations. A broad study from the UK about TGD people's mental health found that almost 90% of respondents had experienced depression (88%) and three quarters had experienced anxiety (McNeil et al., 2012). Several studies have shown that over one third of respondents had attempted suicide (Fish, 2007; McNeil et al., 2012) and over three quarters had experienced suicidality. This should be compared to suicidality experienced by 1%6% of the general population (Winter, et al., 2016).

In particular, waiting for treatment was shown to have a significant negative impact on mental health outcomes, even for young people (Carlile et al., 2021). Individuals with gender dysphoria may experience several different mental health issues, which can be linked to a long history of seeking treatment, and experiencing discrimination (Murad et al., 2010). It is important to identify the centrality of the role of mental health professionals to accessing and receiving health treatment, a situation that is not found elsewhere in healthcare (Ehrensaft, 2017). There are some calls to challenge this gatekeeping (Ettner and Wylie, 2013), with some suggesting that it unfairly pathologises trans and non-binary gender identities, and individual's search for support and appropriate healthcare. What is clear is that for people with gender dysphoria, most of them felt their mental health was better after transitioning, reducing both suicidality and suicide attempts (McNeil et al., 2012).

HIV-Related Challenges

Generally, transgender, and gender diverse individuals have a higher proportion of HIV infection than the general population (Poteat et al., 2016b; Reisner et al., 2016). This is often combined with a lack of specific resources and attention, creating a 'perfect storm' for this population. Susan Buchbinder (2016), from the San Francisco Department of Public Health, argued that there is probably no population, which is both more heavily impacted by HIV, and less discussed around the world, than transgender people (Buchbinder, 2016).

It is difficult to identify with any certainty the prevalence and severity of HIV infections for multiple reasons; the challenges of accurately identifying gender identity of research participants, national differences in societal engagement with TGD people, and policy responses, and missing data from large sections of the world. HIV research often subsumes transfeminine people into the category of men who have sex with men (Poteat et al., 2016a), further obfuscating the prevalence and severity of HIV issues for transgender individuals. Transfeminine people have very high HIV rates (up to 40%) (Poteat et al., 2016a), but this is without data available for much of the world (particularly Sub-Saharan Africa and Eastern Europe/Central Asia). Transfeminine individuals often 'engage in sex work for economic survival and gender affirmation' (Poteat et al., 2016a), with associated significantly greater risk of sexually transmitted infections and violence. In addition, services designed for men who have sex with men are inappropriate for transfeminine individuals and may be less welcoming to transmasculine individuals (Poteat et al., 2016a). When considering the experience of transmasculine people, surprisingly, clinicians often do not outline the risks of unprotected sex with men, meaning a lack of knowledge of risk, behaviour, and treatment options. Importantly, this is an area where intersectionality is a key consideration, as there are some studies that suggest that transfeminine people from minority ethnicities have significantly higher rates of HIV (Institute of Medicine, 2011).

A Personal Perspective

My (JL) experience as a transgender activist supports the description that the most painful discrimination experienced by TGD individuals is manifested via healthcare. If TGD individuals are to be validated in their identities, no place is more important than that of a healthcare environment. It is not uncommon to have one's trans identity outlined during unrelated medical visits (and in the most inappropriate ways). A close (trans) friend of mine found that, after having been released from hospital, following an open-heart surgery, her discharge diagnosis of unstable angina included 'transgender with a history of sex reassignment surgery'. While having x-rays taken of my jaw (because of a car accident), I have been asked whether I had a penis or a vagina – which is wholly unrelated to the issue at hand. Under the guise of curiosity, the subject of a transgender person's body is treated with a levity that, to any cis person, would be reprehensible, if not illegal. Discrimination is, and always will be, an ongoing battle, but it has no place in healthcare. Too often transgender people are asked invasive and irrelevant questions and invalidated by healthcare professionals. When one walks through the healthcare doors, all questions of race, religion, and sex should be discarded if they are not pertinent.

Conclusion

This chapter focused on the health inequalities experienced by transgender, gender-queer, and non-binary individuals. The chapter considered social and structural inequalities which further cause challenges vis-à-vis mental health. The lack of evidence in this area only adds to the challenges in advancing understanding of TDGs' lived experiences, to move forward, and toward a more inclusive and dignified 'for all' system of healthcare. TGD individuals are in the process of navigating the late modern world and complexity of cosmopolitisation, as they stride both 'emancipatory politics' and 'life politics' (Giddens, 1990; 1991; La Placa et al., 2014). Emancipatory politics is the process of liberation from social structures and constraints governing individuals' lives. The process of life politics concerns us more with personal choice and lifestyle, and how individuals construct the authentic self and lifestyle, in response to the flux and instability of the late modern world. The duality of structure and agency can enhance this process on a theoretical level and assist us in understanding the strive for self-determination and equality in healthcare and beyond.

Research Points and Reflective Exercises

TDG individuals face continuous discrimination and experience stigma on the grounds of their gender identity, which deprives them from making effective use of services. By means of reflection, we invite readers to consider:

1 how does poor understanding and lack of knowledge about TGD challenges lead to discriminatory and exclusionary practice?
2 how this can be combated?

Further Resources and Reading

Gender Creative Kids - https://gendercreativekids.com/
Gendered Intelligence - https://genderedintelligence.co.uk/

The Gender Unicorn - https://transstudent.org/gender/
World Professional Association for Transgender Health – www.wpath.org

References

AB and CD v. Tavistock. (2021). "High Court of Justice Family Division", Courts and Tribunals Judiciary, 26 March. Available at: https://www.judiciary.uk/judgments/ac-v-cd-and-ors/ (Accessed: 1 November 2021).

Bachmann, C. L. and Gooch, B. (2018). *LGBT in Britain: trans report*. London: Stonewall.

BBC News. (2020). "Puberty Blockers: Under-16s 'Unlikely to be able to Give Informed Consent'", BBC News, 1 December. Available at: https://www.bbc.co.uk/news/uk-england-cambridgeshire-55144148 (Accessed: 1 December 2020).

Bell-v-Tavistock. (2020). "Courts and Tribunals Judiciary, Royal Courts of Justice" 1 December. Available at: https://www.judiciary.uk/wp-content/uploads/2020/12/Bell-v-Tavistock-Judgment.pdf (Accessed: 1 December 2020).

Bettcher, T. M. (2014). "Transphobia". *Transgender Studies Quarterly*, 1 (1-2): 249–251. https://doi.org/10.1215/23289252-2400181

Bhanji, N. (2013). "Trans/criptions: Homing Desires, (Trans)Sexual Citizenship and Racialized Bodies". In. S. Stryker and A. Z. Aizura (eds.) *The Transgender Studies Reader 2*. New York: Routledge, 512–526.

Buchbinder, S. (2016). "Introduction to Tonia Poleat's Plenary". *Conference on Retroviruses and Opportunistic Infections (CROI 2016)*. 22-25 February.

Butler, J. (1990). *Gender Trouble: Feminism and the Subversion of Identity*. London: Routledge.

Carlile, A., Butteriss, E., and Sansfaçon, A. P. (2021). "'It's Like My Kid Came Back Overnight': Experiences of Trans and Non-Binary Young People and Their Families Seeking, Finding and Engaging with Clinical Care in England". *International Journal of Transgender Health*, 1-17. doi.org/10.1080/26895269.2020.1870188

Carmichael, P., Butler, G., Masic, U., Cole, T. J., De Stavola, B. L., Davidson, S. and Viner, R. (2020). "Short-Term Outcomes of Pubertal Suppression in a Selected Cohort of 12- to 15-Year-Old Young People with Persistent Gender Dysphoria in the UK. medRxiv, 2020.2012.2001.20241653. https://doi.org/10.1101/2020.12.01.20241653

Clark, B. A., Veale, J. F., Townsend, M., Frohard-Dourlent, H. and Saewyc, E. (2018). Non-Binary Youth: Access to Gender- Affirming Primary Health Care". *International Journal of Transgenderism. Advance online publication*. https://doi.org/10.1080/ 15532739.2017.1394954

Costa, R., Dunsford, M., Skagerberg, E., Holt, M. R., Carmichael, P. and Colizzi, M. (2015). "Psychological Support, Puberty Suppression, and Psychological Functioning in Ado- lescents with Gender Dysphoria". *Journal of Sexual Medicine*, 12: 2206–2214. https://doi.org/10.1111/jsm.1303

Crenshaw, K. (2017). *On Intersectionality: Essential Writings*. New York: New Press.

Downing, J. M. and Przedworski, J. M. (2018). "Health of Transgender Adults in the US, 2014–2016". *American Journal of Preventive Medicine*, 55 (3): 336-344. https://doi.org/10.1016/j.amepre.2018.04.045

Ehrensaft, D. (2017). "Gender Nonconforming Youth: Current Perspectives". *Adolescent Health, Medicine and Therapeutics*, 8: 57-67. https://doi.org/10.2147/AHMT.S110859

Ettner, R. and Wylie, K. (2013). "Psychological and social adjustment in older transsexual people". *Maturitas*. 74(3):226-229. https://doi.org/10.1016/j.maturitas.2012.11.011.

Fish, J., (2007). *Trans People's Health*. London: Department of Health.

Fish, J. and Karban, K. (2015). *LGBT Health Inequalities: International Perspectives in Social Work*. Bristol: Policy Press.

Giddens, A. (1984). *The Constitution of Society*. Cambridge: Polity Press.

Giddens, A. (1990). *The Consequences of Modernity*. Cambridge: Polity Press.

Giddens, A. (1991). *Modernity and Self-Identity: Self and Society in the Late Modern Age*. Cambridge: Polity Press.

Giddens, A. and Sutton, F. (2021). *Sociology*, 9th edn. Cambridge: Polity Press.

Gillick v West Norfolk and Wisbech AHA. (1986) AC 112 ((HL)).

Government Equalities Office. (2018). "Trans People in the UK". Available at: https://assets.publishing.service.gov.uk/government/uploads/system/uploads/attachment_data/file/721642/GEO-LGBT-factsheet.pdf (Accessed: 1 November 2020).

Greenhalgh, H. (2021). "UK Court Rules in Favour of Parental Consent in Trans Treatment Row", Reuters, March 26. Available at: https://www.reuters.com/article/britain-lgbt-legal/uk-court-rules-in-favour-of-parental-consent-in-trans-treatment-row-idUSL8N2LO43Q (Accessed: 1 November 2020).

Hendley, A. (2019). "I Supported Trans Ideology Until I Couldn't Anymore", Feminist Current, April 10, 2019. Available at: www.feministcurrent.com/2019/04/10/i-supported-trans-ideology-until-i-couldnt-anymore/ (Accessed: 1 November 2020).

Hopkins, P. (1996). "Gender Treachery: Homophobia, Masculinity, and Threatened Identities". In L. May, R. Strikwerda and P. D. Hopkins (eds.) *Rethinking Masculinity: Philosophical Explorations in Light of Feminism*. Lanham, MD: Rowman and Littlefield, 95–116.

Hughto, J. M. W., Reisner, S. L. and Pachankis, J. E. (2015). "Transgender Stigma and Health: A Critical Review of Stigma Determinants, Mechanisms, and Interventions". *Social Science and Medicine,* 147: 222-231. https://doi.org/10.1016/j.socscimed.2015.11.010

Institute of Medicine (U.S.). 2011. *The Health of Lesbian, Gay, Bisexual, and Transgender People: Building a Foundation for Better Understanding*. Washington, DC.: National Academies Press.

Joshi, M., Rahill, G.T., Carrington, C., Mabie, A. and Salinas-Miranda, A. et al. (2021) "They are not satisfied until they see our blood": Syndemic HIV risks for trans women in urban Haiti, *International Journal of Mental Health,* 50:4, 337-367. doi:10.1080/00207411.2021.1891364

Kenagy, G. P. (2005) "Transgender Health: Findings from Two Needs Assessment Studies in Philadelphia". *Health and Social Work*, 31 (1): 19–26. https://doi.org/10.1093/hsw/30.1.19

La Placa, V., Knight, A. and McNaught, A. (2014). "Conclusion". In A. Knight, V. La Placa and A. McNaught (eds.) *Wellbeing: Policy and Practice*. Banbury: Lantern, 109-113.

Matsuno, E. and Budge, S. (2017). "Non-Binary/Genderqueer Identities: A Critical Review of the Literature". *Current Sexual Health Reports*, 9 (3): https://doi.org/10.1007/s11930-017-0111-8

McDermott, E. and Roen, K. (2012). "Youth on the 'Virtual' Edge: Researching Marginalized Sexualities and Genders Online. *Qualitative Health Research*, 22: 560-570. https://doi.org/10.1177/1049732311425052

McNeil, J., Bailey, L., Ellis, S., Morton, J. and Regan, M. (2012). "Trans Mental Health Study 2012", Scottish Transgender Alliance, September 2021. Available at: http://www.scottishtrans.org/wp-content/uploads/2013/03/trans_mh_study.pdf (Accessed: 11 May 2021).

Murad, M. H., Elamin, M. B., Garcia, M. Z., Mullan, R. J., Murad, A., Erwin, P. J. and Montori, V. M. (2010). "Hormonal Therapy and Sex Reassignment: A Systematic Review and Meta-Analysis of Quality of Life and Psychosocial Outcomes". *Clinical Endocrinology*, 72 (2): 214–231. https://doi.org/10.1111/j.1365–2265.2009.03625.x

Pearce, R., Erikainen, S. and Vincent, B. (2020). "TERF Wars: An Introduction". *The Sociological Review*, 68 (4): 677–698. doi.org/10.1177/0038026120934713

Pentaris, P. (2021). *Death, Grief and Loss in the Context of COVID-19*. London: Routledge.

Poteat, T., German, D. and Flynn, C. (2016a). "The Conflation of Gender and Sex: Gaps and Opportunities in HIV Data Among Transgender Women and MSM". *Global Public Health*, 11 (7-8): 835–848. https://doi.org/10.1080/17441692.2015.1134615

Poteat, T., Scheim, A., Xavier, J., Reisner, S. and Baral, S. (2016b). Global Epidemiology of HIV infection and Related Syndemics Affecting Transgender People". *Journal of Acquired Immune Deficiency Syndromes (1999)*, 72 (3): S210. https://doi.org/10.1097/QAI.0000000000001087

Rai, S. S., Peters, R. M. H., Syurina, E.V., et al. (2020). "Intersectionality and Health-Related Stigma: Insights from Experiences of People Living with Stigmatized Health Conditions in Indonesia". *International Journal for Equity in Health*, 19 (1): 206. https://doi.org/10.1186/s12939-020-01318-w

Raymond, J. G. (1994). *The Transsexual Empire: The Making of the She-Male*. New York: Teachers College Press.

Reisner, S. L., Greytak, E. A., Parsons, J. T. and Ybarra, M. L. (2014). "Gender Minority Social Stress in Adolescence: Disparities in Adolescent Bullying and Substance Use by Gender Identity". *Journal of Sex Research,* 52 (3): 243-256. https://doi.org/10.1080/00224499.2014.886321

Reisner, S. L., Poteat, T., Keatley, J., Cabral, M., Mothopeng, T., Dunham, E. and Baral, S. D. (2016). "Global Health Burden and Needs of Transgender Populations: A Review". *The Lancet*, 388(10042): 412-436. https://doi.org/10.1016/S0140-6736(16)00684-X

Scheim A, Kacholia V, Logie C, et al. (2020). Health of transgender men in low-income and middle-income countries: a scoping review. *BMJ Global Health,* 5: e003471

Schilt, K. and Westbrook, L. (2009). "Doing Gender, Doing Heteronormativity: 'Gender Normals,' Transgender People, and the Social Maintenance of Heterosexuality". *Gender and Society*, 23: 440–464. doi.org/10.1177/0891243209340034

Smythe, V. (2018). "I'm Credited with Having Coined the Word 'Terf'. Here's How it Happened", The Guardian, 28 November. Available at: https://www.theguardian.com/commentisfree/2018/nov/29/im-credited-with-having-coined-the-acronym-terf-heres-how-it-happened (Accessed: 1 November 2021).

Taylor, A. B., Chan, A., Hall, S. L., Saewyc, E. M. and the Canadian Trans and Non-B. (2020). *Being Safe, Being Me 2019: Results of the Canadian Trans and Nonbinary Youth Health Survey*. Vancouver, Canada: Stigma and Resilience Among Vulnerable Youth Centre, University of British Columbia.

Tewksbury, R. (2015). "Sexual Deviance". In G. Reitzer (ed.) *The Blackwell Encyclopaedia of Sociology*. https://doi.org/10.1002/9781405165518.wbeoss091.pub2

Thorne, N., Witcomb, G. L., Nieder, T., Nixon, E., Yip, A. and Arcelus, J. (2018). "A Comparison of Mental Health Symptomatology and Levels of Social Support in Young Treatment Seeking Transgender Individuals Who Identify as Binary and Non-Binary". *The International Journal of Transgenderism*, 20 (2-3): 241–250. https://doi.org/10.1080/15532739.2018.1452660

Thornton, J. (2021). "Court Upholds Gillick Competence in Puberty Blockers Case". *The Lancet*, 398(10307): 1205-1206. https://doi.org/10.1016/s0140-6736(21)02136-x

Wagaman, M. A. (2014). "Understanding Service Experiences of LGBTQ Young People Through an Intersectional Lens". *Journal of Gay and Lesbian Social Services,* 26 (1): 111-145. https://doi.org/10.1080/10538720.2013.866867

Winter, S., Diamond, M., Green, J., Karasic, D., Reed, T., Whittle, S. and Wylie, K. (2016). "Transgender People: Health at the Margins of Society. *The Lancet,* 388 (10042): 390-400. https://doi.org/10.1016/S0140-6736(16)00683-8

20

THE SOCIAL CONSTRUCTION OF LONELINESS AND GLOBAL PUBLIC HEALTH

Vincent La Placa and Julia Morgan

Introduction

Loneliness and its link to, for example, mental health have become important to global public health and research in the social sciences. Often referred to as the 'epidemic' of loneliness, it is increasingly perceived as a global health, wellbeing, and social issue. This chapter will explore the issue of loneliness, as a global public health issue, and consider current literature on the groups most likely to experience loneliness. The chapter proceeds to argue for a study of loneliness 'in its own right' and suggests some strategic directions for further research, such as use of broader theoretical frameworks, especially the social constructionist approach, and qualitative orientated approaches.

Loneliness and Global Public Health

Loneliness and links to, for instance, mental health have become increasingly central to global public health and social sciences. Often referred to as the 'epidemic' of loneliness, it is increasingly recognised as a global health, wellbeing, and social issue. It is also perceived to assume a critical determinant of global health that not only causes individuals significant stress but that can also have physiological effects, such as reducing lifespan, similarly to activities, like tobacco use (Mental Health Foundation 2017; Victor and Yang, 2018). Whilst globalisation would suggest a more inter-connected society, broader social changes, and the 2020-2021 global pandemic, suggest greater disconnection and isolation has occurred. Globally, most people who require mental health care lack access to high-quality mental health services. Stigma, human resource shortages, fragmented service delivery models, and lack of research infrastructure contribute to the contemporary mental health treatment gap (Wainberg et al., 2017).

DOI: 10.4324/9781003128373-20

Research around loneliness can be complex and multifaced in that it can be deconstructed and defined differently throughout the literature (Yanguas et. al., 2018). Age UK (2015) identifies 'isolation' as separation from social or familial contact, community involvement, or access to services, but 'loneliness' is perceived as an individual's personal, subjective feeling, of not having such things. Furthermore, whilst social isolation is framed as an objective circumstance, perceived in terms of the quantity of social relationships, loneliness is a socially constructed phenomenon. Some definitions perceive loneliness as unidimensional to the extent that it is unitary, differing only in intensity, and is the result of deficits, in various relationships. Other studies define loneliness as 'multidimensional' in that it can comprise subtypes. For example, it might emphasise a distinction between 'emotional loneliness', seen as absence or lack of a close, intimate emotional attachment, and 'social loneliness', an absence of an engaging social or collective network, such as meaningful friendships, and integration within local communities. Neither are there any agreed theoretical frameworks for locating loneliness, with much of the literature biased (although not exclusively) towards psychology and statistical-orientated methods (La Placa and Oham, 2019). Definitions of loneliness are often impacted by how societies socially construct views of loneliness, as well as the available language and cultural frames, with which to construct this.

Nevertheless, increasingly, research is explaining loneliness with recourse to wider social determinants, for example, living alone, and lack of social relations with significant others and networks (Sharabi et al., 2018). Morrison and Smith (2018) identified the absence of stable and close relationships, attachment, social integration, and reassurance of worth, as key determinants of loneliness. Restricted face-to-face communication, the result of growing use of the internet, and other information technologies were also identified as prevalent (Morrison and Smith, 2018). Sagan (2018) has argued that loneliness is primarily caused by the dominance of neo-liberal thought and restructuring of relations between people in contemporary capitalism, which engender atomisation, lack of interaction, and, therefore, higher rates of mental illness, globally.

Imrie (2018) perceived increasing global urbanisation and weakened infrastructure as reducing opportunities for people to develop relations, arguing for urban development, which fostered inclusivity, and opportunities for people to meet. Loneliness is frequently linked to enhanced physiological risks for a variety of physical and mental conditions: high blood pressure, heart disease, obesity, a compromised immune system, anxiety, depression, cognitive decline, Alzheimer's, and even death (Cacioppo and Cacioppo, 2018). Wu (2020) contends that the global pandemic of 2020-2021 will increasingly impact upon loneliness and isolation, given global lockdowns.

Loneliness is often stigmatised, not treated seriously, or trivially ignored (Cacioppo and Cacioppo, 2018), but the rapidly increasing number of older adults globally, increased likelihood of premature mortality, and the detrimental effects of loneliness, such as depression, means the issue has assumed global significance.

There is increasing recognition that tackling loneliness is a preventative measure that enhances the quality of life and reduces long-term costs for health and social care (Ali, 2017).

Governments and global health organisations have been confronted by similar challenges (Goossens et al., 2015; Cacioppo and Cacioppo, 2018). Issues of loneliness are highly cultural variables, but it might be that in the future, continued globalisation and urbanisation mean that low- and middle-income countries will begin to experience public health and wellbeing challenges like high-income countries. As loneliness and social isolation become increasingly global public health and wellbeing issues, Governments from Australia and Denmark to Japan are formulating policies and initiatives around it. For example, in the USA, in 2017, the Senate Committee on Ageing met to discuss loneliness; and Mike Lee, a Republican senator from Utah, established the social capital project, researching the network of relationships in people's lives, which can contribute to resolving issues around loneliness (La Placa and Oham, 2019). Similarly, the World Health Organization lists 'social support networks' as a determinant of health (Wilkinson and Marmot, 2003). The chapter now continues to consider loneliness in the global population.

Loneliness in the Global Population

Much of the literature on loneliness focuses on older people (Kaye and Singer, 2018) and is characterised by contested definitions and theories used to explore it. As numbers of older people globally augment, the proportions experiencing loneliness have amplified, leaving more older people experiencing loneliness. For example, demographic and family changes entail that there are fewer older people with families to provide care and support. The risk of dementia increases considerably with age, with effects on health and wellbeing. Wu (2020) argues that the 2020-2021 global pandemic will impact sharply on older people across the globe. This is not only due to weaker immune systems and enhanced likelihood of experience of chronic conditions but also the fact that globally, for instance, nursing and residential care homes have been especially affected, with high levels of morbidity and mortality, than other settings. In long-term care facilities, visits from family and friends were prevented, to minimise the risk of spreading COVID-19. Globally, older people were instructed to self-quarantine, and distance themselves from others, who might risk infecting them, beyond care settings, further reducing social activities. Wu (2020) suggests raising global awareness of the health impact of social isolation and loneliness of older people across the healthcare workforce and formulating innovative technology-based interventions to marshal resources from families, community-based networks, and assets, to address loneliness in older adults.

Less considered are children and younger adults (Loades et al., 2020). They often experience various and predictable transitions, connected to puberty, schooling, barriers to adequate participation in social activities, through to issues around bullying, and use of social media, which can trigger loneliness. The effects of loneliness on mental health of young adults are apparent in much of the evidence base (Mishra et al., 2018). Loneliness often co-occurs with depression, anxiety, and self-harm, and lonely individuals are more likely to seek assistance from healthcare services for mental health difficulties, compared to individuals, not lonely. For young people, navigating decisions around, for instance, education, developing relationships, or deciding when to start a family, and the precariousness caused by the global pandemic, can compound pressure on existing stressful decisions and during an already critical developmental stage in transitions to adulthood.

The experience of loneliness is critical in terms of gender, particularly, men, although literature in this regard is more limited and contradictory, compared to women. Barreto et al. (2021) argue that although women are socialised to develop more significant and pro-active social networks, potentially safeguarding them from loneliness, it is also clear that women tend to exhibit longer lifespans than men and are, therefore, more likely to be affected by widowhood or likely to assume the role of caregiver. This may suggest that women can experience more loneliness than men, particularly in older age. As a result, Barreto et al. (2021) assert the importance of exploring loneliness, through a multifaceted perspective, which considers the social construction of gender on loneliness, across different age groups, and cultures.

Literature suggests that the social and cultural construction of men's emotional reticence often constitute a barrier to discussing loneliness and to developing loneliness-preventing relationships (Bergland, Tveit and Gonzalez, 2016; Franklin et al., 2019). Neville et al. (2018) report that unpartnered men of lower socio-economic status, with limited social networks, and mental health difficulties were more likely to be lonely. Similarly, using a 'gender-relations' approach (which perceives gender as socially produced and constructed through everyday social practices, as opposed to a fixed set of essential characteristics which people possess), Mckenzie et al. (2018) ascertained that social constructs of masculinity played a part in men's experience of loneliness. Men were more likely to experience difficulties in mobilising support from existing social connections, as well as the need to be perceived as independent, and in less need of social support. This enables men to retain their masculine status and social standing with other men. Barreto et al. (2021) suggest that men are more reluctant than women to admit feeling lonely and that men who do are more stigmatised than women, who admit to similar feelings.

The globalisation of lesbian, gay, and bisexual (LGB), and transgender and non-binary studies has precipitated a growing focus on global discrimination against sexual and gender minorities (Garcia et al., 2020; Eres et al., 2021). This has led researchers and practitioners to focus upon heightened risks of social isolation and loneliness, which LGB, non-binary, and trans people often confront, given internalised homophobia and trans-phobia and external discrimination. It has also precipitated an increased concentration on research that can elucidate pathways and processes, which predict health or that promote, for instance, resiliency and wellbeing among sexual and gender minorities. Much of the literature explores loneliness through the lens of 'minority stress theory', like the 'psychological mediation framework', which emphasises the significance of stigma, prejudice, and discrimination, which foster a hostile and stressful social environment, and translates into mental health issues (Kuyper and Fokkema, 2010). Ratanashevorn and Brown (2021) argue that loneliness for LGB, non-binary, and trans people is compounded by marginalisation, discrimination, and alienation in society and social networks. Experiences of increased loneliness often led to other harmful mental health outcomes, such as substance abuse, HIV, and suicide. They argue for more emphasis on loneliness through existential therapy to help alleviate it and aid LGB, non-binary, and trans people to adjust. The chapter will now proceed to consider further directions in loneliness research.

Further Research into Loneliness

Loneliness now constitutes a significant research and policy issue in global health, largely because of its link to negative mental health outcomes. This has accentuated the limited resources and policies towards global mental health previously, in comparison to the burden it engenders, generally. Others have argued for a deeper understanding, rooted in structured and unequal relationships in society, which further cause stress to already marginalised people (Sagan, 2018) and are less grounded in individual psychology.

Wainberg et al. (2017) argue that two momentous events in 2016 influenced the international development community and led to increased action in relation to addressing mental health globally. The first event was the World Bank's endorsement of mental health as a global development priority. The second was the inclusion of mental health in the United Nation's Sustainable Development Goals, which will influence global and national agendas for the near future, according to Wainberg et al. (2017). The commitment to a global mental health approach was further cemented by the World Health Organization (2019), which has also formulated the 'Special Initiative for Mental Health (2019–2023): Universal Health Coverage for Mental Health'. The Initiative looks to promote mental health policies, advocacy, and human rights, and scale up services across community-based, general health, and specialist settings.

The authors assert that the growing trend towards elevating loneliness as a new and critical issue in social science and global public health will undoubtedly be welcomed by mental health advocates, and those working in, for instance, counselling and the psychological sciences. However, we identify two issues in need of being addressed as a result. The first represents the requirement to ensure that the study of, and responses to, loneliness remains an endeavour that maintains the concept/idea within its only contours and frames of study and not be solely subsumed under 'mental health studies' and psychology. The second refers to issues around the theoretical and strategic direction of loneliness research, for instance, the need to use and develop adequate theoretical and definitional frameworks and types of research, which also captures the cross-cultural dimension of it.

Whilst the growth in loneliness as a public health issue is to be welcomed, the authors believe that the study of loneliness should not be simply substituted by or completely subsumed under concepts of mental health, stress, and stressful environments only (despite the strong link). Loneliness needs to be considered as a study, and issue in its own right, if future researchers are to be able to, for example, capture its root causes, its effects on different groups, and the diverse global, social, and cultural constructions of it. This we believe also mitigates against one-size-fits-all approaches towards interventions, as well as protecting against the study of loneliness as synonymous with mental health studies only, often through a proximal and psychological approach; although, of course, as this chapter has demonstrated, not exclusively.

For example, La Placa and Oham (2019) found that much of the research on young adults, mental health, and loneliness was often biased towards biomedical and psychological frameworks and did not inherently locate it within perspectives, which focus on how it is socially constructed, and within wider determinants. Therefore, the symbolic and discursive nature of loneliness was often negated. Leigh-Hunt et al. (2017) conducted a systematic review of literature focused on loneliness and highlighted consistent evidence connecting loneliness to negative cardiovascular and psychological health outcomes, suggesting overemphasis on the psychological and clinical elements. They also found that more evidence was required regarding associations with cancer, health behaviours, and the impact of wider determinants, such as experience of the life-course, and the wider socio-economic consequences of loneliness.

Rather, we perceive the study of loneliness as something which encompasses and is located within, for example, branches of sociology, economics, and psychology and which strands the social sciences broadly. Neither is there a one-size-fits-all approach to addressing loneliness, and the requirement to tailor interventions, to match the needs of individuals, specific groups, or the degree of loneliness experienced, as well as health inequalities strategies, will be enhanced by a broad approach. As the field of loneliness in public health abounds, the authors also feel that research should be more clearly directed, with an emphasis on developing adequate definitional and theoretical frameworks, as well as an enhanced focus on qualitative research. La Placa and Oham (2019) also found that much evidence was biased towards psychology compared with social determinants and their link to experiences and interpretations of loneliness. Also, there was little effort to distinguish 'health' from 'wellbeing', largely because of bias towards positivist frameworks, which negated the social and symbolic construction of loneliness.

As a result, we would concur that further loneliness research needs to utilise more holistic concepts of 'wellbeing', 'quality of life', and 'happiness', and definitional references beyond only the 'physical', to capture detail, and multiple perspectives. We would also concur with their finding that the evidence needs broader theoretical frameworks to encompass specific research and guide intervention developments, for instance, minority stress theory, and the gender-relations approach. We also argue that the social constructionist perspective is useful, which would perceive loneliness and isolation within language, culture, and available individual, and social representations around relationships, and break down experiences into distinct categories of loneliness, as well as the link to wider determinants (Stein and Tuval-Mashiach, 2015). Ozawa de-Silva and Parsons (2020) contend that loneliness is a social, relational, affective, and inter-subjective reality, distinct from the physical reality of social isolation, enhancing the usefulness of Social Constructionism. For a more detailed focus on social constructionist theory, please refer to Chapter 2.

We also posit that the association between mental health and loneliness studies often lends research to more quantitative orientated approaches, grounded in positivism, and proximal categories, as well as large literature reviews of the (often statistical) evidence, when more qualitative research is needed, to expand and enhance current evidence. Qualitative methods will enable an in-depth understanding of the research subject and supply more detailed interpretivist data to generate practice-based policy.

Conclusion

This chapter has explored the issue of loneliness as a global public health issue and considered current literature on the groups most likely to experience loneliness. The chapter argued for a study of loneliness, in its own right, and suggested some strategic directions for further research.

Research Points and Reflective Exercise

With reference to the discussions in this chapter, begin to reflect upon the following:

- Why is loneliness a significant global public health issue?
- What interventions may alleviate loneliness?
- How far do you think that loneliness as a concept differs cross culturally?

Further Resources and Reading

La Placa, V. and Oham, C. (2019). "Loneliness and Young People Experiencing Mental Health Difficulties: Evidence and Further Research". *PEOPLE: International Journal of Social Sciences,* 5 (2): 1024-1039. https://doi.org/10.20319/pijss.2019.52.10241039

References

Age UK. (2015). *Promising Approaches to Reducing Loneliness and Isolation in Later Life*. London: Age UK.

Ali, N. (2017). *Public Health England: Recognising the Impact of Loneliness: A Public Health Issue*. London: Public Health England.

Barreto, M., Victor, C., Hammond, C., Eccles, A., Richins, M. T. and Qualter, P. (2021). "Loneliness Around the World: Age, Gender, and Cultural Differences in Loneliness". *Personality and Individual Difference*, 169: 110066. https://doi.org/10.1016/j.paid.2020.110066

Bergland, A. M. G., Tveit, B. and Gonzalez, M. T. (2016). Experiences of Older Men Living Alone: A Qualitative Study. *Issues in Mental Health Nursing*, 37 (2): 113–120. https://doi.org/10.3109/01612840.2015.1098759

Cacioppo, J. T., and Cacioppo, S. (2018). "The Growing Problem of Loneliness". *The Lancet*, 391, 246. https://doi.org/10.1016/S0140-6736(18)30142-9

Eres, R., Postolovski, N., Thielking, M. and Lim, M. H. (2021). "Loneliness, Mental Health, and Social Health Indicators in LGBTQIA+ Australians". *American Journal of Orthopsychiatry*, 91 (3): 358–366. https://doi.org/10.1037/ort0000531

Franklin, A., Barbosa Neves, B., Hookway, N., Patulny, R., Tranter, B. and Jaworski, K. (2019). "Towards an Understanding of Loneliness among Australian Men: Gender Cultures, Embodied Expression and the Social Bases of Belonging". *Journal of Sociology*, 55 (1): 124–143. https://doi.org/10.1177/1440783318777309

Garcia, J., Vargas, N., Clark, J. L., Magaña Álvarez, M., Nelons, D. A. and Parker, R. G. (2020). "Social Isolation and Connectedness as Determinants of Well-Being: Global Evidence Mapping Focused on LGBTQ Youth". *Global Public Health*, 15 (4): 497-519. https://doi.org/10.1080/17441692.2019.1682028

Goossens, L., Verhagen, M., van Roekel, E., Cacioppo, J. T., Cacioppo, S. and Boomsma, D. I. (2015). "The Genetics of Loneliness: The Quest for Underlying Mechanisms and Developmental Processes". *Perspectives on Psychological Science*, 10: 213–222. https://doi.org/10.1177/1745691614564878

Imrie, R. (2018). "'The Lonely City': Urban Infrastructure and the Problem of Loneliness". In O. Sagan and E. D. Miller (eds.) *Narratives of Loneliness: Multidisciplinary Perspectives from the 21st Century*. London: Routledge, 140-152.

Kaye, L. W. and Singer, C. M. (2018). *Social Isolation of Older Adults: Strategies to Bolster Health and Well-Being (Critical Topics in an Aging Society)*. New York: Springer.

Kuyper L. and Fokkema, T. (2010). "Loneliness Among Older Lesbian, Gay, and Bisexual Adults: The Role of Minority Stress". *Archives of Sexual Behavior*, 39 (5): 1171–1180. https://doi.org/10.1007/s10508-009-9513-7

La Placa, V. and Oham, C. (2019). "Loneliness and Young People Experiencing Mental Health Difficulties: Evidence and Further Research". *PEOPLE: International Journal of Social Sciences,* 5 (2): 1024-1039. https://doi.org/10.20319/pijss.2019.52.10241039

Leigh-Hunt, N., Bagguley, D., Bash, K., Turner, V., Turnbull, S., Valtorta, N. and Caan, W. (2017). "An Overview of Systematic Reviews on the Public Health Consequences of Social Isolation and Loneliness". *Public Health*, 152: 157-171. https://doi.org/10.1016/j.puhe.2017.07.035

Loades, M. E., Chatburn, E., Higson-Sweeney, N., Reynolds, S., Shafran, R., Brigden, A., Linney, C., Niamh McManus, M., Borwick, C. and Crawley, C. (2020). "Rapid Systematic Review: The Impact of Social Isolation and Loneliness on the Mental Health of Children and Adolescents in the Context of COVID-19". *Journal of the American Academy of Child and Adolescent Psychiatry*, 59 (11): 1218-1239. https://doi.org/10.1016/j.jaac.2020.05.009

McKenzie, S. K., Collings, S., Jenkin, G. and River, J. (2018). "Masculinity, Social Connectedness, and Mental Health: Men's Diverse Patterns of Practice". *American Journal of Men's Health*, 12 (5): 1247–1261. https://doi.org/10.1177/1557988318772732

Mishra, S. K., Deo Kodwani, A., Kumar, K. K. and Jain, K. K. (2018). "Linking Loneliness to Depression: A Dynamic Perspective". *Benchmarking: An International Journal*, 25: 2089-2104. https://doi.org/10.1108/BIJ-10-2016-0158

Morrison, P. S. and Smith, R. (2018). "Loneliness: An Overview" In O. Sagan and E. D. Miller (eds.) *Narratives of Loneliness: Multidisciplinary Perspectives from the 21st Century*. London: Routledge, 11-25.

Neville, S., Adams, J. and Montayre, J. (2018). "Loneliness in Men 60 Years and Over: The Association With Purpose in Life". *American Journal of Men's Health*, 12 (4): 730–739. https://doi.org/10.1177/1557988318758807

Ozawa de-Silva, C. and Parsons, M. (2020). "Towards an Anthropology of Loneliness". *Transcultural Psychiatry*, 57 (5): 613-622. https://doi.org/10.1177/1363461520961627

Ratanashevorn, R. and Brown, E. C. (2021). "'Alone in the Rain(bow)': Existential Therapy for Loneliness in LGBTQ + Clients". *Journal of LGBTQ Issues in Counseling*, 15 (1): 110-127. https://doi.org/10.1080/15538605.2021.1868375

Sagan, O. (2018). "Narratives of Loneliness and Mental Health in a Time of Neoliberalism". In O. Sagan and E. D. and Miller (eds.) *Narratives of Loneliness: Multidisciplinary Perspectives from the 21st Century*. London: Routledge, 89-100.

Sharabi, A., Levi, U. and Margalit, M. (2018). "Children's Loneliness, Sense of Coherence, Family Climate and Hope: Development Risk and Protective Factors". In A. Rokach (ed.) *Loneliness Updated: Recent Research on Loneliness and How it Affects Our Lives*. London: Routledge, 65-87.

Stein, J. Y. and Tuval-Mashiach, R. (2015). "The Social Construction of Loneliness: An Integrative Conceptualization". *Journal of Constructivist Psychology*, 28: (3): 210-227, https://doi.org/10.1080/10720537.2014.911129

The Mental Health Foundation. (2017). *Loneliness: The Public Health Challenge of Our Time- A Policy Briefing by the Mental Health Foundation and Age Scotland*. London: Mental Health Foundation.

Wainberg, M. L., Scorza, P., Shultz, J. M., Helpman, L., Mootz, J. J., Johnson, K. A., Neria, Y., Bradford, J. M. E., Oquendo, M. A. and Arbuckle, M. R. (2017). "Challenges and Opportunities in Global Mental Health: A Research-to-Practice Perspective". *Current Psychiatry Reports*, 19, 28. https://doi.org/10.1007/s11920-017-0780-z

Wilkinson, R. and Marmot, M. (2003). *The Social Determinants of Health: The Solid Facts*. Europe: World Health Organisation (WHO).

World Health Organization (WHO). (2019). "The WHO Special Initiative for Mental Health (2019-2023): Universal Health Coverage for Mental Health". World Health Organization. Available at: https://apps.who.int/iris/handle/10665/310981 (Accessed: 8 July 2020).

Wu, B. (2020). "Social Isolation and Loneliness Among Older Adults in the Context of COVID-19: A Global Challenge". *Global Health Research and Policy*, 5: 27. https://doi.org/10.1186/s41256-020-00154-3

Victor, C. R. and Yang, K. (2018). "The Prevalence of Loneliness Among Adults: A Case Study of the United Kingdom". In A. Rokach (ed.) *Loneliness Updated: Recent Research on Loneliness and How it Affects Our Lives*. London: Routledge, 88-107.

Yanguas, J., Pinazo-Henandis, S. and Tarazona-Santabalbina, F. J. (2018). "The Complexity of Loneliness". *Acta bio-medica: Atenei Parmensis,* 89 (2): 302–314. https://doi.org/10.23750/abm.v89i2.7404

21

GLOBAL ORAL HEALTH AND INEQUALITIES

Charlotte Jeavons and Bal Chana

Introduction

Oral diseases are a global public health issue. They are among the most prevalent diseases in the world and have a considerable effect on people's quality of life. Oral diseases also create a significant economic burden for society (Peterson et al., 2005). Of all oral diseases, the most common are dental caries, periodontal disease, and cancers of the oral cavity, including the lips. Worldwide, oral diseases affect 3.9 billion people and untreated caries in adults was found to be the most prevalent condition in the Global Burden of Disease Study (UN, 2011; Marcenes et al., 2013; Global Burden of Disease Collaborative Network, 2016). They also share common risk factors with other non-communicable diseases (NCDs), which have increased sharply in low- and middle-income countries (LMICs). Poor oral health can indicate low socio-economic status, poverty, and lack of access to services, with oral health inequality increasing. This chapter will focus on health inequalities and the burden of oral disease globally, also linking it to the process of the globalisation of health and lifestyle.

Common Oral Diseases

The term 'oral disease' covers a wide range of conditions that affect the hard and soft tissues of the oral cavity. These include congenital anomalies, cranio-facial disorders, trauma, and various infections and diseases such as oral cancers. However, the most prevalent on a global scale are dental caries (tooth decay) and periodontal disease (gum disease). Sharing a common inflammatory pathway means periodontal disease is associated with other chronic diseases, including diabetes (Chapple and Genco, 2013), cardiovascular diseases (Lockhart et al., 2012), low birth weight and premature babies (Piscoya et al., 2012), and dementia (Daly

DOI: 10.4324/9781003128373-21

et al., 2017). In older adults periodontal disease has been causally linked to aspiration pneumonia (Awano et al., 2008). Caries is also associated with sepsis (Pine et al., 2006). Both dental caries and periodontal disease can cause unremitting pain and suffering, but both are preventable through good oral hygiene and low sugar diet (Levine and Stillman-Low, 2018). These are considered global public health priorities (Pitts et al., 2017; Peres et al., 2019).

The primary risk factors for major chronic and NCDs frequently cluster in the same individuals (Georgios et al., 2015). Multiple behavioural risk factors have been associated with increased (oral) disease risk, for example, smoking, alcohol intake, and low consumption of fruits and vegetables. Similarly, to general health, there is a clear socio-economic gradient to health behaviours with increased clustering of health-compromising behaviours experienced by those lower down the gradient. Therefore, a common risk factor approach better understands biological and behavioural aspects of the aetiology of oral and associated diseases (Watt et al., 2012).

Oral Health Inequalities

A reduction of global oral health inequalities will only be achieved if the underlying causes of social inequalities in structural determinants are tackled. Marmot (2007) has described the social determinants of health as the fundamental structures of social hierarchy and the socially determined conditions these create, in which people grow, live, work, and age. In short, they are the causes of the causes, where the social becomes the biological, because the lived experience of socio-economic disadvantage results in poor (oral) health. Muirhead et al. (2020) argue that theoretical frameworks in oral health research are lacking, and it has been slow to use theories, such as intersectionality and perspectives which, for example, focus on gender inequality in oral health. Social Constructionism has often been negated too, as much of the research derives from deductive quantitative methods, outside of social sciences, where social theories are perceived as secondary (Muirhead et al., 2020).

However, the World Health Organization's (WHO) social determinants framework is highly influenced by social science theories of power and control, especially Critical Public Health (Levine and Stillman-Lowe, 2018). The theory challenges dominant discourses and approaches in public health and questions the status quo with reference to social determinants, social gradients, and who defines public health 'problems and issues. It deconstructs fundamental assumptions by considering them within the context of the social and cultural milieus in which they are constructed, and challenges existing inequalities, and why they exist as such. Critical Public Health frameworks also demonstrate how significant determinants relate to one another, and to the mechanisms, involved in generating inequalities in population (oral) health. Changing the distribution of power within society requires political processes that empower disadvantaged communities and increases accountability and responsibility from those in authority.

Critical Public Health theory seeks to embed these approaches strategically, and design new and innovative policies and interventions, to address inequality and social exclusion. Muirhead et al. (2020) assert that enhanced use of critical perspectives like intersectionality theory would show which intersections predispose people to enhanced risk of poor oral health and protective factors. Adopting intersectionality would identify populations, more likely to be a target of stigma, experience exclusion from dental services, disengage from services, and illuminate more broadly the influence of social gradients, and health inequalities.

Social gradients are apparent in oral health in most countries, and these have been widely reported in high-income nations. However, much less is known about LMICs, but available evidence shows high levels of oral health inequality in, and between, LMICs (Do, 2012). Measurement of inequalities in LMICs using the Human Development Index (HDI), Gross Domestic Product (GDP) for urban and rural communities, education levels, and occupation enables analysis of socio-economic indicators, as a proxy for oral health. These indicators comprise structural and intermediary determinants (Watt and Sheiham, 2012). Structural determinants are the socio-economic and political context that create social hierarchies, which then determine the socio-economic position of individuals. Intermediary determinants outline how individual socio-economic position influences health by creating individual circumstances. For example, people living in LMICs with low socio-economic positions are born, live, work, and age in less favourable circumstances, than those in high-income countries (HICs), due to the economic and political context of their country of birth and its global position.

Regardless of country, poorer people are more vulnerable to oral disease because of increased exposure to risk factors and inadequate access to oral health services (Peterson et al., 2005). It is the common biological, behavioural, psychological, environmental, and socio-economic risk factors that determine the global pattern of general and oral health inequalities. How oral health relates to socio-economic inequality has been extensively described in literature and some recent studies have demonstrated a causal relationship between socio-economic status and oral health (Matsuyama et al., 2017). For example, the association between low educational background and caries experience is significantly higher in countries with high HDI scores relative to countries with low index scores (Schwendicke et al., 2015). Another example of how levels of oral disease mirror the social-economic gradient was demonstrated by Klinge and Norlund (2005), who showed that socio-economic circumstances are associated with poor periodontal health.

Dental caries was traditionally low in low-income countries until recently (Do, 2012). Caries has changed from a disease of affluence to one of deprivation on a global scale. The dental caries experience of children living in countries with high levels of HDI or GDP has seen a significant improvement, while child oral health for those living in low-income countries remains unchanged, thus increasing the level of inequality between child oral health in LMICs and HICs. The increasing consumption of soft drinks and of obesity in several LMICs indicates an upward trend in caries in those countries. There is a similar unequal global distribution in the rate of periodontal disease. A key risk factor for periodontal disease is tobacco use, including smoking, which has increased sharply in many low-income countries (Hosseinpoor et al., 2011) Conversely HICs are witnessing a reduction in smoking rates because of successful public health policies (Petersen and Ogawa, 2012), and so the level of periodontal disease between LMICs and HICs is diverging, further increasing oral health inequalities globally. Other oral diseases such as cancers, facial deformities, and dental trauma are also more common in LMICs than in HICs (Petersen et al., 2005).

Extreme oral health inequalities exist for the most marginalised groups, for example, the homeless, prisoners, refugees, Indigenous groups, and those with long-term disabilities (Peres et al., 2019). Homeless people, living in HICs, have more untreated dental caries, more severe tooth loss, and are more likely to experience dental pain, than the general population (Parker et al., 2011). Prisoners have extremely poor oral health. Boyer et al. (2002) reported that prisoners in the USA had 8.4 times more untreated caries than non-institutionalised adults. There is little evidence about people who are homeless or prisoners in LMICs, although the oral health gradient will broadly adhere to the social gradient for each individual LMIC, with people in these groups, located at the bottom. Poorly resourced or limited availability of services in many LMICs is likely to exacerbate the problem. Indigenous peoples globally are especially vulnerable to oral diseases, even if living in a HIC, where general population oral health is good. Early childhood caries in Indigenous people has been reported to range from 68 to 90% and with increased severity (Parker et al., 2010). Adults from Indigenous groups have also been shown to have poorer oral health and higher treatment needs (Schroth et al., 2009).

Indigenous populations often live in remote or rural communities, meaning accessing dental care is not easy or straightforward. Some people with disabilities display specific oral health problems, related to their disability, while others live with restrictions to their actions to maintain good oral hygiene and access care (Faulks et al., 2012). When a person has high general health needs, their oral health is often not prioritised, which further compounds existing problems. Sadly, often those people in most need, because of ill health, personal circumstances, or place of birth, are often the people, who receive least assistance.

Moreover, the primary risk factors for major chronic and NCDs frequently cluster in the same individuals (Georgios et al., 2015; Tonetti et al., 2017). Multiple behavioural risk factors have been associated with increased (oral) disease risk, for example, smoking, alcohol intake, and low consumption of fruits and vegetables. Similarly, to general health, there is a clear socio-economic gradient to health.

The Burden of Oral Disease

The global burden of oral disease is high. The Global Burden of Disease study (2016) reported that 3.5 billion people worldwide live with oral disease with untreated caries, severe periodontal disease, edentulism (complete tooth loss), and severe tooth loss (having between one and nine teeth remaining) featuring prominently (Kassebaum et al., 2017). The International Agency for Research reported cancers of the lip and oral cavity were among the top 15 most common cancers in the world (Bray et al., 2018). In 2015, oral disease expenditure was US $356.80 billion in direct costs and US $187.61 billion in indirect costs, while €90 billion was spent by EU member states, making this the third highest expenditure in the EU, behind diabetes, and cardiovascular disease (Righolt et al., 2018).

Lifetime prevalence of caries has decreased in the past four decades, but this reduction has largely been experienced by people living in HICs (Frencken et al., 2017). This is mostly due to the widespread availability and use of fluoride toothpaste. But when caries prevalence is viewed globally, the burden remains relatively unchanged. Untreated caries in deciduous teeth affected 9% of the global child population in 2010, which remained unchanged since 1990 (Marcenes et al., 2013). In 2010 the age-standardised global incidence was 15,205 cases per 1000,000, which was slightly but non-significantly less than 15,437 cases per 100,000 in 1990 (Marcenes et al., 2013).

By 2015, the prevalence of untreated caries in deciduous teeth had improved to 7.8% of the global child population, but the age-standardised prevalence estimates were similar to 1990. Untreated caries peaked in 2015 among children aged one to four years old (Kassebaum et al., 2017). For many of these children, treatment under general anaesthesia is the only option (Peres et al., 2019). Not only can this be traumatic, but often it is only available in HICs. A 4% reduction in the global prevalence of untreated caries occurred in adults with permanent dentition between 1990 and 2017, from 31,407 cases in 1990, decreasing to 30,129 cases per 100,000 (Kassebaum et al., 2015). Access to oral care is financially challenging for adults, lower down the social-economic gradient, and often individuals wait until the pain is severe, or if serious infection, such as sepsis develops, before seeking emergency care. Globally, adult oral pain is the most common contributor to poor quality of life (Slade et al., 1998).

Prevalence of severe periodontal disease also remains largely unchanged since 1990, although there has been a slight improvement. In 1990, prevalence was estimated at 11.2%, and by 2010, this had decreased to 10.8% of people, worldwide (Kassebaum et al., 2014). Epidemiological studies of periodontal disease are a challenge due to the various measurement tools used globally, and problems of coverage, and, as a result, figures are estimates. Incidence of cancer of the lip and oral cavity was 500,550 in 2018, with 177, 384 total deaths, of which 67% were males. The major risk factors for oral cancers are tobacco and alcohol consumption and areca nut (betal quid) chewing (Jethwa and Khariwala, 2017; Mehrtash et al., 2017). Oral cancer has the highest incidence of all cancers in Melanesia and South Asian males (Bray et al., 2018). It is the leading cause of cancer-related mortality for males in India and Sri Lanka. For males in LMICs, with a low HDI, oral cancer is the fourth highest of all cancers (Bray et al., 2018). In many HICs, the human papilloma virus infection is responsible for increasing oropharyngeal cancers (Mehanna et al., 2013) and prevalence is greater among men and older age groups from poorer backgrounds (Conway et al., 2015).

The globalisation and convergence of health, illness, and lifestyles assume an increasing part in the burden of oral disease and have become a particular focus for Critical Public Health perspectives. Critical perspectives have emerged, especially to focus on economic and commercial relationships between high- and low- to middle-income countries and the production of global inequalities in health and illness, as a result. Since the 1960s, there has been a gradual increase in the production and consumption of sugar (Kearney, 2010). Marketing of tobacco products has become heavily restricted in many HICs, but much less so in LMICs. Conversely, economic development in many LMICs has improved the lives of millions of people, lifting them out of poverty, but has also led to adverse dietary changes and use of tobacco products (Kearney, 2010; Watt et al., 2018). Multinational corporations have re-orientated their products and marketing from the near-saturated markets of HICs to also target the new opportunities emerging in LMICs (Peres et al., 2019). Please refer to Chapter 3 for a more detailed focus on the globalisation of health and wellbeing.

Commercial determinants of health are defined as strategies and approaches used by the private sector to promote products and choices that are injurious to health (Kickbusch et al., 2016). The WHO Director General has stated that the effort to impede NDCs goes against the business interests of powerful economic operators (Chan, 2013; WHO, 2015). From this information, it is clear to see that while the overall global burden of oral disease may not have reduced significantly, the pattern of disease is moving and clustering in LMICs. There are many complex reasons for this, including poorly resourced, or very limited services, increasing consumption of food and drinks containing free sugars, poor access to fluoride, use of tobacco, and smoking.

Conclusion

Oral diseases are a major public health problem but are often underestimated and poorly understood. Research lacks sufficient social sciences theoretical frameworks to adequately elaborate on health inequalities, the unfair global burden of oral disease, and their interaction with other diseases of the body. The development of, for instance, Critical Public Health, and Intersectionality theory may begin to address this, given the prevalence of oral disease, its negative effects, and the social and structural determinants that cause it. Oral diseases are intricately linked to socio-economic status and wider social and commercial determinants. They disproportionately affect poorer and marginalised groups. Oral disease is preventable. Treatment alone will not solve this global problem. More attention is required to tackle the social and commercial determinants, if the burden of disease experienced and inequalities caused are to be reduced.

Research Points and Reflective Exercise

With reference to the discussions in this chapter, begin to reflect upon the following:

- What is the coverage of oral health services in your own country or region?
- How is dental care financed in your own country or region?
- What dental public health initiatives have your country implemented and do these differ from other countries?
- Identify an area of oral health knowledge that either requires further development, or that you want to research, and decide how you plan to address this.

Further Reading and Resources

Challacombe S., Chidzonga M., Glick M., Hodgson T., Magalhães, M., et al. (2011). "Global Oral Health Inequalities: Oral Infections–Challenges and Approaches". *Advances in Dental Research*, 23: 227-236. https://doi.org/10.1177/0022034511402081

Sheiham A., Cohen A., Marinho V., Moysés, S., Petersen, P. E., et al. (2011). "Global Oral Health Inequalities: Task Group—Implementation and Delivery of Oral Health Strategies". *Advances Dental Research*. 23: 259-267. https://doi.org/10.1177/0022034511402084

Watt R. (2012). "Social Determinants of Oral Health Inequalities: Implications for Action". *Community Dental Health*, 40: 44-48. https://doi.org/10.1111/j.1600-0528.2012.00719.x

References

Awano, S, Ansai., T, Takata., Y, Soh I., Akifusa, S., et al. (2008). "Oral Health and Mortality Risk from Pneumonia in the Elderly". *Journal of Dental Research,* 87 (4): 334-349. https://doi.org/10.1177/154405910808700418.

Boyer, E. M., Nielsen-Thompson, N. J. and Hill, T. J. (2002). "A Comparison of Dental Caries and Tooth Loss for Iowa Prisoners with Other Prison Populations and Dentate US Adults". *Journal Dental Hygiene,* 76 (2): 141–50. https://doi.org/10.4103/2141-9248.139365

Bray, F., Ferlay, J., Soerjomataram, I., Siegel, R. L., Torre, L. A., et al. (2018). "Global Cancer Statistics 2018: GLOBOCAN Estimates of Incidence and Mortality Worldwide for 36 Cancers in 185 Countries". *CA Cancer Journal for Clinicians,* 68: 394-424. https://doi.org/10.3322/caac.21492

Chan M. (2013). "WHO Director-General Addresses Health Promotion Conference", 10 June. Available at: https://www.who.int/director-general/speeches/2013/%20health_promotion_20130610/en (Accessed: 30 December 2021).

Chapple, I. L. and Genco, R. (2013). "Diabetes and Periodontal Diseases: Consensus Report of the Joint EFP/AAP Workshop on Periodontitis and Systemic Diseases". *Journal of Periodontology,* 84: S106–112. https://doi.org/10.1902/jop.2013.1340011

Conway, D. I., Brenner, D. R., McMahon A. D., Macpherson, L. M. D., Agudo, A., et al. (2015). "Estimating and Explaining the Effect of Education and Income on Head and Neck Cancer Risk: INHANCE Consortium Pooled Analysis of 31 Case-Control Studies From 27 Countries". *International Journal of Cancer,* 136 (5): 1125-1139. https://doi.org/10.1002/ijc.29063

Daly, B., Thompsell, A., Sharpling, J., Rooney, M., Hillman, L. et al. (2017). "Evidence Summary: The Relationship Between Oral Health and Dementia". *British Dental Journal*, 223 (11): 846–53. 24. https://doi.org/10.1038/sj.bdj.2017.992

Do, L G. (2012). "Distribution of Caries in Children: Variations Between and Within Populations". *Journal of Dental Research*, 91 (6): 536-543. https://doi.org/10.1177/0022034511434355

Faulks, D., Freedman, L., Thompson, S., Sagheri, D. and Dougall, A. (2012). "The Value of Education in Special Care Dentistry as a Means of Reducing Inequalities in Oral Health". *European Journal of Dental Education*, 16: 195–201. https://doi.org/10.1111/j.1600-0579.2012.00736.x

Frencken, J. E., Sharma, P., Stenhouse, L., Green, D., Laverty, D., et al. (2017). "Global Epidemiology of Dental Caries and Severe Periodontitis— A Comprehensive Review". *Journal Of Clinical Periodontology*, 44: S94–105. https://doi.org/10.1111/jcpe.12677

Georgios, A. W., Aida, J. and Alzahrani, S. (2015). "The Role of Psychosocial and Behavioural Factors in Shaping Oral Health Inequalities". In R. G. Watt, S. Listl, M. Peres and A. Heilmann (eds.) *Social Inequalities in Oral Health: From Evidence to Action*. London: ICOHIRP, 18-19.

Global Burden of Disease Collaborative Network. (2016). *Global Burden of Disease Study 2015 (GBD 2015) Population Estimates 1970-2015*. Seattle: Institute for Health Metrics and Evaluation (IHME).

Hosseinpoor, A. R., Parker, L. A., Tursan d'Espaignet, E. and Chatterji, S. (2011). "Social Determinants of Smoking in Low- and Middle-Income Countries: Results from the World Health Survey". *PLoS One*, 6 (5): e20331. https://doi.org/10.1371/journal.pone.0020331

Jethwa, A. R. and Khariwala, S. S. (2017). "Tobacco-Related Carcinogenesis in Head and Neck Cancer". *Cancer and Metastasis Reviews*, 36 (3): 411-423. https://doi.org/10.1007/s10555-017-9689-6

Kassebaum, N. J., Bernabé, E., Dahiya, M., Bhandari, B., Murray, C. J. L., et al. (2014). "Global Burden of Severe Periodontitis in 1990–2010". *Journal of Dental Research*, 93: 1045–1053. https://doi.org/10.1177/0022034514552491

Kassebaum, N. J., Bernabé, E., Dahiya, M., Bhandari, B., Murray, C. J. L., et al. (2015). "Global Burden of Untreated Caries: A Systematic Review and Metaregression". *Journal of Dental Research*, 94: 650–658. https://doi.org/10.1177/0022034515573272

Kassebaum, N. J., Smith, A. G. C., Bernabé E., Fleming, T. D., Reynolds, A. E., et al. (2017). "Global, Regional, and National Prevalence, Incidence, and Disability-Adjusted Life Years for Oral Conditions for 195 Countries, 1990–2015: A Systematic Analysis for the Global Burden of Diseases, Injuries, and Risk Factors". *Journal of Dental Research*, 96: 380–387. https://doi.org/10.1177/0022034517693566

Kearney J. (2010). "Food Consumption Trends and Drivers". *Philosophical Transactions of The Royal Society B Biological Sciences*, 365 (1554): 2793-2807. https://doi.org/10.1098/rstb.2010.0149

Kickbusch, I., Allen, L. and Franz, C. (2016). "The Commercial Determinants of Health". *The Lancet Global Health*, 4: e895–896. https://doi.org/10.1016/S2214-109X(16)30217-0

Klinge B. and Norlund, A. (2005) "A Socio-Economic Perspective on Periodontal Diseases: A Systematic Review". *Journal Of Clinical Periodontology*, 32: 314–325. https://doi.org/10.1111/j.1600-051X.2005.00801.x

Levine, R. and Stillman-Lowe, C. (2018). *The Scientific Basis of Oral Health Education*, 8th edn. Switzerland: Springer Nature.

Lockhart, P. B., Bolger, A. F., Papapanou, P. N., Osinbowale, O., Trevisan, M., et al. (2012). Periodontal Disease and Atherosclerotic Vascular Disease: Does the

Evidence Support an Independent Association? *Circulation,* 125 (20): 2520–2544. doi 10.1161/CIR.0b013e31825719f3

Marcenes, W., Kassebaum, N. J., Bernabe, E., Flaxman, A., Naghavi, M., et al. (2013). "Global Burden of Oral Conditions in 1990-2010: A Systematic Analysis". *Journal of Dental Research,* 92 (7): 592-597. https://doi.org/10.1177/0022034513490168

Marmot, M. (2007). "For the Commission on Social Determinants of Health. Achieving Health Equity: From Root Causes to Fair Outcomes". *The Lancet,* 370 (9593): 11. https://doi.org/10.1016/S0140-6736(07)61385-3

Matsuyama, Y., Aida, J., Tsuboya, T., Hikichi, H., Kondo, K. et al. (2017). "Are Lowered Socioeconomic Circumstances Causally Related to Tooth Loss? A Natural Experiment Involving the 2011 Great East Japan Earthquake". *American Journal of Epidemiology,* 186: 54–62. https://doi.org/10.1093/aje/kwx059

Mehanna, H., Beech, T., Nicholson, T., El-Hariry, I., McConkey, C., et al. (2013). "Prevalence of Human Papillomavirus in Oropharyngeal and Nonoropharyngeal Head and Neck Cancer--Systematic Review and Meta-Analysis of Trends by Time and Region". *Head and Neck,* 35 (5): 747-755. https://doi.org/10.1002/hed.22015

Mehrtash, H., Duncan, K., Parascandola, M., David, A., Gritz, E. R., et al. (2017). "Defining A Global Research and Policy Agenda for Betel Quid and Areca Nut". *The Lancet Oncology,* 18 (12): e767-e775. https://doi.org/10.1016/S1470-2045(17)30460-6.

Muirhead, V. E., Milner, A., Freeman, R., Doughty, J. and Macdonald, M. E. (2020). "What is Intersectionality and Why is it Important in Oral Health Research?" *Community Dentistry and Oral Epidemiology,* 48 (6): 464-470. https://doi.org/10.1111/cdoe.12573

Parker, E. J., Jamieson, L. M., Broughton, J., Albino, J., Lawrence, H. P., et al. (2010). "The Oral Health of Indigenous Children: A Review of Four Nations". *J Paediatr Child Health,* 46: 483–486. https://doi.org/10.1111/j.1440-1754.2010.01847.x

Parker, E. J., Jamieson, L., Steffens, M., Cathro, P. and Logan, R. (2011). "Self-Reported Oral Health of a Metropolitan Homeless Population in Australia: Comparisons with Population-Level Data". *Australian Dental Journal,* 56: 272–277. https://doi.org/10.1111/j.1834-7819.2011.01346.x

Peres, M. A., Macpherson, L. M. D., Weyant, R. J., Daly, B., Venturelli, R., et al. (2019). "Oral Diseases: A Global Public Health Challenge". *The Lancet,* 394: 249-260. https://doi.org/10.1016/S0140-6736(19)31146-8

Petersen, P. E. and Ogawa, H. (2012). "The Global Burden of Periodontal Disease: Towards Integration with Chronic Disease Prevention and Control". *Periodontology 2000,* 60 (1): 15-39. https://doi.org/10.1111/j.1600-0757.2011.00425.x

Petersen, P. E., Bourgeois, D., Ogawa, H., Estupinan-Day, S. and Ndiaye, C. (2005). "The Global Burden of Oral Diseases and Risks to Oral Health". *Bulletin of the World Health Organisation,* 83 (9): 661-669. https://pubmed.ncbi.nlm.nih.gov/16211157/

Pine, C., Harris, R., Burnside, G. and Merrett, M. C. W. (2006). "An Investigation of the Relationship Between Untreated Decayed Teeth and Dental Sepsis in 5-Year-Old Children. *Br Dent J,* 200 (1): 45–47. https://doi.org/10.1038/sj.bdj.4813124

Piscoya, M. D., Ximenes, R., Silva, G. and Jamelli, G. (2012). "Maternal Periodontitis as a Risk Factor for Prematurity". *Peadeatrics International,* 54 (1): 68-75. https://doi.org/10.1111/j.1442-200X.2011.03502.x

Pitts, N. B., Zero, D. T., Mash, D. T., Ekstrand, K., Weintraub, J. A., et al. (2017). "Dental Caries". *Nature Reviews Disease Primers,* 3: 17030. https://doi.org/10.1038/nrdp.2017.30.

United Nations. (2011). *Political Declaration of the High-level Meeting of the General Assembly on the Prevention and Control of Non-Communicable Diseases. Resolution A/66/L1.* New York: United Nations.

Righolt, A. J., Jevdjevic, M., Marcenes and Listl, S. (2018). "Global-, Regional-, and Country-Level Economic Impacts of Dental Diseases in 2015". *Journal of Dental Research,* 97: 501–507. https://doi.org/10.1177/0022034517750572

Schroth, R. J., Harrison, R. L. and Moffatt, M. E. K. (2009). "Oral Health of Indigenous Children and the Influence of Early Childhood Caries on Childhood Health and Well-being". *Pediatric Clinics of North America,* 56: 1481–1499. https://doi.org/10.1016/j.pcl.2009.09.010

Schwendicke, F., Dörfer, C. E., Schlattmann, P., Page, L. F., Thomson, W. M., et al. (2015). "Socioeconomic Inequality and Caries: A Systematic Review and Meta-Analysis". *Journal of Dental Research,* 94: 10–18. https://doi.org/10.1177/0022034514557546

Slade, G. D., Strauss, R. P., Atchison, K. A., Kressin, N. R., Locker, D., et al. (1998). "Conference Summary: Assessing Oral Health Outcomes—Measuring Health Status and Quality of Life". *Community Dental Health,* 15: 3–7. https://pubmed.ncbi.nlm.nih.gov/9791607/

Tonetti, M. S., Jepsen, S., Jin, L. and Otomo-Corgel, J. (2017). "Impact of the Global Burden of Periodontal Diseases on Health, Nutrition and Wellbeing of Mankind: A Call for Global Action". *Journal Of Clinical Periodontology,* 44: 456–462. https://doi.org/10.1111/jcpe.12732

Watt R. (2012). "Social Determinants of Oral Health Inequalities: Implications for Action". *Community Dental Health,* 40: 44–48. https://doi.org/10.1111/j.1600-0528.2012.00719.x

Watt, R. G., Mathur, M. R., Aida, J., Bönecker, M., Venturelli, R., et al. (2018). "Oral Health Disparities in Children". *Pediatric Clinics of North America,* 65: 965–979. https://doi.org/10.1016/j.pcl.2018.05.006

Watt, R. G. and Sheiham, A. (2012). "Integrating the Common Risk Factor Approach into a Social Determinant Framework". *Community Dentistry And Oral Epidemiology,* 40: 289–296. https://doi.org/10.1111/j.1600-0528.2012.00680.x

World Health Organisation. (2015). Guideline: sugars intake for adults and children. Geneva: World Health Organization, 2015. Available at: https://www.who.int/publications/i/item/9789241549028 (Accessed: 28January 2022)

22

HEALTH PROTECTION AND GLOBAL APPROACH TO NEGLECTED COMMUNICABLE DISEASES

Maria Jacirema Ferreira Gonçalves,
Anny Beatriz Costa Antony de Andrade, and
Amanda Rodrigues Amorim Adegboye

Introduction

Neglected communicable diseases (NCDs) are prevalent in tropical and subtropical regions, caused by various pathogens, for example, viruses, bacteria, protozoa, and parasitic worms (helminths), affecting more than one billion people globally. This chapter aims to discuss neglected diseases (e.g., Chagas Disease, Dengue, and Leishmaniasis) in the global context, including health inequalities, public health surveillance, and research. The focus is on a diverse group of communicable diseases that are more prevalent in tropical and subtropical countries, but which are not restricted to such regions. These diseases continue to be a significant hindrance to poverty reduction and socio-economic development, particularly in low- and middle-income countries.

Definition of NCDs

NCDs are prevalent in tropical and subtropical regions, caused by various pathogens, for example, viruses, bacteria, protozoa, and parasitic worms (helminths). They are less prevalent in temperate climates, in which the cold season controls the vector's population by forcing hibernation (Farrar et al., 2014). NCDs include a diverse set of disease/s groups with a singular commonality that is their impact on impoverished communities. Together they affect more than one billion people with devastating health, social and economic consequences (WHO, 2020a). The concept of neglected diseases encompasses social, political, economic, and cultural dimensions.

There is no international consensus definition for NCDs. Overall, NCDs are a group of infectious diseases, including 17 parasitic, bacterial, and viral infections that predominantly affect the poorest and most vulnerable populations,

DOI: 10.4324/9781003128373-22

and contribute to the poverty cycle, social exclusion, and inequalities. This is because this group of diseases has a major impact on maternal and child health, productivity, and generates stigma (WHO, 2009). The World Health Organization classifies the following diseases and disease groups as NCDs: Buruli ulcer; Chagas disease (American trypanosomiasis); dengue and severe dengue; Dracunculiasis (Guinea-Worm disease); Echinococcosis; foodborne trematode infections; human African trypanosomiasis (sleeping sickness); leishmaniasis; leprosy; lymphatic filariasis; mycetoma, chromoblastomycosis, and other deep mycoses; onchocerciasis (river blindness); rabies; scabies and other ectoparasite; schistosomiasis; soil-transmitted helminth infections; snakebite envenoming; taeniasis/cysticercosis; trachoma; vector-borne diseases, yaws, and Endemic Treponematoses (WHO, 2020b). Beyond these NCDs, the PLoS Neglected Tropical Diseases also consider the relevance of co-infections between NCDs and HIV/AIDS, Malaria, and Tuberculosis (TB), and the nutritional links underlying neglected diseases (Hotez, 2017). The seven most common NCDs include three helminth infections: Ascariasis, Hookworm, Trichuriasis, Schistosomiasis, Lymphatic Filariasis, Onchocerciasis, and Trachoma. Mortality from these diseases is relatively low. However, morbidity is extremely high.

Why Are They Neglected?

The existence of NCDs is a barrier to the right to health and to development of communities and countries (WHO, 2017a). It is observed that the geographical distribution of NCDs correlates with poverty, exclusion, and inequality, mainly in areas where social and health indicators are less favourable (WHO, 2009). Their common characteristics are high endemicity in rural areas, or non-planned urban areas in low-income countries, in addition to the scarcity of research for the development and innovation of technologies and pharmacological therapies (Fonseca et al., 2020). These diseases can impair child growth, intellectual development, and labour productivity of the population. Despite their social impact, NCDs do not attract monetary incentives for innovation of treatments and prevention, especially development of new drugs. This lack of investment is due to their low prevalence and because they affect less affluent populations, usually in low-income regions (WHO, 2017b). Since NCDs occur more frequently in deprived regions, they contribute significantly to the poverty and health inequality cycle (Hotez, 2017).

The appropriateness of the term 'neglected diseases' is questionable. Perhaps the most appropriate term would be 'neglected conditions', assuming the term 'condition' is capable of encompassing, not only the disease in the nosological aspect, but situations that lead to, or are involved in the illness process, including the context in which the health events occur (Gondim de Oliveira, 2018). Historically, NCDs were often called 'tropical diseases'. However, this term reinforces a geographic determinism of these conditions. Although 'tropical diseases' are constrained in the lines between the tropics (more prevalent in tropical and subtropical regions), the neglected conditions embody social, political, and economic dimensions (Morel, 2006), which proceed beyond geographic boundaries. Furthermore, the use of the term 'communicable' may not be appropriate to certain neglected conditions. For example, snakebite envenoming is a non-communicable life-threatening disease. However, it is a neglected condition, as most victims live in the world's poorest communities. Agricultural workers, working children, rural dwellers, herders, fishermen, hunters, and people living in poorly constructed houses constitute high-risk groups. It is also observed that there is lack of investment to produce antivenoms drugs and other therapeutical agents to treat people affected by this condition (WHO, 2021). Many victims have limited access to education and healthcare and rely on traditional treatments (Williams et al., 2019).

Public Health Surveillance

The prevalence of NCDs is closely related to the characteristics of the environment where the population live. Responses to NCDs occur unevenly worldwide. The existence of public health surveillance and policies that guarantee access to services are critical for tackling NCDs (Gondim de Oliveira, 2018; Fonseca et al., 2020). Public health surveillance includes the ongoing, systematic collection, analysis, and interpretation of health-related data, essential to planning, implementation, and evaluation of public health practice, closely integrated with the timely dissemination of data to those responsible for prevention and control (Thacker and Birkhead, 2008).

Surveillance is considered one of the main actions of health services to prevent the occurrence or avoid the spread of infections, notification, and monitoring of cases, and contacts of NCDs. Surveillance activities should also involve environmental and social factors, in addition to including vector control, and other biological factors, as well as food safety (Morse, 2012; Dubeux, 2019). Adequate evaluation of implemented surveillance measures can assist in the decision-making for the adoption of low-cost interventions and wide population coverage, such as the interruption of the transmission chain and monitoring of NCDs (Liang et al., 2014).

Surveillance should inform various strategies for the successful control of NCDs. In the case of human Chagas disease, for example, surveillance should consider 1) community engagement in the control of vector proliferation, 2) mapping of proliferation areas, 3) seroepidemiological surveys, 4) donor serology blood, 5) timely diagnosis of pregnant women during prenatal care and neonatal screening, 6) early diagnosis of the general population, and 7) timely specific treatment and epidemiological investigation of cases in the region.

Social and Economic Burden of NCDs

NCDs compromise the performance of those affected in activities related to work and education and have a significant impact on the development and economic growth of endemic regions. NCD-incurred deaths are not immediately per-ceived, compared to cases of maternal mortality, due to haemorrhage or death of young adults in automobile accidents. However, NCDs can significantly con-tribute to health and social inequalities. The burden of these diseases varies across countries based on their political, economic, social, and cultural systems that affect the country health and well-being (Kirigia and Mburugu, 2017). The im-pacts caused by NCDs should not be only evaluated by the death counts, but by the severity of infections, its incidence and prevalence, and associated morbidity, as some of these conditions can lead to disability, and reductions in the econom-ically active population in the region (Lenk et al., 2016). NDCs accounts for more than 57 million Disability Adjusted Life Years (DALYs) globally (Ochola et al., 2021).

The NCDs precipitate loss in revenue due to their impact on agricultural and industrial productivity, costing billions of dollars every year to low-income economies, and affecting the wage potential of individuals in poverty (Ochola et al., 2021). In 2015, about 67,860 deaths from NCDs were recorded in the African continent, resulting in the loss of Int $ 5,112,472,607 (Kirigia and Mbu-rugu, 2017). Madagascar, for example, loses an estimated US$9 million annually in economic productivity due to NCDs, equivalent to 0.29% of its annual Gross Domestic Product (GDP). Similar impacts are observed in Cameroon (US$33 million), Central African Republic (US$16 million), Chad (US$13 million), Senegal (US$8 million), and Burundi (US$3 million). The impact of NCDs has consequences for human capital development, economic growth, and the achievement of the Sustainable Development Goals (SDGs) (Sorgho et al., 2018).

It is also important to consider the social stigma associated with certain NCDs, particularly those causing visible disfiguring ulcers or swelling, such as Buruli ulcer, Leprosy, and Lymphatic Filariasis. Stigma leads to social exclusion, reduced quality of life and well-being, and mental health difficulties. Addressing the social underpinnings of NCDs, and removal of the systemic and structural barriers that create health inequalities, is paramount in the SDGs era to achieve the goal of 'Leaving no one Behind' (WHO, 2015). Data from the World Health Organization indicate that currently one in five people are affected by NCDs, totalling more than 1.7 billion individuals globally. NCDs cause about 185,000 deaths per year, in addition to severe disability, disfigurement, blindness, and malnutrition. Although NCDs are endemic in 149 countries, less than 1% of new drugs approved were for NCDs between 1975 and 2011 (WHO, 2015).

Social and Environmental Determinants of NCDs

The occurrence of NCDs is the result of a complex relationship between intrin-sic and extrinsic factors, which are subdivided into socioeconomic and environ-mental characteristics (Mackey et al., 2014). It is not an exclusive condition for low- and middle-income countries, since some high-income countries may also have areas of social vulnerability, and difficult access to health services, causing

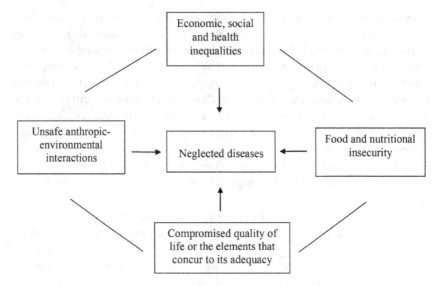

FIGURE 22.1 Factors associated with the occurrence of neglected diseases and their relationships.

different ways of coping with diseases (Barata, 2012). The context in which these diseases remain is permeated by situations that favour or disregard their existence. These situations are listed below (Figure 22.1), which, if they are adequately addressed, may limit the progress of NCDs, and even reverse the situation, leading to the exclusion from the list of NCDs.

The low investment in structural issues, like social and economic inequalities, perpetuates the existence of favourable environments for the development of NCDs, especially those of an infectious and contagious nature. It is necessary to consider that it is not only the development of actions directly related to the disease, but also the importance of the entire context where the population is resident. The provision of basic sanitation, access to education and healthcare services, and social policies for the reduction of poverty and social inequality must be recognised as important preventive actions in the occurrence of NCDs (Bertolozzi et al., 2020).

Interaction between NCDs and Nutrition

As described previously, the process of determining NCDs is complex and involves multi-level factors, ranging from the distal (e.g., social environmental, economic factors, policies, living conditions, and sanitation) to proximal factors (e.g., genetic, physiological, and nutritional factors) (Ehrenberg and Ault, 2005). To fully understand the different patterns of the occurrence of NCDs, it is paramount to consider all factors including individual attributes. Individual factors such as nutritional status have a direct impact on the immune response that is vital for fighting infections (Hall et al., 2012).

The interaction between NCDs and nutrition is based on competition for nutrients. Infectious organisms (e.g., parasites, viruses, or bacteria) use the host, in this case, a human body, as a source of all nutrients, required by the infectious organisms to live, grow, reproduce, and spread (Hall et al., 2012). However, the impact of infectious organisms goes beyond nutrient requirements. The impact involves the host response to the pathogenic organism leading to an increase in metabolic rate, loss of appetite, immune response cascade, and pathological tissue changes (Farhadi and Ovchinnikov, 2018). Additionally, fever leads to increased energy and micronutrient requirements. These responses are host protective mechanisms against acute infections. However, when the host is faced with chronic or recurrent infections, these reactions can cause undernutrition, particularly when the nutritional status of the host is already compromised (Solomons, 2007). Undernutrition, on the other hand, increases susceptibility to infections, the severity of the disease, and the ability to recover (Katona and Katona-Apte, 2008; Hall et al., 2012) creating a vicious cycle. Therefore, the temporal relationship between NCDs and malnutrition is not yet fully established in terms of what comes first (Figure 22.2).

Intestinal parasites, due to lack of access to clean water, sanitary food handling, and effective hygiene, can cause a reduction in food intake, malabsorption, and endogenous nutrient loss (Katona and Katona-Apte, 2008). NCDs not only exacerbate the risk of malnutrition, but it can also affect growth and cognitive development. Intestinal worm infections have been associated with low IQ, anaemia, undernutrition,

The spiral of Malnutrition and Infection

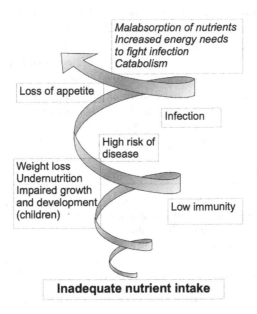

FIGURE 22.2 Spiral of malnutrition and infection.

and stunted growth (low height for age) (Guan and Han, 2019). While it is known that parasites can lead to malnutrition, the degree to which malnutrition itself can lead to increased parasite infestation is not clearly understood. However, the conditions often coexist and therefore they should be considered together.

Targeted Interventions

Globally, health policy needs to prioritise the management of NCDs to curb its socially deleterious effects such as:

- Global Health Initiatives: Involving cooperation between countries, especially between those with a low human development index and middle and high-income countries (Banati and Moatti, 2008);
- Research and innovation: Fostering research and innovation with a focus on the control, elimination, or eradication of NCDs; development, planning, and performance of strategies in vector control; expansion of initiatives aimed at the production and access to medicines (Yamey et al., 2018), for example, Drugs for Neglected Diseases Initiatives – DNDi, Global Alliance for TB Drug Development and UNITAID – Laboratory for Innovative Financing for Development;
- Basics needs: Offer safe water, sanitation, and hygiene, with a focus on overcoming the social gaps and inequalities (Ault, 2007).

Case Study: Tuberculosis

Whilst TB is no longer on the World Health Organization's list of NCDs, in 1993, it declared TB as a global public health emergency, ending a period of prolonged global neglect. However, it remains a public health problem of significant complexity and global concern regarding NCDs. TB affects poor people, currently referred to as neglected populations (de Araújo et al., 2020). Also, the burden of TB is impacted by neglected risk factors (Abdoli et al., 2019). The World Health Organization demands for disease control with the 'End TB Strategy' included three goals with global milestones for 2020 and 2025 (WHO, 2020c). Please see Table 22.1.

TABLE 22.1 TB Facts and Figures

1 80% reduction in the TB incidence rate (new and relapse cases per 100,000 population per year) by 2030, compared with 2015. 2020 milestone: 20% reduction; 2025 milestone: 50% reduction
2 90% reduction in the annual number of TB deaths by 2030, compared with 2015. 2020 milestone: 35% reduction; 2025 milestone: 75% reduction
3 No households affected by TB face catastrophic costs (by 2020) and United Nations Sustainable Development Goals (by 2030), end the epidemic of TB

Globalisation, it is argued, often precipitates people movement, and political instability and war can cause displacement, which both contribute to disease spreading. Therefore, global demands for TB control require coordinated responses across different disciplines and geographic borders.

The main challenges for national TB control programmes are:

- Adequate and active surveillance for case detection follow-up;
- Guarantee of successful outcomes with priority to high rates of cure and low rate of treatment default;
- Adherence to treatment regime to avoid antibiotics resistance.

TB is explained by the epidemiological triad (Figure 22.3) also known as the traditional model of infectious disease composed of three elements: an external agent, a susceptible host, and an environment that brings the host and agent together.

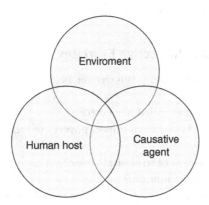

FIGURE 22.3 The epidemiological triad for tuberculosis.

The environment is the most complex factor intricate in the global TB burden since it represents the context in which humans live, including physical, social, economic, and cultural conditions. These conditions, including crowded living, poor dwelling conditions, low income and poverty, lack of access to healthcare, food insecurity, and low education, produce the ideal environment for TB endemicity and qualify it as a neglected condition (Orcau et al., 2011). Like NCDs, TB has a history of poor investments in new drugs development.

Conclusion

In conclusion, NCDs are largely preventable. However, these conditions do not attract vital global public health policy inclusion and investment for driving sustainable efforts to reduce their medical and societal burden. This is mostly attributable to the demographics of the affected populations and their lack of political voice. Initiatives to tackle NCDs must be incorporated within national and regional health plans and aligned with global commitments to achieving universal health coverage and the SDGs. These initiatives should be based on four pillars 1) ensuring that safe and effective treatment is accessible and affordable for all; 2) empowering regional, national, and local communities to take proactive action; 3) strengthening health systems to deliver better outcomes; and 4) building a strong global coalition of partners to build advocacy, mobilise resources, coordinate action, and ensure that implementation of the roadmap is successful (Williams et al., 2019). Finally, when combating NCDs, it is necessary to consider that investing in preventive measures may be more cost-effective than just providing curative care for sick populations and those with chronic conditions resulting from NCDs (Fitzpatrick et al., 2017).

Research Points and Reflective Exercises

With reference to the discussions in this chapter, begin to reflect upon the following:

1 Why are some diseases called neglected?
2 How do NCDs and conditions impact poverty reduction strategies and economic development?
3 How far is the concept of structural violence (Chapter 12) helpful in understanding NCDs and conditions?
4 Reflect upon what more needs to be done to reduce NCDs and conditions.

Further Resources and Reading

Houweling, T. A. J, Karim-Kos, H. E., Kulik, M. C., Stolk, W. A., Haagsma, J. A., et al. (2016). "Socioeconomic Inequalities in Neglected Tropical Diseases: A Systematic Review". *PLOS (Public Library of Science) Neglected Tropical Diseases,* 10 (5): e0004546. https://doi.org/10.1371/journal.pntd.0004546

World Health Organization. (2013). *Sustaining the Drive to Overcome the Global Impact of Neglected Tropical Diseases: Second WHO Report on Neglected Diseases.* Geneva: World Health Organization.

References

Abdoli, A. and Mofazzal Jahromi, M. A. (2019). "Neglected Factors Affecting the Burden of Tuberculosis". *Archives of Medical Research,* 50 (1): 19–20. https://doi.org/10.1016/j.arcmed.2019.03.007

de Araújo, R. V., Santos, S. S., Sanches, L. M., Giarolla, J., El Seoud, O., et al. (2020). "Malaria and Tuberculosis as Diseases of Neglected Populations: State of the Art in Chemotherapy and Advances in the Search for New Drugs. *Memórias do Instituto Oswaldo Cruz*, 115: e200229. https://doi.org/10.1590/0074-02760200229

Ault, S. K. (2007). "Pan American Health Organization's Regional Strategic Framework for Addressing Neglected Diseases in Neglected Populations in Latin America and the Caribbean". *Memórias do Instituto Oswaldo Cruz*, 102 (1): 99–107. https://doi.org/10.1590/S0074-02762007005000094

Banati, P. and Moatti, J.-P. (2008). "The Positive Contributions of Global Health Initiatives". *Bulletin of The World Health Organization*, 86 (11): 820. https://doi.org/10.2471/BLT.07.049361

Barata, R. B. (2012). *Como e Por Que as Desigualdades Sociais Fazem mal à Saúde?* 21st edn. Rio de Janeiro: Fiocruz.

Bertolozzi, M. R., Takahashi, R. F., França, F. O. de S. and Hino, P. (2020). "The Incidence of Tuberculosis and its Relation to Social Inequalities: Integrative Review Study on PubMed Basew", *Escola Anna Nery* 24 (1): e20180367. https://doi.org/10.1590/2177-9465-EAN-2018-0367

Dubeux, L. S. (2019). "Evaluation of the Program to Combat Neglected Diseases in Controlling Schistosomiasis Mansoni in Three Hyperendemic Municipalities, Pernambuco, Brazil, 2014. *Epidemiologia e servicos de saude,* 28 (2): e2018085. https://doi.org/10.5123/S1679-49742019000200008

Ehrenberg, J. P. and Ault, S. K. (2005). "Neglected Diseases of Neglected Populations: Thinking to Reshape the Determinants of Health in Latin America and the Caribbean". *BMC Public Health*, 5 (1): 119. https://doi.org/10.1186/1471-2458-5-119

Farhadi, S. and Ovchinnikov, R. (2018). "The Relationship Between Nutrition and Infectious Diseases: A Review". *Biomedical and Biotechnology Research Journal (BBRJ)*, 2 (3): 168. https://doi.org/10.4103/bbrj.bbrj_69_18

Farrar, J., Hotez, P. J., Junghanss, T., Kang, G., Lalloo, D. et al. (2014). *Manson's Tropical Infectious Diseases*, 23rd edn. Philadelphia: Elsevier Saunders.

Fitzpatrick, C., Nwankwo, U., Lenk, E., de Vlas, S. J. and Bundy, D. A. P. (2017). "An Investment Case for Ending Neglected Tropical Diseases". In: K. K. Holmes, S. Bertozzi, B. R. Bloom and P. Jha (eds). *Major Infectious Diseases*. Washington DC: The International Bank for Reconstruction and Development / The World Bank.

Fonseca, B. P., Albuquerque, P. C. and Zicker, F. (2020). Neglected Tropical Diseases in Brazil: Lack of Correlation Between Disease Burden, Research Funding and Output". *Tropical Medicine and International Health*, 25 (11): 1373–1384. https://doi.org/10.1111/tmi.13478

Gondim de Oliveira, R. (2018). "Sentidos das Doenças Negligenciadas na Agenda da Saúde Global: O Lugar de Populações e Territórios". *Ciência and Saúde Coletiva*, 23 (7): 2291–2302. https://doi.org/10.1590/1413-81232018237.09042018

Guan, M. and Han, B. (2019). Association Between Intestinal Worm Infection and Malnutrition Among Rural Children Aged 9–11 Years Old in Guizhou Province, China". *BMC Public Health*, 19 (1): 1204. https://doi.org/10.1186/s12889-019-7538-y

Hall, A., Zhang, Y., MacArthur, C. and Baker, S. (2012). "The Role of Nutrition in Integrated Programs to Control Neglected Tropical Diseases. *BMC Med,* 10: 41. https://doi.org/10.1186/1741-7015-10-41

Hotez, P. J. (2017.) "The Poverty-Related Neglected Diseases: Why Basic Research Matters". *PLOS Biology*, 15 (11): e2004186. https://doi.org/10.1371/journal.pbio.2004186

Katona, P. and Katona-Apte, J. (2008). "The Interaction Between Nutrition and Infection". *Clinical Infectious Diseases*, 46 (10): 1582–1588. https://doi.org/10.1086/587658

Kirigia, J. M. and Mburugu, G. N. (2017). The Monetary Value of Human Lives Lost Due to Neglected Tropical Diseases in Africa. *Infectious Diseases of Poverty*, 6: 165. https://doi.org/10.1186/s40249-017-0379-y

Lenk, E. J., Redekop, W. K., Luyendijk, M., Rijnsburger, A. J. and Severens, J. L. (2016). "Productivity Loss Related to Neglected Tropical Diseases Eligible for Preventive Chemotherapy: A Systematic Literature Review". *PLOS Neglected Tropical Diseases*, 19. https://doi.org/10.1371/journal.pntd.0004397

Liang, S., Yang, C., Zhong, B., Guo, J., Li, H. et al. (2014). "Surveillance Systems for Neglected Tropical Diseases: Global Lessons from China's Evolving Schistosomiasis Reporting Systems, 1949–2014". *Emerging Themes in Epidemiology*, 11 (1): 19. https://doi.org/10.1186/1742-7622-11-19

Mackey, T. K., Liang, B. A., Cuomo, R., Hafen, R., Brouwer, K. C., et al. (2014). "Emerging and Reemerging Neglected Tropical Diseases: A Review of Key Characteristics, Risk Factors, and the Policy and Innovation Environment". *Clinical Microbiology Reviews*, 27 (4): 949–979. https://doi.org/10.1128/CMR.00045-14

Morel, C. (2006). "Innovation in Health and Neglected Diseases". *Cadernos de Saúde Pública*, 22 (8): 1522–23. https://doi.org/10.1590/S0102-311X2006000800001

Morse, S. S. (2012). "Public Health Surveillance and Infectious Disease Detection". *Biosecurity and Bioterrorism: Biodefense Strategy, Practice, and Science*, 10 (1): 6–16. https://doi.org/10.1089/bsp.2011.0088

Ochola, E. A. Karanja, D. M. S., Elliott, S. J. (2021). *"The Impact of Neglected Tropical Diseases (NTDs) on Health and Wellbeing in Sub-Saharan Africa (SSA): A Case Study of Kenya"*. *PLOS Neglected Tropical Diseases,* 15 (2): e0009131. https://doi.org/10.1371/journal.pntd.0009131

Orcau, À., Caylà, J. A. and Martínez, J. A. (2011). "Present Epidemiology of Tuberculosis: Prevention and Control Programs". *Enfermedades Infecciosas y Microbiología Clínica*, 29: 2–7. https://doi.org/10.1016/S0213-005X(11)70011-8

Solomons, N. W. (2007). Malnutrition and Infection: An Update. *British Journal of Nutrition*, 98 (S1): S5–S10. https://doi.org/10.1017/S0007114507832879

Sorgho, G., Lavadenz, F. and Matala, O. O. T. (2018). "A Call to Support Francophone African Countries to End the Tremendous Suffering from NTDs", World Bank. Health, Nutrition and Population Global Practice. Available from: https://pdfs.semanticscholar.org/4bf6/605eaaafa490e9f547318bfe66e5322ab450.pdf (Accessed: 1 November 2020).

Thacker, S. B. and Birkhead, G. S. (2008). "Surveillance". In M. B. Gregg (ed.) *Field Epidemiology*. Oxford: Oxford University Press.

World Health Organization. (2009). *Neglected Tropical Diseases, Hidden Successes, Emerging Opportunities*. Geneva: World Health Organization.

World Health Organization. (2015). *Investing to Overcome the Global Impact of Neglected Tropical Diseases: Third WHO Report on Neglected Tropical Diseases 2015*. Geneva: World Health Organization.

World Health Organization. (2017a). *Integrating Neglected Tropical Diseases into Global Health and Development: Fourth WHO Report on Neglected Tropical Diseases*. Geneva: World Health Organization.

World Health Organization. (2017b). *Ten Years In Public Health, 2007–2017*. Geneva: World Health Organization.

World Health Organization. (2020a). *Ending the Neglect to Attain the Sustainable Development Goals: A Road Map for Neglected Tropical Diseases 2021–2030*. Geneva: World Health Organization.

World Health Organization. (2020b). "Control of Neglected Tropical Diseases". Available at: https://www.who.int/teams/maternal-newborn-child-adolescent-health-and-ageing/maternal-health/about/control-of-neglected-tropical-diseases (Accessed: 30 November 2020).

World Health Organization. (2020c). *Global Tuberculosis Report*, 1st edn. Geneva: World Health Organization.

World Health Organization. (2021). "Snakebite". Available at: https://www.who.int/-health-topics/snakebite#tab=tab_1 (Accessed: 20 August 2021).

Williams, D. J., Faiz, M. A., Abela-Ridder, B., Ainsworth, S. and Bulfone, T. C., et al. (2019). "Strategy For A Globally Coordinated Response To a Priority Neglected Tropical Disease: Snakebite Envenoming". *PLOS Neglected Tropical Diseases*, 13 (2): e0007059. https://doi.org/10.1371/journal.pntd.0007059

Yamey, G., Batson, A., Kilmarx, P. H. and Yotebieng, M. (2018). "Funding Innovation In Neglected Diseases". *BMJ*, k1182. https://doi.org/10.1136/bmj.k1182

23

CONCLUSION

Social Sciences Perspectives on Global Public Health

Vincent La Placa and Julia Morgan

Global public health is increasingly perceived as a speciality field within its own right across teaching, education, and research in public health, and its approaches to populations and individuals. Public health is associated with the populations of a specific country or community with a spotlight on, for example, prevention and solutions to health challenges, be it lifestyles, or wider determinants (Karkee et al., 2015). Global health puts the emphasis upon issues which can include, but also eclipse, national boundaries, affecting populations globally, because of, for instance, globalisation processes, global pandemics, and other momentous events, which necessitates cooperation between countries and national institutions (Shelton et al., 2018). As a result, global health is perceived as increasingly interdisciplinary, enveloping health prevention, promotion, and healthcare, with contributions from various disciplines. These often assume the forms of, for instance, sociology, psychology, and behavioural sciences, through to law, economics, history, biomedical, and environmental science, and public and social policy and theory (Karkee et al., 2015).

As this book identifies, the social sciences have made discerning contributions to global public health, individual, and population health. By focusing upon specific disciplines, theories, concepts, ideas, and aims, the social sciences can identify and address common and persistent themes, relevant to global public health, beyond traditional biomedical approaches. It has also demonstrated a unity between public health and global public health and illustrated how teaching, education, and research approaches often need to stride both disciplines, given increasing social and economic developments cross the globe (Shelton et al., 2018). Through application of social sciences perspectives, it is also noticeable that many solutions can be proposed in terms of enhancing global public health and wellbeing policy and practice. The rich and detailed contributions of social sciences research to individual and population global public health have been

DOI: 10.4324/9781003128373-23

displayed in the current book, which has sought to detail a variety of relevant and interesting topics and which have proceeded beyond traditional biomedicine and positivistic approaches (which, of course, remain salient and complimentary to the book's approach).

The book, among many other things, has significantly highlighted (1) the role of social sciences and theory in application to global public health, (2) the place of social sciences in highlighting the ever-increasing importance of health inequalities across a wide spectrum, and (3) the eclectic nature of social sciences perspectives in, for example, making links between public health and global public health, and its place in developing core public health skills, and competencies.

Interestingly, the significance of social theory, and its ability to contribute to the realm of global public health, is apparent, particularly across the current book. The current shift towards social sciences across public health encourages a focus upon the social and economic and individual determinants of health, broadly encompassing 'objective' and 'subjective' dimensions, and the inter-relations between them, as outlined in Chapters 2, 3, and 15. Social theories are systematic, reflective, and holistic elucidations on how social systems function, operate, and change and can be applied to broadly explain, for example, the workings of health and social systems, healthcare, and social contexts, within which people construct health and wellbeing, as well as those within which healthcare practitioners work. Not only are they a tool of explanation and revision but also assist in understanding solutions to health and healthcare challenges, through an eclectic comprehension of how broader social systems operate, and the barriers and enablers they exhibit as a result. This is illustrated throughout the book with a host of authors developing and applying social perspectives to more effectively, understand social practices, health beliefs, social systems, and contemporary issues, beyond traditional biomedicine.

The book also demonstrates that the articulation and role of health inequalities across a range of behaviours and contexts, which application of social sciences perspectives, assists to highlight and explain, beyond traditional approaches (Chapters 10 and 11, particularly the relation between climate change and health inequalities). Though high- and low-income countries are increasingly converging, occurrences and experiences of, for example, disease patterns and healthcare, health status, and health experiences, be it maternal health or mental health, are characterised by significant disparities within and between countries. These can often be explained with reference to wider economic, structural, and ethnic patterns of inequalities but also in the enablers and constraints built into wider social systems, affecting how individuals and groups respond to and change behaviours and practices within them. Through articulation and application of social sciences perspectives, the book has focused upon the roles of, for instance, stigma and marginalisation, social support and networks, socioeconomic position, and armed conflict in, for example, generating and prolonging health inequalities, and disparities in responses to them (Chapters 18 and 21).

By focusing on the global determinants of health through the social sciences, the book has generated insight and demonstrated the development of divergent approaches and orientations to public health training, research, and development, enabling practical thought and application (Chapters 4 and 19). As such, the book will assist students and practitioners to further develop and cement core public health skills and competencies, especially in application of theory and social sciences approaches. This includes knowledge of, for example, the diversity of infrastructural and environments which determine the global health environment (Chapter 7), but also competencies in, for instance, health equity and minorities (Chapters 5 and 20), professional collaboration and networking (Chapters 9 and 22), ethical reasoning (Chapter 6), and core design and implementation of public health interventions (Chapter 8).

The book also highlights the eclectic nature of social science perspectives across global public health, and the diverse approaches which can be used to frame research and develop solutions in an increasing late modern world, as well as the link between public and global health. It has enabled perspectives which cut across both dimensions, as well as articulating the uniqueness and relevance of focusing upon social science perspectives (Chapters 12 and 13). Similarly, it enables students and practitioners to connect the links, and think about how their current public health competencies can be developed and aligned, with the global health dimension highlighted across the book, as well as the ever-increasing contribution of social sciences to public health.

The book is predicated upon the idea that social sciences perspectives explain and develop how, for example, individuals, communities, and societies, are subject to change, with reference to broader processes such as, for instance, globalisation, and the transformation from traditional to modern societies, and emergent social and psychological changes, which emerge, as a result. Such changes also highlight innovative ideas, discourses, social arrangements, and relations, which emerge too (Knight et al., 2014) and, as such, occur upon and affect global public health. For instance, potential processes of social and economic de-globalisation, intensified by the global pandemic, and the Russian war against Ukraine in February 2022, may entail that global public health studies need to shift the focus to countries and communities, more vulnerable to dislocation of food supplies, higher food, and fuel prices, and therefore, detrimental effects on health and wellbeing. De-globalisation and 'globalisation through equilibrium' do not necessarily render global public health any less important or the ability of the social sciences to explain its causes and consequences. Global health perspectives will need to change but the importance of approaching health through a global lens will not recede, but may well be transformed (like globalisation, similarly).

Resulting global and social conflict may trigger more population movements with resulting changes in how public health is approached, with reference to, for instance migrants and refugees (Chapters 14, 16, and 17). Never has the link between social science (and its capacity to explain the social world) been more important in explaining and understanding health and wellbeing, healthcare interventions, health inequalities, and what Habermas (1990/1992; La Placa and Corlyon, 2014) deemed, the 'unfinished project of modernity' (the requirement to rethink practices to create 'stability' and 'happiness' in the face of insecurity and momentous change). It is to this effect that this book was written and to widen the appeal of social sciences within global public health in a changing world and environment.

References

Habermas, J. (1990). *The Philosophical Discourse of Modernity: Twelve Lectures*. Cambridge: Policy Press.

Habermas, J. (1992). *The Structural Transformation of the Public Sphere: An Inquiry into a Category of Bourgeois Society*. Cambridge: Policy Press.

Karkee, R., Comfort, J. and Alfonso, H. (2015). "Defining and Developing a Global Public Health Course for Public Health Undergraduates". *Frontiers in Public Health*, 3: 66. https://doi.org/10.3389/fpubh.2015.00166

Knight, A., La Placa, V. and McNaught, A. (2014). *Wellbeing: Policy and Practice*. Banbury: Lantern.

La Placa, V. and Corlyon, J. (2014). "Social Tourism and Organised Capitalism: Research, Policy, and Practice. *Journal of Policy Research in Tourism, Leisure, and Events*, 6 (1): 66–79. https://doi.org/10.1080/19407963.2013.833934

Shelton, R. C., Hatzenbuehler, M. L., Bayer, R. and Metsch, L. R. (2018). "Future Perfect? The Future of the Social Sciences in Public Health". *Frontiers in Public Health*, 5 (357). https://doi.org/10.3389/fpubh.2017.00357

INDEX

Note: **Bold** page numbers refer to tables; *Italic* page numbers refer to figures.

Abiyamo Maternal and Child Health Insurance Scheme 74
Àbíyè (Safe Motherhood) programme 70–71
abstract systems theory 23
accessibility of health services 80, 122, 149–154, 162, 200, 211
active agency and actions 12
active pharmaceutical ingredients (APIs) 21
Adegboye, Amanda Rodrigues Amorim 3, 4
Adjaye-Gbewonyo, Kafui 3
adolescence 119; communicable diseases, poverty 124; contemporary issues 121–124; COVID-19 pandemic 121–122; Life-Course Theory 120–121; malnutrition 122–123; mental health and wellbeing 123; rights-based approach 121; SDGs 125; SDOH 120; sexual and reproductive health 123–124; social and structural determinants 124–125; theoretical approaches 119–121; treatments and prevention services 125
Afolabi, M. O. 53
agency 1, 8, 11, 12, 17, 24, 25, 64, 91, 112, 120, 132–135, 145, 163, 180
agentic dying: hospices and homes 143–144; palliative care 139–141; quality of dying 141; quality of life 141; Reimagining Global Health 139; self-reflection 144–145; social imaginary 141, 142; total pain 142

American Heart Association study 44
antenatal care (ANC) 70, 71
APIs *see* active pharmaceutical ingredients (APIs)
Applerouth, S. 7
applied ethics 51
armed conflicts: and children's mental health 129–130; culturally responsive interventions 132–134; defined 129; psychosocial support interventions 131–132
assets-based approach 81, 82
Atkinson, P. 10
atmospheric aerosol loading 89
autonomy 50, 53, 144–145

Banke-Thomas, Aduragbemi 3
Barna, Stefi 3
Barreto, M. 192
Barry, C. 10
Beauchamp, T. L. 53
beneficence 50, 53
Bentham, Jeremy 52
Berger, P. L. 10
Bernheim, R. G. 53
Biden, Joe 21
Biehl, J. 150, 151
biodiversity loss 89
biological diversity 92
biopower 8
Bourdieu, P. 112

Boyer, E. M. 201
Brown, E. C. 193
Buchbinder, S. 184

capitalism 23
Capitalocene 91
Cash, R. 20–21
Castoriadis, C. 139, 141, 144, 145
Caulfield, T. 152
Chana, Bal 3–4
chemical pollution 89
Child Friendly Spaces (CFSs) 131–133
children 2, 3, 25, 111, 170, 191, 200, 202, 210; armed conflict and mental health 129–135; communicable diseases, poverty 124; contemporary issues 121–124; COVID-19 pandemic 121–122; Life-Course Theory 120–121; malnutrition 122–123; mental health and wellbeing 123; migration 158–159, 163; rights-based approach 121; SDGs 125; SDOH 120; sexual and reproductive health 123–124; social and economic needs 125; stigmatisation of 78; theoretical approaches to 119–121; treatments and prevention services 125
Childress, J. F. 53
Choak, Clare 3
Chuckuoma, Julia Ngozi 3
climate and ecological emergency 88–90
climate change 22, 33, 51, 83, 89, 98, 99, 103, 104, 121, 221
cognitive-behavioural technique 132
collective order 6
Collins, P. H. 62, 63
colonisation 90–91
community-based interventions 132
contraception 24
cosmopolitanism 180–181, 185
COVID-19 2, 17, 18, 28, 39–40, 42, 43, 45, 65, 79, 161, 182–184; care-led recovery 32–33; ethics 55–56; feminist approaches 31–32; GFC 29, 30; and health and wellbeing 20–22; mHealth technologies and applications 101; mortality rate 30; vaccine inequality 30–31
Crenshaw, K. 44, 150
critical pedagogy, teaching and learning: and global health 59–61; identity 61; power 62–63; radical pedagogical practice 63–65; risk 61–62
critical public health 5, 7–8, 22
Critical Race Theory 112
cultural competency 173–174
cultural diversity 92

culturally responsive interventions 132–134
culturally sensitive dietary intervention 174
cultural violence 112, 113

Dawson, A. 51, 54
Deane, Kevin 3
Deccan Development Society 94
deductive-nomological conditions 6
de-globalisation 17, 21–22, 54, 222
degrowth perspective 34
demand-side interventions 68–69
deontology 50, 52
Desfor Edles, L. 7
Diderichsen, F. 120
dietary acculturation: cultural competency 173–174; culturally sensitive dietary intervention 174; dietary change and patterns 170; global consumption 169; health implications of 173; immigrants and minority communities 173–174; migrant *vs.* immigrant 169; nutrition transition 170; post-migration dietary patterns 171–173, *172*; social isolation 172–173; ultra-processed foods 171; urbanisation 170
Dijkstra, R. F. 102
disciplinary power 63
Djordjevic, C. 142, 144
Doughnut Model 92, *93*
duality of structure 11
dynamic qualities 6

Eborieme, Ejemai 3
economic migrants **159**
economics *see* Health Economics
ecosystem integrity 92–93
Ehrenreich, B. 9
emancipatory politics 185
emotional loneliness 190
empowerment 63
Engels, F. 40
English, D. 9
environmental threats 93
epistemology 12, 13
ethics: autonomy 50, 53; beneficence 50, 53; COVID-19 55–56; deontology 50, 52; framework 53; global health inequalities 54–55; global public health 50–52; individual liberty 55–56; justice 50, 53; lockdowns 55–56; non maleficence 50, 53; principles 53; public health 50–51; utilitarianism 50, 52; virtue ethics 50, 52
evidence-side interventions 68–69
external social structures 12

fair-trade organisations 80
faith-based social enterprises 79–80
Farmer, P. 139, 145
Federal Ministry of Health (FMOH) 69
Feldman, R. 130
Female Genital Mutilation (FGM) 24
femicide 113
feminism 5, 8–10, 22; 'radical' and 'liberal' 8
feminist critical theory 113
FGM see Female Genital Mutilation (FGM)
fiscal policy measures 29
foreign land: action 165; migration 154–
    160; OFWs 164; refugee and migrant
    health inequalities 160–161; refugees and
    migrants, barriers to 162–163; socio-
    ecological perspective 161–162
Foucault, M. 8, 150
foundationalism 23
Freire, P. 59, 60, 63
functionalism 22

Galloway, L. 80
Galtung, J. 111
Gandhi, V. 3
Gawande, A. 141, 143
gender-relations approach 192
genders 8–10, 32, 33, 38, 39, 43, 44, 95,
    111–113, 124, 150, 192, 193, 195, 199;
    health inequalities 182–183; HIV-related
    challenges 184; mental health challenges
    183–184; and sexual orientation 179;
    Tavistock Inquiry 181–182; trans
    affirming 180–181
GFC see Global Financial Crisis (GFC)
Giddens, A. 7, 11, 179, 180–181
Gilbert, P.A. 173
Gilligan, J. 112
Giroux, H. 59, 60
Global Exchange for Social Investment
    (GEXSI) 82
Global Financial Crisis (GFC) 29–30
global freshwater 89
global inequalities: discrimination
    43–44; health and social inequalities
    38–39; intersectionality 44; materialist
    explanations 42–43; measuring
    and addressing 40–41; psychosocial
    mechanisms 43; social determinants and
    poverty 42–43; social gradients 39–40;
    social selection vs. social causation
    41; socio-political frameworks 44–45;
    structural determinants 44–45
globalisation 2, 3, 6, 9, 11, 13, 45, 121, 169,
    180, 189, 191, 215, 220, 222; capitalism
    23, 25; and colonisation 90–91, 95;

COVID-19 20–22; Feminist frameworks
    24; functionalism 22; and global health
    17–18; global wellbeing 18–20, 20;
    health and lifestyle 198, 203; and
    industrialisation 90–91, 95
global solidarity 54, 56
Global Steering Group for Impact (GSG)
    83
Gonçalves, Maria Jacirema Ferreira 4
Greenhalgh, T. 12
green healthcare infrastructure 100
Green New Deal 33–34
Green Revolution 94

Hari, J. 64
health economics 28; feminist approaches
    31–33; Keynesian 28–30; planetary
    health 33–34; political 30–31
health inequalities 1–4, 7, 8, 10, 18, 21,
    22, 38, 39, 79, 110–111, 174, 179–181,
    221, 223; discrimination 43–44; ethics
    of 54–55; genderqueer 182–184; global
    oral 198–203; healthcare services 150,
    154; intersectionality 44; materialist
    explanations 42–43; non-binary
    individuals 182–184; poverty 42–43, 209;
    psychosocial mechanisms 43; refugee
    and migrant health 158–165, **159**;
    social determinants 42–43; and social
    inclusion 91; social selection vs. social
    causation 41; socio-political frameworks
    44–45; structural determinants 44–45;
    transgender 182–184
health rangers 70–71
Healthy Foundations Life-stage
    Segmentation model 12
hegemonic power 63
heterogeneity 18
Heubber, P. 143
Holocene 88
Honwana, A. 133, 134
hooks, b. 59, 60, 63
Horkheimer, M. 7
Hunter, D. 51, 54

IASC see Inter-Agency Standing
    Committee (IASC)
IDP see internally displaced person (IDP)
illness prevention 103
Imrie, R. 190
incentive-based schemes 74
industrialisation 90–91
Inter-Agency Standing Committee (IASC)
    131
internally displaced person (IDP) **159**

internal social structures 12
international migrants **159**
International Organization for Migration (IOM) 158
interventions 5, 18, 28, 40–41, 46, 125, 130, 152, 182, 191, 200; carbon-reducing 103; culturally sensitive dietary 174; global health issues 11; market-based 33; maternal health 68–75, 72; mental health and trauma 132–134; person-centred healthcare 12; psychosocial 129, 131–132; public health 1, 3, 13, 19–20, 52, 78, 80, 98, 222–223; targeted 214; urban greening 103; violence prevention 110, 114
intimate partner violence (IPV) 8, 110, 113
invisibilisation 149–150
IOM *see* International Organization for Migration (IOM)
IPV *see* intimate partner violence (IPV)

Jeavons, Charlotte 3–4
Jong, Christie-de 3

Kakar, S. 143
Kantian ethics 52, 56
Kaplan, G. 39
Kass, N. E. 53
Kawachi, Ichiro 3
Kerr, T. E. A. 64
Keynes, John Maynard 29
Keynesian economics 28–30
Keynesian Health Economics 28–30
Khokhar, S. 173
King, Martin Luther Jr. 142
Kleinman, A. 59
Klinge B. 200
Knight, A. 3, 6, 20
Kumar, A. 25

land system change 89
La Placa, V. 3, 4, 6, 12, 13, 194
Leigh-Hunt, N. 194
lesbian, gay, and bisexual (LGB) 192
Life-Course Theory 120–121
life politics 185
lifestyle diseases 18
loneliness: in global population 191–193; and global public health 189–191
low-and middle-income countries (LMICs) 121, 123, 124, 198, 200–201, 203; *see also* maternal health interventions
low carbon medical practices 100–102
Lucas, Robert 29
Luckmann, T. 10
Lynch, J. 39

Mackay, K. 52
macro approach 6
magic money tree 30
Malagi, H. E. 154
male violence 113
malnutrition: adolescence 122–123; children 122–123; and infection 213, *213*
Marcuse, H. 7
marginalisation 149–150
market-based interventions 33
market failure 78
Marmot, M. 199
Martin, J. S. 82
Marx, K. 7, 31, 112
Marxism 22
maternal health interventions: Àbíyè (Safe Motherhood) programme 70–71; demand-side interventions 68–69; evaluation of 74–75; evidence-side interventions 68–69; MSS 69–70, 73, 74; supply-side interventions 68; TyDI framework 71–74, 72
McKenzie, S. K. 192
McNaught, A. 19–20, 20
meditation-relaxation intervention 131
Mehmet, N. 3
mental health 9, 12, 24, 43, 81, 83, 122, 189, 192–195, 211, 221; armed conflict, children 129–130; challenges 183–184; and psychosocial support interventions 131–132; of refugees and migrants 160; and trauma based interventions 132–135; and wellbeing 123
mental health and psychosocial support (MHPSS) 131–132
meta-ethics 50–51
micro approach 6
Midwives Service Scheme (MSS) 69–70, 73, 74
migration: children 158–159, 163; foreign land 154–160
Mill, John Stuart 52
Millennium Development Goals 91
mindfulness-informed interventions 131
minority stress theory 193
monopsony capitalism 25
Montgomery, C. 9
moral significance 54
Moreno-Leguizamon, C. 3, 142
Morgan, Julia 3, 4
Morrison, P. S. 190
Muirhead, V. E. 199, 200
Murphy, L. B. 55

Narayan, D. 9
Narrative Exposure Therapy 131
Nation, M. 114
National Primary Health Care
    Development Agency 72–73
neglected communicable diseases (NCDs)
    4, 198, 199, 201; characteristics 209;
    definition 208–209; and nutrition
    212–214, *213*; prevalence 210; public
    health surveillance 210; social and
    economic burden 210–211; social
    and environmental determinants
    211–212, *212*; surveillance 210; targeted
    interventions 214; TB facts and figures
    214, **214,** 215; tropical diseases 209–210
Neoclassical Economics 34
neoliberal ideologies and practices 18
Neville, S. 192
Nigeria Demographic and Health survey
    (NDHS) 70, 71
nitrogen and phosphorous cycle 89
nomadic peoples: barriers, healthcare
    access 150–153; healthcare provision
    153–154; health inequalities 149–150;
    invisibilisation 149–150; marginalisation
    149–150; quality of services 152
non maleficence 50, 53
Norlund, A. 200
normative ethics 51
not-for-profit organisations 78
Novicevic, M. 82
nutrition: dietary acculturation 170; NCDs
    212–214, *213*
Nyamtema, A. S. 68

ocean acidification 89
Oham, C. 3, 194
Okechukwu, Abidemi 3
Okeke, E. N. 75
ontological security 12
oral health: burden of 201–203; inequalities
    199–201; LMICs 198, 200–201, 203;
    NCDs 198, 199, 201; oral diseases 198–
    199; prevalence 202; quality of life 198
Overseas Filipino Workers (OFWs) 164
Owens, Philip 64
Ozawa de-Silva, C. 195

palliative care services 139–146
Palmer, P. 59
Parsons, J. T. 195
Patel, V. 20–21
patient empowerment 102–103
patriarchy 8–10
Pearce, R. 181
personal protective equipment (PPE) 21

person seeking asylum **159**
Pingali, P. 170
planetary boundaries framework 89
planetary health 33–34; and anthropocene
    88–95, *93*; Health Economics 33–34
political economy approach 80
political Health Economics 30–31
post-colonial perspectives 18
post-migration dietary patterns 171–173,
    172
postmodernism 22
PPE *see* personal protective equipment
    (PPE)
Primary Health Centres (PHCs) 69
PSS *see* psychosocial support (PSS)
psychiatric illness 10
psychosocial support (PSS) 131
psychosocial support interventions 131–132
public health surveillance 210
public health wellbeing 17, 19, 21, 24, 92,
    125, 189, 222–223
Pupavac, V. 133

quality of dying 141
quality of life 93, 141
Quandt, S. A. 172

racialised violence 114
Randall, J. 3
Ratanashevorn, R. 193
Raworth, K. 92
Raymond, J. G. 181
RECONEMPACT 65
refugee and migrant health: barriers to
    162–163; inequalities 158–165
refugees **159**
Reimagining Global Health 139
Renault, E. 91
representational theories 6
Rich, A. C. 9
Roe, Danielle J. 3

Sagan, O. 190
Saunders, D. C. M. 141–143, 145
Savulescu, J. 56
Schumpeter, J. A. 79
SDOH *see* social determinants of health
    (SDOH)
SEEDS *see* Sowing Empowering and
    Engaging Discussions on Substances
    (SEEDS)
self-reflection 144–145
Sellschopp, A. 143
Sengedorj, Tumendelger 3
SEP *see* socioeconomic position (SEP)
SES *see* socioeconomic status (SES)

sexual and reproductive health 123–124
sexual harassment 9
sexual violence 8
SHE *see* Sustainable Health Enterprises
   (SHE)
Shibli, H. 152
Shumba, Constance 3
Smith, R. 190
social 21–25, 34, 60–61, 64–65, 110–115,
   158–165, 172; anthropological aspects
   139–146; constructionism 10–11;
   contract 55; determinants and poverty
   42–43, 53, 54, 88; entrepreneurs and
   enterprise 78–81; entrepreneurship
   81–82; exclusion 150, 209; factors
   43; and global public health 1–4,
   220–223; gradients 39–40, 200, 201;
   human and social capital development
   82–83; inequalities 38–39, 45–46, 199;
   innovation 81–82; justice 18, 20, 54, 62,
   121, 124–125, 149–151, 154; loneliness
   189–195; NCDs 210–212; reproduction
   32; selection *vs.* causation 41; structural
   inequalities 179–185; structuration
   theory 11–12; structure 1, 2, 6, 11, 12,
   55, 91, 180; suffering 7–8, 91; theories
   and public health 5–7; theory 2, 5–7, 13,
   139, 221; wellbeing 18–19
social capital 82
social construction 189–193
social constructionism 5, 10–11
social contract 55
social determinants of health (SDOH) 3,
   13, 39, 42, 43, 81, 83, 95, 98, 110, 111,
   119, 120, 160, 164, 171, 199
social enterprise 78–81; human and social
   capital development 82–83
social entrepreneurs 78–81
social entrepreneurship 81–83
social exclusion 150
social gradients 39–40, 200, 201
social imaginary 141, 142
social impact 83
social innovation 81–82
social isolation 191
social loneliness 190
social reality 10
social reproduction 32
social suffering 7–8, 91
social theory 2, 5–7, 13, 139, 221
societal failure 78
socio-ecological conceptual framework
   161–162

socio-ecological drivers, illness 92
socio-economic determinants 1
socio-economic policies 92
socioeconomic position (SEP) 39
socioeconomic status (SES) 39–41
Sorensen, M. 103–104
Sowing Empowering and Engaging
   Discussions on Substances (SEEDS)
   64–65
Sternberg, T. 151
stipulative conditions 6
Stones, R. 12, 23
stratospheric ozone depletion 89
structural violence 3, 60, 91, 111–115, 145
structuration theory 5, 11–12
structure 113, 199; and action 7, 12; agency
   dualism 162; demystification of 64;
   duality of 11; global economic system
   45; globalisation 22; hegemonic power
   63; social 1, 2, 6, 11, 12, 55, 91, 180;
   structure-agency approach 161
supply-side interventions 68
Sustainable Health Enterprises (SHE) 81
Sutton, F. 180–181
Syria Relief 131

Tanveer, F. 55, 56
targeted interventions 214
Tavistock inquiry 181–182
Theory-Design-Implementation (TyDI)
   framework 71–74, 72
time-space distantiation 11
Tomlinson, J. 17
Torre, C. 133
toxic masculinity 9
Trans-Exclusionary Radical Feminists
   (TERFs) 180
transfeminine 184
transgender and genderqueer (TGD):
   discrimination 184–185; gender critical
   and trans affirming 180–181; health
   outcome 179; health-related stigma 180;
   language 179; needs 179; non-binary
   individuals 182–184; structuration 179;
   Tavistock inquiry 181–182;
   TERFs 180
tropical diseases 209–210
Trump, Donald 21, 42

UK Office of National Statistics 9
ultra-processed foods 171
United Nations' Sustainable Development
   Goals (UNSDGs) 19

UN Sustainable Development Goals
(SDGs) 91–92, 94, 111
unsustainable health system: climate change
98–99; Critical Public Health 99; green
healthcare infrastructure 100; low carbon
medical practices 100–102; zero-carbon
health system 99–100, *100*
urban greening 103–104
urbanisation 170
utilitarianism 50, 52, 56

Vancouver Network of Drug Users
(VANDU) 64
Villermé, Louis René 40
violence: cultural 112, 113; femicide 113;
male 113; and public health 109–111;
racialised 114; structural 111–114; youth
114–115
virtue ethics 50, 52

Wainberg, M. L. 193
Waldhausen, J. H. 101
Wallerstein, I. 6
Western-focused mental health 133
Wild, H. 151
Wilunda, C. 152–153
Wu, B. 190, 191

youth violence 114–115

zero-carbon health system 99–100, *100*
Zoetti, P. A. 114

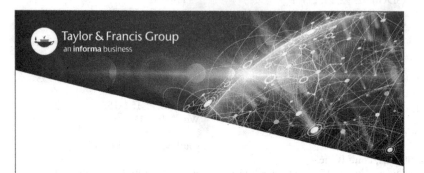

Printed in the United States
by Baker & Taylor Publisher Services